A CROWDED SILENCE

LI LANNI

Translated by Tsien Yee Yu

ACA Publishing Ltd

A CROWDED SILENCE

LI LANNI

Translated by
TSIEN YEE YU

ACA PUBLISHING LTD

Published by
ACA Publishing Ltd.
University House
11-13 Lower Grosvenor Place,
London SW1W 0EX, UK
Tel: +44 (0)20 7834 7676
Fax: +44 (0)20 7973 0076
E-mail: info@alaincharlesasia.com
Web: www.alaincharlesasia.com

Beijing Office
Tel: +86(0)10 8472 1250
Fax: +86(0)10 5885 0639

Author: Li Lanni
Translator: Tsien Yee Yu
Editors: Samantha C. Allen and David Lammie
Cover art: Daniel Li

Published by ACA Publishing Ltd in association with the People's Literature Publishing House

© 2018, by People's Literature Publishing House, Beijing, China

ALL RIGHTS RESERVED. NO PART OF THIS PUBLICATION MAY BE REPRODUCED IN MATERIAL FORM, BY ANY MEANS, WHETHER GRAPHIC, ELECTRONIC, MECHANICAL OR OTHER, INCLUDING PHOTOCOPYING OR INFORMATION STORAGE, IN WHOLE OR IN PART, AND MAY NOT BE USED TO PREPARE OTHER PUBLICATIONS WITHOUT WRITTEN PERMISSION FROM THE PUBLISHER.

The greatest care has been taken to ensure accuracy but the publisher can accept no responsibility for errors or omissions, or for any liability occasioned by relying on its content.

Paperback ISBN: 978-1-910760-32-1
eBook ISBN: 978-1-910760-47-5

A catalogue record for *A Crowded Silence* is available from the National Bibliographic Service of the British Library.

PREFACE

One of my standing principles as a publisher is to never leave my name or any written traces of myself in any published work that comes under my responsibility. However, *A Crowded Silence* by Li Lanni is an exception to this rule. Moved and overwhelmed by her work, which came as a revelation to me, I cannot help but come forward to say a few words. Superior to other literary works in its forcefulness and intensity, this book left me speechless and in a state of stupefaction. It was not until much later that I finally understood: Even the most outstanding literary work cannot be compared to the spiritual depth, wealth, and practical implications of Li Lanni's book. For it is a cry from the heart of life and from the soul! What is more precious than our life and soul? It is our duty to cherish, protect and nurture them.

As well as providing practical guidance, this book is also an answer to the questions of our times. It is a testament of courage and intelligence. According to World Health Organisation estimation, 10.4 percent of the world population suffers from depression, meaning that one out of ten people is affected. It is on the top of the list of mental illnesses worldwide. What about the situation in China? Unable to find any reliable statistics, I must wonder if my two following suppositions are correct. One: The level of research regarding depression and its treatment is inadequate in China. And two: As part of the "global village," even if the rate of depression in China does not reach 10.4 percent, it is unlikely to be much lower. More troubling is the fact that around 90 percent of those with depression have no idea that they have a mental illness, let alone seek adequate treatment. Their first reaction would be, as Li Lanni recounts in her book: "What, me? Depressed? You must be joking!" Even if they do realise that they suffer from depression, lacking in-depth knowledge of their condition, they choose to remain silent and escape from their reality.

Li Lanni has bravely come forward to tell of her struggle with depression, which she fought against ceaselessly for five long years. She lays bare her soul in her book, which is comprised of four sections: "Diary," "Notes," "Correlations" and "Complementary Notes." She says: "Depression plunges you into pain and suffering. Staying alive is more difficult than letting yourself die, but light is at the end of the tunnel. You hold the key and power to change your condition for the better."

It is a book of courage and tenacity. Li Lanni descended into depression in 1998, and underwent three surgical interventions, followed by five cycles of chemotherapy. For the last five years, she has been taking antidepressants: Seroxat, buspirone, etc. Several times, her inner torment and suffering pushed her to the brink of suicide. Life was a thousand-fold more painful than death.

But Li Lanni fought her way out of the darkness and found the strength to live. Not only has she broken the taboo surrounding physical and mental illnesses, but, as a patient herself, she has also become something of an expert on the matter.

A Crowded Silence makes us acutely aware of our own ignorance in regards to mental illness. Among the millions of people who suffer from depression, Li Lanni may be just another drop in the ocean. But among the published works that are available today, there are few that recount the experience of a patient hit with a "double whammy" of cancer and depression. Li Lanni's past is full of pain. Time and time again, she delves into her memories, stirring up sadness and despair, which forced her time and time again to put aside her writing before picking up the thread again. She fought to bring her book to completion. In my ignorance, I made constant and relentless demands on her to edit her texts, insisting, almost without pity, on countless modifications. I plead guilty to such insensitivity. She never once refused the proposed changes. Her experience has taught her that life and death are but one and the same thing. To her, writing, publication, fame and worldly prestige are all irrelevant. But she continues to write, obstinate and single-minded in her efforts to tell of her subjective experience, thus bringing help and moral support to all her brothers and sisters who are trapped in the purgatory of depression.

The wealth and depth of this book goes beyond that of an ordinary literary work. The "Diary" section acts as a self-help guide; the "Notes" section explores her family history and her own past to root out the causes of her depression; "Correlations" is a collection of the different points of view on depression; and "Complementary Notes" provides additional information on the previous sections. The four parts come together to form what I call an exceptional literary work. But to Li Lanni, the essence of her book is not in its title nor its contents, but in her attempt to explore the causes of her depression, the different pathological symptoms of the disease and therapeutic methods. With stark, brutal honesty, she examines, under glaring daylight, the myriad aspects of depression: biological, pathological, psychological, historical, familial, social and cultural. Enough. Anything else would be superfluous.

To my mind, *A Crowded Silence* is about whether, when you are faced with mental illness, you can open your heart and let the sun come in to dispel the fog and darkness. The sun rises every day, and there will be a day when it reaches your corner, no matter how small and insignificant you may feel. Just like Lanni says...

Pan Kaixiong

1st May 2008

ABOUT LI LANNI

6th June to 27 th July 2003

Me? Depressed? Impossible. Everybody I know say I am cheerful and optimistic. If I am depressed, then who wouldn't be in this province?

My head is floating in front of me. My limbs are trembling, as if dangling from the carcass of a headless frog. All my insides have been gutted out – my brain, blood, a shred of skin from my forehead, eyeballs… They're floating in mid-air. I never understood Picasso, but now I am one of his paintings

28th June to 17th July 2003

Zhang Guorong,[1] his face… eternal, youthful…is staring at me from the television screen, his eyes wrinkled at the corners, a smile playing on his lips, the look in his eyes – mischievous, anxious and weary. He says: "It's April Fool's Day, won't you come and play a game of death with me? Who wants to play? Come on!"

I'm hanging onto the edge of the rooftop of a skyscraper; dangling in mid-air, I am about to fall. I don't know how long I can last, nor when I can climb back up onto the roof. The weight of my body is hinged upon the three fingers of one hand. I just want to let go.

18th July to 30th July 2003

We have all experienced events that have changed our destinies and our mental states. Once we are diagnosed with depression, we should try to remain level-headed and go through our mental life with a fine-toothed comb. At which stage of our lives did problems begin to surface? In which part of ourselves are the hidden wounds? Where are the blockages? How deep are the fissures?

As I was drawing up the will, I was lucid and at peace. No sadness, no worries, no regrets. There is nothing much to say in the face of death.

31st July to 27th October 2003

As children, they had difficult relationships with their mothers. These mothers were the first generation of career women in China. They're usually attractive, hold a professional title, are ambitious about their political careers, are extremely professional, keep their homes in good order, wear the trousers in their marriage and are slightly obsessive about cleanliness. The boundaries between their private and public lives are clear cut, and they're more caring and considerate to people outside the family than to their own children.

For these women, their maternal archetype conflicts with the maternal figure of our society and our consciousness. History created this phenomenon. They must go through the pain of "mental re-education."

29th October to 17th November 2003

All day long, she would clean the chairs, floor and windows. She rubbed the mat until it was in tatters; and she scrubbed the window frames until the paint came off. When she disciplined my brother and me, she made sure all the windows were closed, so that no one could see or hear us. At the time, my little brother was only 5 or 6 years old, but he was already wise to her ways. She only needed to throw a glance at the windows and he would shut them, put the latch down and draw the curtains, not letting a single shred of light through.

Suddenly the bank note blew up into a red paper cut the size of a towel, making it almost impossible to stick the pieces together. As if under a spell, the more difficult the task was, the more obsessed I became. Fatso came over to see me when she finished work. She watched curiously, as I tried to stick the pieces together. As if driven by insanity, I couldn't stop.

18th November to 1st December 2003

I was at the crossroads, waiting for the lights to turn green. Suddenly, in my mind, I saw the portable computer that was lying on my desk in Guangzhou. On its black surface was Einstein's face. That all-too-familiar face: tousled white hair, deep wrinkles, an enigmatic expression, eyes full of intelligence and a mischievous smile on his lips. Laughing, he said to me: "Why don't you come over?"

When I try to write about my experience in Shenzhen, my memory becomes a blank. I see nothing but a hazy mist before me: grey fog, shadowy lakes.

Depression is your punishment.

This thought has a life of its own, becomes uncontrollable and slips from my grasp. It springs out of the blue, leaps in front of me, shouting: "Li Lanni, are you capable of finishing this book? I doubt it very much. If you relapse into depression, it'll finish you off, won't it? And if you dropped dead? If you were given the choice, would you let yourself die? Don't think, just answer me! Li Lanni, if your cancer spreads to your brain, you'll never finish this book. Face the truth. You're scared of going back to the hospital for a check-up. You can't bear the thought of going through another operation.

12th April to 12th May 2004

Plagued by hallucinations and by my own obsessive-compulsive behaviour, I heard voices of people who had committed suicide. They said: "Why don't you leave? Come. Quickly, come. There's nothing here for you."

I do my best to stay alive. All my energy is channelled into just staying alive. It's harder to live than to die.

13th May to 7th August 2004

All life is precious, be it sick, disabled or dying.

To be plagued with cancer and depression is part of my destiny. I need to go through the experience in order to put it into words. It is like that glaring scar on my neck. The otolaryngologist took a photo of it as an example of a botched operation to show to medical students. The purpose is to help others live in health and happiness.

WE WENT THROUGH FIRE AND WATER,
BUT YOU BROUGHT US TO A PLACE OF ABUNDANCE.

Book of Psalm 66:12
Old Testament, Bible

FOREWORD

Today is Friday 26th August 2005. The time is 11:20 am. I haven't opened my diary since 7th August 2004.

I've often wanted to turn on my computer, but the mere thought of being confronted with my diary gives me chest pains, nausea, and I feel dizzy.

Why?

Am I running away from myself?

Pull yourself together, Li Lanni. Your brain is swamped with voices and shadows. They belong to people with depression who have taken their own lives. Shut the door. Take a deep breath.

Do you feel better? You are shivering inside.

You went through three operations for cancer and four and a half cycles of chemotherapy. Since April 2003, you've been on antidepressants: Seroxat, buspirone and alprazolam. Every day you can't help but think how it's harder to live than to die.

This thought goes round and round in your head every single day.

You are alone, lost in the wilderness. Turn towards the light. You'll be guided through the valley of death.

People often ask you: What do you write about?

Nothing.

What do you do all day long?

Nothing.

But I think to myself: I stay alive. It's all I can do.

ONE

Diary
Friday, 6th June 2003 12:15 pm

Today I drew up a daily schedule for the therapy to treat my depression. Also started my diary. It will help me on my road to recovery.

I've read many publications by English and German psychologists and they all say that keeping a diary helps patients untangle their thoughts and change a negative mindset to a positive one.

In his book, an American pastor, writer, and education specialist, Norman Vincent Peale, quoted the following verse from the Bible: "I can do all things through Christ who strengtheneth me."[1] He believes strength lies in positive thinking.

Made appointments with a psychiatrist and a physician in Traditional Chinese Medicine for this afternoon. I pray that everything will go smoothly. I've already jotted down my questions, in case I get nervous and forget.

I was sceptical of diary writing as a form of therapy. The word "write" makes me anxious, because I feel I am not up to the task. But the Bible says: "He [...] increases the power of the weak."[2] I am pleased with what I've achieved so far today. Mustn't give up.

Don't force yourself too much on the first day. Starting a diary is already an achievement.

Well done, Li Lanni. You can do it.

Notes

I have a glowing tan this summer. Every day at half-past midday, I go out and sit in the sun for about 45 minutes. It's a kind of light therapy for depression.

For many years, I've avoided the sun. All the beauty books say this: To have a beautiful white complexion and to prevent premature aging, avoid exposing yourself to the devastating effects of UV rays. A celebrity beauty once gave this pertinent advice: Limit your exposure to sunlight as much as possible and stay indoors between 10 in the morning and 4 in the afternoon. She said that if we do get a tan during the holidays, it would take up to five years for our complexion to go back to being clear and white again.

Chinese people like to "hide a hundred imperfections with a stroke of white." Today's urbanites, intentionally or not, are drifting away from the sun and nature. We must be careful not to let it lead us into the death valley of depression. According to a World Health Organisation estimation, 10.4 percent of the world's population suffer from depression; in other words, one in ten are affected.

The most terrifying hidden side of depression is suicide.

Susan Aldridge, a professor at Cambridge University, points out: 15 percent of those suffering from severe depression commit suicide.[3]

Depression has no age. Ursula Nuber, a German psychologist, cites the following example: A national survey conducted in the United States shows that 34 percent of students between eighth and tenth grade have thought about suicide at some point in time.[4]

In Northern Europe, England, and New York, 15 to 30 percent of the adult population has experienced severe depression once in their lives.

The number of people suffering from depression in Asia and its high suicide rate are a great cause for concern. China's overall suicide rate constitutes almost half of that of the world's population.

Psychologists warn that we are currently facing an epidemic of depression.

Until 23rd December 2002, I knew nothing about depression. And I didn't care.

In the spring of that year, Ququ and I were travelling to Jianggang on the express train when she received a phone call that left her in a state of shock. "Yang Ganhua has committed suicide," she said.

Yang Ganhua, a well-known writer from Guangdong, was also the vice president of the Association of Writers of the Provinces of China. He was a sociable and popular man. Apparently, the night before he died, he was at a Communist Party meeting discussing his work with the Writers' Association, and there was nothing unusual about his behaviour. He died peacefully. In a suicide note of about 100 words, he said his death was no one's fault and gave his last instructions with the utmost serenity.

Ququ said: "I saw him recently. He said he was ill. I asked him what with, but he didn't answer, so I didn't insist."

Passengers on the lower bunk were playing Tractor poker.[5] Sitting on the upper bunk, Ququ and I stared at each other without a word. A sadness came over me. I had goose bumps all over, my skull was tingling, and a rush of cold air brushed against my skin.

"You can be cured of an illness, can't you? Why did he do it? I went through a lymph node dissection and chemotherapy for my cancer. I survived, didn't I?" I said.

In April of this year, I thought back to what I had said about Yang Ganhua at the time and felt ashamed of myself. Because I had undergone surgery and chemotherapy, I had, to my mind, endured untold suffering. I thought I had sailed across vast oceans, but in fact I had only stepped over a small stream.

Back in Guangzhou, people couldn't stop talking about Yang Ganhua's suicide. No one knew what kind of illness he had, except that it was something peculiar that had to do with depression. He had a stable family life, good relations with his colleagues in his unit, and didn't appear to have any problems. So people sighed in disbelief: Why would he be depressed and put an end to his life?

The first time I heard a doctor pronounce the word "depression" was on the morning of 23rd December 2002. The nameplate on his desk said he had a PhD in medicine.

"It's probable that you suffer from depression," Dr Li said.

Me? Depressed? Impossible. Everyone I know says I am cheerful and optimistic. If I am depressed, then who wouldn't be, in this province?

The doctor explained to me what depression was, but I wasn't listening. All I wanted was for him to prescribe me some sleeping pills.

I had walked into the psychiatric department at the North Shenzhen Hospital. At the reception desk, a nurse with a small face and small mouth had told me that according to the new hospital rules, sleeping pills were available only on prescription by a psychiatrist. "Bad luck," I thought. "I'm not hanging around to see a doctor. I'm getting out of here now." But, as luck would have it, the waiting room was empty. The doctor would have all the time and patience in the world for me.

26th to 28th September 2005

Correlations

Excerpts from my psychiatric records

Date: 23/12/2002

Chief complaint: Sleep disturbance

History of present illness: Due to stress at work, the patient started to experience sleeping disorders in 1996: difficulty falling asleep, excessive dreaming, light sleep and waking up with the feeling of not having slept. At the same time, she reports feeling worried, anxious and fearful. Other symptoms: exhaustion, chest pressure, slow heartbeat, dryness in mouth, cold limbs, dizziness, headaches and nausea. In August or September 1998, she was admitted to the emergency ward with the following symptoms: tightness in the chest, dyspnea and intense sensation of cold. The electrocardiogram showed no anomaly. The above symptoms disappeared after 30 minutes. The dynamic electrocardiogram was normal. Quality of sleep has improved in the last 2 years, but she experiences early-morning awakenings around 4 am and finds it difficult to go back to sleep again. Excessive dreaming, even nightmares. She denies feeling depressed but admits to being anxious.

Complementary Note

When I'm writing the "Diary" section, I am a cancer patient.

When I'm writing "Notes," I am a literary writer. This section is written mostly in essay form. While writing about myself, I also tried to provide background information on history, society, and the times we're living in. It's an indirect way to follow the roots of my depression.

"Correlations" are extracts from the books which have helped me on my road to recovery and which may be of interest to my readers. I have also included some of my medical records for cancer and depression and the results of my medical exams. I want others who are ill, like myself, to know this: it's possible to live with illness in your life. Life and death can coexist.

"Complementary Notes" provide additional information to "Correlations."

TWO

Diary
Monday, 9th June 2003 12:20 pm

The thought of all the things that are waiting for me to do makes me nervous and anxious.

Relax. Be happy as you live each passing day.

Li Lanni, try to remember the things that have made you happy these last couple of days.

My consultation with the psychologist, Dr Gong, went well. He told me not to follow medical textbooks to the letter and that increasing the dosage of alprazolam could lessen my fatigue and regulate my mood. The Chinese physician, Dr Chen, said I must tonify my body before my problems related to Heat and Humidity[1] could be treated.

Saw my niece for the first time. Li Jiaen is one month old. She is very cute and looks just like my brother Fanding when he was a baby. I was exhausted when I got home.

Watched the Sunday service at the Crystal Cathedral in California on television. The Reverend Robert H. Schuller quoted from the Bible: "You are the light of the world."[2]

Lord, I ask you to drive the sins and darkness from my body, heart, and soul. Shine your light upon me, that I may be of service to you, that I may be your vessel and shine your divine light onto the world.

I read *The Power of Positive Thinking*[3] by Dr Norman Vincent Peale, who is a pastor, writer, and educator. In his book, he teaches us how to pray and suggests ways of cultivating our strengths and positive states of mind.

I'm sitting in front of the computer. Words are stuck inside me. Ninety-nine percent of my channels of communication are blocked, letting only superficial and trivial things through. I suspect I may have a touch of dementia.

Talked to Mother this afternoon and told her about my appointment with the psychologist. She was very negative, as usual. She has this habit of contaminating others with her negativity, dragging them down with her. Just talking to her wears me out.

I mustn't let myself be affected by her.

If you're not happy, how can you make others happy? If you don't feel good within yourself, how can you give and receive love?

I can smell the Chinese herbal decoction that is simmering in the kitchen. The trouble with me is that I am incapable of doing only one thing at a time. A psychologist, whose name I forget, said to reduce stress, you must concentrate on one thing at a time. The Bible says something similar.

This afternoon, I fell asleep while praying. Reciting verses from the Bible worked wonders and I felt myself opening up to a divine force.

Notes

Rereading my diary, it strikes me as odd that in June 2003, I made no mention of SARS[4] and the Iraq War. These two major events affected the whole world and yet there was no trace of them in my inner world. Is it because I am selfish? No. Even the most selfish among us must deal with reality, especially during the SARS epidemic. We all had to look out for ourselves. So did I just forget about them? No. Keeping a diary helps dispel negative thoughts and unveil my inner unhappiness.

I remember. Before the SARS outbreak, I was lost. Lost in a kind of emptiness.

The edge of desolation. My body, heart, and soul were scattered and lost in the valley of death. In a wasteland. Endless. Infinite. Where there was no sun, no moon. I was no longer of this world. I was lost in a desolate wilderness. I had eyes but could not see. I had ears but could not hear. I had a mouth but could not speak. I was crawling, fumbling. I touched the face of death. It was beautiful, smooth, fresh, youthful and firm, with a smile playing on its lips.

Between April and June, I was locked up within myself. I was afraid to go out. I shunned contact with people. I could not listen to music nor watch television and refused to answer the phone. I didn't even want to see my only brother, Fanding, who lived close by. I was looking forward to the birth of my niece and was hoping to be waiting outside the delivery room to see her. But I could not make it. My brain, body and limbs were completely disconnected. I dreaded hearing the phone ring, a knock at the door or the sound of footsteps. I was so afraid that I would lock myself in the study and curl up in a corner. I didn't even know what I was afraid of. My soul had left my body. In fact, I was incapable of feeling my own body. I was like a doll that had been torn into a thousand pieces, impossible to put together again.

No, don't go out onto the balcony. Twelve storeys high. It's a pity that the anti-burglary net is such an eyesore. It gets in my way. I have this maddening urge to fly into the sky, break through the net and fly like a butterfly, float like a sheet of paper. Is it going to hurt when I touch the ground? I would like to fly in broad daylight, under a clear sky... A glimpse of the balcony would stir up this impulse in me to fly. Like being caught in a tug-of-war, I pull my eyes away, but it pulls me back again. My fingers cling tightly onto the door frame or the back of a chair. I close my eyes, go back into the sitting-room or into the corner of the study. A demonic force is pushing me. I curl up, my back against the corner. I see the shadow of a strange beast lurking inside me. It's roaring, pacing up and down inside my chest, waiting to break loose. It roars furiously, ready to burst out, destroying everything in its path. It stalks inside my chest, round and round and round, wearing down my resistance.

I've flipped through about a dozen books on depression but am too tired and lack the concentration to read them properly. I leafed through a few pages today, slumped on a chair, on the sofa, or on the floor. In one of the books, doctors and psychologists, who themselves suffer from depression, gave a description of the different kinds of symptoms. They also included the experiences of writers, politicians, prominent journalists and people from all walks of life. But in my view, none of them were able to clearly describe their feelings. No one who has fallen into a deep depression can express his or her pain. Our nervous system prevents us from doing this. And what we do manage to say is shallow, inadequate and incapable of capturing the most terrifying aspect of depression in all its nakedness. Words fail to encompass the depths of this experience.

People often ask me: "What's it like to suffer from depression?" I am at a loss for words.

People ask me this question so often that, just to shut them up, I answer: "It's worse than cancer."

6th to 9th October 2005

Correlations

Excerpts from a histopathology report from the Oncology Hospital

Name: Li Lanni

Case Number: 105921

Clinical Diagnosis: Post-operative histopathology for cancer of the thyroid – right lobe

Date: 21/02/2000

Histopathology Report:

<u>Lower deep jugular chain nodes:</u> Metastasis of papillary carcinoma. Its structure corresponds to papillary thyroid carcinoma.

<u>Middle deep jugular chain nodes</u>: Metastasis of papillary carcinoma. Its structure corresponds to papillary thyroid carcinoma.

<u>Upper deep jugular chain nodes</u>: Metastasis of papillary carcinoma. Its structure corresponds to papillary thyroid carcinoma.

<u>Supraclavicular lymph nodes</u>: No sign of cancer.

Complementary Notes

I didn't read the histopathology report of my lymphadenectomy. Could make neither head nor tail of it.

However, two months after the operation, when a doctor friend of mine saw the huge scar on my neck, he urged me to read the post-operative report. It was only then that I realised how serious my operation was. To rule out the possibility of metastasis to the brain, lungs and bone, I immediately had a CT-scan and a radioisotope scan of the brain, neck and chest. This was followed by five cycles of chemotherapy. It destroyed my entire body: nervous system, immune system, respiratory system, secretion system, blood system, kidneys, skin, hair, organs, viscera and even my voice.

I didn't tell my friends about my lymphadenectomy and I found the surgeon who operated on me without going through my social network.

THREE

Diary
Friday, 20th June 2003

I am a woman blessed. At times I am touched by the Holy Spirit, and in that split second I know that under God's protection, I will someday recover my health.

A LIST OF HAPPY AND UNHAPPY THINGS IN MY LIFE.

HAPPY THINGS:

- All my basic medical expenses (medication and tests) are covered.
- I've been on antidepressants for the last three months. The worst is behind me and the side effects are subsiding.
- Even though I am on sick leave, I still receive my monthly salary, which is sufficient for my everyday needs.
- Staying at home means I do not get myself tangled up in complicated social relationships.
- Because I am sick, people are more tolerant and less demanding of me at work and in general. It takes the pressure off.
- My parents enjoy a stable life and my brother is happily settled in his family life.
- My husband is in good health, his career is going smoothly, and he takes good care of me.
- My friends care about me and think I'm easy-going.
- I am independent and haven't become a burden on others.

Tired. Have headache and feel nauseous.

NOTES

When I reactivate the memories on the uppermost layers of my consciousness, it triggers the alarm bell in my nervous system. It's probably due to an imbalance in my brain's neurotransmitters and cerebral fluid. Warning: I had another dream about depression.

I was in a lively place. Doctors were presenting a report and were deep in discussion with journalists. I was about to sneak out when the security guards stopped me at the door. A stern-looking man, like a university professor, told me to follow him and said I must help a student. There was a crowd outside a room, and someone told me to look inside. A young, thin, sick-looking man in his 20s was sitting on a bed. The people standing next to me said it was my job to prepare him psychologically for death and to tell him not to be afraid, etc. I said I didn't know him and that they should find someone else more suitable.

"It's too late," the doctor said. "He's in the final stages of cancer. He has a month to live at the most."

"Why me?" I asked.

"Because you're going to die before him," he replied. "He'll listen to you."

"But if I remember correctly, I'm supposed to die in the second half of this year," I said, confused.

"No, you've got it mixed-up. You'll die in the next few days. Aren't you ready for it? It'll be painless. We'll give you some powerful analgesics. People compliment me on my work all the time. Families don't have to worry..."

I couldn't listen to him anymore. Damn, I got my dates wrong. Was there anything to prepare? Did I have enough time?

I hate these last-minute changes. I had resigned myself to the fact that I wasn't going to die before the end of the year and now I had to reverse my state of mind and brace myself for death.

Realising I was afraid, I chided myself: "Li Lanni, what're you scared of? Six months, what difference does it make? If you must die, then you must. It's your destiny and will come as a release. Heaven is a beautiful place." But I was upset. Why were the others being so casual about my death? They're worried about the student and regret his death but are completely indifferent to mine. I'm going to die first, so why should I be the one to comfort him? Yes, I understand. Because I'm going first, it's my task to teach him, to show him the way.

Relieved, as if a weight had been lifted off my shoulders, I walked towards the room. The dream became blurred. End of dream. Woke up tired.

In her book, Dr Aldridge describes the feelings of people who suffer from major depression. Certain passages make me go: "Yes, yes, it's like that. Almost, but not quite..."

Some examples:

A successful television producer said: "You lose all sense of priority, because nothing seems to make sense anymore, devoid of relevance... You wake up in the morning drowned in fear, like waves of sea water gushing into the hull of a sinking ship. You're completely incapacitated, unable to get out of bed, unable to get through the day. What am I afraid of? I can't tell you... Those who haven't suffered from depression can't understand the fear."

A biologist said: "Depression is more frightening than seeing my wife die from cancer. It fills me with shame to say that I suffered more from depression than from my wife's death, but it was my inner reality."

Leo Tolstoy was haunted by thoughts of suicide during his depressive episodes: "Look at me, I am blessed in my life, and yet every night when I undress for bed, I make sure I put the rope outside the bedroom to stop me from hanging myself. I go hunting without my rifle, in case I'm unable to resist the temptation to end my life."[1]

Before reading Dr Aldridge's book, I was unaware that Tolstoy suffered from depression. It has shed a light on a habit I have with knives. After using the fruit knife, I invariably put it back in its sheath. Even when it's late at night and the sheath is nowhere to be found, I put it beneath a thick book, mindful of its sharp blade. Often when I am alone at home, I am very conscious of the presence of that blade. I try to ignore it or go into another room, but the image of a knife cutting deep into the skin, exposing the veins, goes round and round in my mind.

The temptation is irresistible.

12th October 2005

Correlations

Excerpts from the Oncology Hospital's Discharge Report

Name: Li Lanni

Date of Discharge: 24/02/2000

Post-operative Diagnosis: Metastatic papillary thyroid cancer (right side)

Procedure: Following pre-operative examinations, cervical lymph node dissection was carried out under local anaesthesia on 20th December.

Status at Discharge: Surgical incision healed. Pathology results are compatible with clinical diagnosis.

Complementary Notes

My operation happened almost by chance. Just after the New Year in 2000, a doctor in Guangzhou discovered a small lump in my neck and I was admitted immediately into hospital.

"But I don't have my personal belongings with me and I don't have much cash," I said, alarmed.

"You can use your credit card and have your family bring you your things," the doctor said.

I was operated on after two days of routine medical examinations. The stiches were taken out, leaving a spectacular red lumpy scar on my neck. You couldn't miss it, and I decided it had a symbolic meaning. I returned to Shenzhen with the hospital's discharge report. Apparently, I couldn't apply for reimbursement for expenses incurred outside of Shenzhen. Worried that I might have another operation in Guangzhou in a couple of years' time, I made inquiries at the Social Security Department, where a good part of my day was spent waiting in line. The woman at the counter glanced at the discharge form and threw it back at me.

"You can't claim!" she said in her shrill voice.

"I'd like to know," I said, trying my best to be polite, "if the next time a doctor decides I must have an emergency operation, what are the necessary formalities to file a claim for a refund?"

"You can't claim!" she repeated, as if I hadn't uttered a single word. "Too many people have cancer."

Then she ignored me.

FOUR

Diary
Saturday, 21st June 2003

The time is 11:15 am. Therapy begins.

A LIST OF THE NOT-SO-HAPPY THINGS:

- I feel as if I am walking on glass. Every day I have the same aches and pains: dizziness, nausea, stomach ache, bloated abdomen, fatigue and lassitude. The side effects of the medications are killing me.
- I am sick and tired of seeing doctors. It drains me, and people are patronising. A waste of time, energy and money. My patience is wearing thin.
- It's impossible to read and think, let alone write. What a waste.
- (Just drank some Chinese herbal decoction. Tasted so bitter.) Emotional wounds are hard to heal. Childhood wounds begin in the family. The deeper and more hidden they are, the more difficult it is to express them. You pretend they don't exist or that they no longer affect you. But it's burying your head in the sand. How can you escape from your own subconscious?
- Can't control my negative thoughts, nor feelings of insecurity and self-blame.

That's why I am down in the dumps.

Why does my head hurt every time I switch on the computer? Is it a mental blockage?

Answer: I am anxious when I switch on the computer because of my dissatisfaction with my own writing and my fear that it's only a heap of junk. Fatigue and feelings of inferiority overwhelm me. My constant self-reproach puts me under tremendous pressure, and to escape from it, my nervous system sends out signals which are then converted into headaches.

How about that for an explanation?

But things are never that simple.

I am tired of having to always analyse my thoughts.

Exercise: Relax. Re...lax.

I can't. Today's frenetic pace of life has dulled my ability to relax and let myself go.

Notes

According to Dr Gong, I am too sensitive and I always find excuses not to join in. The members of the "Chinese Women's Association" have criticised me for this: Every time they plan an excursion, Li Lanni is the first to say yes, but when the time comes, she spoils the fun, claiming she is too busy and can't go.

Stop...

Li Lanni, you're going round in circles. You avoid talking about what makes you unhappy and you refuse to analyse the reasons. What are you afraid of?

I don't know. I don't want to talk about it. Don't make me. Or I'll tear my hair out, strand by strand. Enough.

There are complex reasons behind each of the nine happy and five unhappy things on my lists.

Sadness. Bitterness.

Only meaningless words, devoid of emotion, come to me.

When I woke up this morning, my brain was exhausted, as if it had spent all night wandering around by itself.

For some time now, I have felt that there are three different people in me. My physical body participates in my everyday life, but my mind often drifts during the day; at night my soul has a life of its own. It's like I live in three different worlds. What I experience in my daydreams and in my dreams at night are far more distressing than what I go through in my real life.

I started having lots of dreams when I was in primary school. The people and landscapes were very clear and would linger for a long time after I woke up. Long dreams left me exhausted. They were clear and realistic, had a beginning and an end. It was quite confusing, because on days when my life seemed real, I would forget my dreams, but on other days when my life seemed unreal, my dreams would come back clearly and appear almost tangible. I thought everyone had dreams like mine. When I grew up, I talked about it with my friends. They said: "Our dreams are vague, scattered and incoherent. We can't remember them afterwards. Are your dreams really that complicated? How can you remember everything in such detail? Are you joking or just making it up?" This was how I knew that other people dreamt differently. Not wanting to be misunderstood, I told myself never to talk about my dreams again. It was pointless.

This is my diary. I can talk to my heart's content about things I cannot normally say.

Had a dream last night...No...Early this morning, because I don't normally switch off the lights until one in the morning.

I was in Hong Kong for an assignment with a few women colleagues (the bit before was blurry). We were staying in a rather basic international youth hostel with shared toilets and bathrooms. The men and women's sections were separated by a canvas, like the "changing rooms" you'd find in market places. Just outside the rooms and next to a canteen was a courtyard, where the personnel washed the dishes and cleaned the vegetables. To go outside onto the streets, you had to cross a wet, muddy, foul-smelling courtyard and then pass through the canteen. On my way out, I noticed a fish lying on the ground next to a basin. It was about a foot long and looked like a mackerel, but shorter, wider, and prettier. It had bright silvery scales. Out of curiosity, I picked it up to take a closer look and put it back down on the ground. Later, in the middle of a meeting, my head was aching, my eyes were prickling, and my cheeks felt uncomfortable. I went back to the youth hostel alone, and as I was crossing the courtyard, I caught myself in the mirror above the wash basin. My complexion had turned grey and my naturally thin face had become so round and bloated, like a fish bladder filled with water, that the skin was just a thin transparent ashen-grey film. I resembled a gigantic Chaozhou cake. I was horrified. The person in the mirror wasn't me. Luckily, I have slit eyes. My eyelids weren't swollen, which meant I was still vaguely recognisable. My head, face and body were itching and hurting, and I could not breathe properly. Since I could neither lie down nor stand up, I sat up on the bed, my back leaning against the wall.

What kind of strange disease did I have? How come I looked so ghastly? Who could help me? I knew I could return to Shenzhen for treatment, but I would run into problems at customs because I looked nothing like the photograph in my passport. I looked at myself again in the mirror. My eyelids were now swollen, and my eyes were mere slits on my face. No one would recognise me, so how could I prove that I am me at customs? I was in a state panic.

(After this, my colleagues returned to the youth hostel and tried to find a solution, but it would take too long to explain. This torture left me physically and mentally exhausted. To make a long story short, I'll jump to the last part of the dream.)

A middle-aged doctor from Hong Kong who no one knew arrived. He asked me what I had done that morning and where I had been. He examined me, thought for a while and said: "It's an allergy."

"Have you any idea of what might have caused the allergy?" he asked, looking at me. "Think."

I thought hard and remembered the silvery fish.

"Yes, it must be the fish," he said.

"Should I go to a hospital for an allergy shot?" I asked, relieved that it was only an allergy. I was used to injections.

"No, it won't be necessary. Just take the fish and rub it on your face until the inflammation subsides."

Was he a qualified doctor? Were Hong Kong doctors ethical? How long had that fish been dead? How long had it been lying there next to the basin? It must stink by now, or maybe someone had thrown it away. Just the thought of rubbing it on my face made me nauseous. Wouldn't it aggravate the inflammation and damage my skin? The doctor made no effort to convince me and left without a word. I told myself that I would only do it if the fish was still there.

The dead fish was still there.

I picked it up and rubbed it all over my face, again and again. It was revolting, and I felt so stupid and helpless. After a while, I looked in the mirror again, and to my surprise, the inflammation had subsided a little. I clutched the fish even tighter and rubbed it even harder against my face: here and there, round and round, up and down, until it reverted back to how it was before. But my initial excitement then turned into panic. My head, face, hands and body stank of fish. I needed to clean myself from head to toe, but the women's bathroom was closed for repairs. I wanted to use the men's, but there were still people inside. Panic. Panic. I was dying for a wash. Like an athlete at a 100-metre sprint, I was ready to dash into the bathroom at the first opportunity. I couldn't wait anymore. Panic. If only I could rid myself of that stink.

13th October 2005

Correlations

Excerpts from my medical report from the Department of External Consultation at the Oncology Hospital

Date of Examination: 12/05/2000

Post-operative examination for lymph node dissection in papillary thyroid carcinoma:

Residual tissue mass on right side of neck is homogeneous. Below the sternocleidomastoid muscle on the right, presence of a lymph node measuring 1 x 0.6 cm. A smaller lymph node measuring 0.5 x 0.5 cm is visible on left side of neck.

Comment: Post-operative report of cervical lymph node dissection in papillary thyroid cancer: as indicated above.

Date: 16/05/2000

Conclusion of the otolaryngologist: LN[1] on right and left side of neck measure 0.5 cm.

- Thyroxine
- Mifurol: take 2 tablets once daily for 5 cycles. Each cycle is 21 days.

Complementary Notes

Mifurol is a cancer treatment. One chemotherapy cycle lasts for 21 days, followed by a seven-day break before the next cycle begins. In total, there were five cycles.

The post-operative report mentioned the presence of suspicious lymph nodes after my cervical lymph node dissection (right side). I asked an otolaryngologist: "Is it because the lymph node dissection wasn't thorough enough, or is it a relapse?" He answered: "Both are possible. We'll keep an eye on it. If the lymph node grows to three centimetres, we'll do another operation." What a mess. I was operated on in February and already in May another operation was looming on the horizon.

What I didn't realise was that chemotherapy would be far more devastating than surgery.

FIVE

Diary
Sunday, 22nd June 2003 10:50 am

The time is 4:50 pm. Therapy begins.

Felt completely drained before getting out of bed this morning. As if my heart had stopped beating.

Emotionally and mentally, I am at rock bottom. It's been ages since chemotherapy started and it's going *so* slowly. Is it going to drag on forever?

When I eat, my stomach hurts; I have nightmares and insomnia; zero energy for a social life, let alone sports or travelling. Sometimes watching television or listening to music just wipes me out. So miserable.

Negative thoughts contaminate my mind. I must stop them from wreaking havoc on my life.

"This is the day the Lord has made; let us rejoice and be glad."[1]

Get a grip on yourself. Stay calm. You can do it.

Go on. Stretch out your hand. Pick up the glass of water and the pills. Healthy people have no idea how much energy it takes just to bring a glass of water to your lips and pop a couple of pills into your mouth.

Overcame my despondency. Got out of bed.

Drew the curtains back and saw the foul weather outside. Heavy rain. Felt reassured, because dreary weather always makes me gloomy. All I need to do is maintain a stable mood, hold out until the weather improves and I'll be back on my feet again.

Once out of bed, I kept reciting in my head: "If God is for us, who is against us?"[2] It's a technique recommended by the American professor Norman Vincent Peale in his book *The Power of Positive Thinking*.

His other methods are:

1. Stay calm and listen to the voice of God in your heart.
2. Find your strength in God and learn to follow His rhythm.
3. Make a habit of being happy.
4. Slow down and learn to relax.
5. Let your subconscious be immersed in faith and confidence.
6. Learn to empty your mind of worries and feelings of insecurity.
7. Imagine yourself resting and gathering strength in the arms of God.
8. Give thanks and gratitude in your prayers.

9. Physical exercise can reduce stress.
10. Learn to sit serenely in the sun.

Notes

I wonder if depression sufferers have a kind of "sixth sense." Whenever there was a dramatic change in the weather, a storm, or just before a monsoon or a natural disaster, I would be filled with a sense of foreboding and my body would ache all over. I'd say to myself: "The heavens are sick, do you know that? Yes, I do. The heavens are angry, do you know that?"

The story of Sodom and Gomorrah would come to mind. The people of the cities of Sodom and Gomorrah were treacherous and deceitful; they lived in pride, greed and lust. The wrath of God descended upon them and He rained burning sulphur onto the city and destroyed it.

Man is becoming increasingly disrespectful and destructive towards Mother Nature. She'll rebel and retaliate.

The physically weak are blessed. For they respect our Creator and Mother Nature.

Rereading the "Diary" section, my attention lingered on the sentence: "Learn to sit serenely in the sun."

If you say this to a city office worker, he'll think you're wasting his time and say: "I bust a gut trying to make a living, don't get enough sleep, and you talk to me about 'sitting in the sun.' Where's my next meal coming from? Get real!"

Sitting on a bench in Xiju Gardens and taking in the sun, thoughts were racing around continuously in my head, lost and aimless, unable to halt, like a wild horse galloping, uncontrollable.

I wrote in the "Diary" section: "Only do one thing at a time."

In the past, I was capable of doing several things simultaneously. Like an acrobat with his balancing act holding a pile of dishes in each hand, standing on a heap of bricks, perched on an umbrella, with a stack of crockery sitting on his head and the stem of a flower between my teeth.

While eating breakfast, I could watch television, read the newspaper, listen to music and even talk on the phone. His five senses were on high alert and fully functioning all at the same time. In this day and age, we've made a habit of cramming as much as possible into the shortest span of time. Every minute, every second counts. Life is a race against time.

Some books say the reason behind the rise in the number of people suffering from depression is stress: an unstable and frenetic lifestyle, information overload, and the gap between high expectations and reality.

Is there any point in talking about this? It's like the boy who cried wolf. Who believes him or cares?

We worry about losing our jobs, our houses, our cars. We're ambitious and seek to accumulate resources; we worry about our ever-changing work environments, housing situations, families, even gossip. Who can we trust and turn to in times of need?

As the saying goes: "You never stop learning." But we are drowning in a sea of information. The amount of knowledge and information currently at our disposal is equivalent to all that has been accumulated over the centuries of human existence. What was five weeks in the past is equivalent to one week today.

Knowledge is increasing at an exponential rate. I feel sick and dizzy after spending 20 minutes in a book shop, as if I'm being crushed beneath a mountain of books. Invisible. Silent. Deadly.

Computers, fax machines, emails...all pushing us to go faster and faster. Go, go, go! We live in an age that seeks quick results and immediate gratification.

A hen lays an egg in the morning, we expect it to hatch in the afternoon; the next day the chick matures and lays more eggs; the chicks reproduce; the day after, it becomes a chicken farm; the day after that, it enters Forbes's ranking.

Parents want their children to study in prestigious schools, work in international firms, have an annual income of more than 100,000 yuan, marry a partner of good social standing and have beautiful and intelligent children.

If Bill Gates can succeed, then why can't we?

How dare you "sit serenely in the sun?" How dare you?

14th to 20th October 2005

Correlations

Excerpts from *"Sodom and Gomorrah"*

The Lord said to Abraham:

"The outcry against Sodom and Gomorrah is great and their sin is very grave, I will go down to see whether they have done altogether according to the outcry that has come to me before I destroy the city."

Abraham interceded for the inhabitants of the city and said:

"Suppose there are fifty righteous within the city. Will you then sweep away the place and not spare it for the fifty righteous who are in it?"

And the Lord replied:

"If I find at Sodom fifty righteous in the city, I will spare the whole place for their sake."

Abraham said:

"Oh let not the Lord be angry, and I will speak again but this once. Suppose ten are found there."

The Lord answered:

"For the sake of ten I will not destroy it."

The Lord sent two angels to Sodom and there they found ten righteous. The Lord spared the city.

A story from the Bible

Complementary Notes

There are people who have weaker morals than the inhabitants of Sodom. They are lawless and fear neither God nor man. The reason why their city is still standing and spared from divine fire is because of the 10 righteous that still live there. Many have heard this story, but few heed its warning. They make light of the moral of the story and never tell it to their children. Will there be fewer righteous people in the city? It troubles me greatly.

SIX

Diary
Tuesday, 24th June 2003

I still suffer from Humidity and Deficiency of the Spleen.[1] The Chinese physician said not to force myself to do physical exercise as it might have an adverse effect.

I try to stay optimistic and serene while coping with my daily burden of illness, medication and physical discomfort.

Dr Susan Aldridge, an English psychologist, said in her book *Seeing Red and Feeling Blue: The New Understanding of Mood and Emotion* that it's possible to transform a negative mind set in the space of a few months. This kind of cognitive therapy requires 20 sessions, each lasting 45 minutes.

People with depression criticise themselves constantly:

1. Them:"I'm worthless."
2. The world:"I never do anything right."
3. The future:"I'll never make anything of myself."

Cognitive therapy consists of four steps:

1. Make a list of things to do every day. This will keep the patient active and prevent thoughts from going round in circles.
2. Draw up a list of activities that make the patient feel good or satisfied (no matter how insignificant this activity may be). This will counterbalance the negative thoughts. It will help alleviate feelings of hopelessness and despair and impart a sense of satisfaction and accomplishment.
3. Help the patient understand that his or her negative thoughts are the results of a mental attitude and not a reflection of an objective reality. An obstinate negative thought can be contradicted by an actual fact. For example: The thought "I'm useless" can be countered by: "During business negotiations, I may seem reserved, but my clients appreciate my patience."
4. After an evaluation of the patient's strengths and weaknesses, the therapist then chooses the method most suitable for him or her.

The therapy aims to make long-lasting changes to the patient's negative ways of thinking.

Additional tips:

1. Take vitamin B6 and cod liver oil.
2. Eat fish and bananas; drink coffee.
3. Walk for one hour every day. Results can be felt after just five days. Outdoor activities help reduce anxiety and ward off morbid thoughts.
4. Get up at the same time every day; make sure you have good quality sleep.
5. Listen to rhythmic music that promotes a sense of well-being.
6. Keep a diary to sort out your thoughts.
7. Watch movies; go to the theatre.
8. Do any activities that you find interesting as much as possible. This helps you relax.
9. Take a time-out. Switch off your mobile phone; get a housekeeper.
10. Organise your day using post-it notes to help take the pressure off.

I started my cognitive therapy on 6th June.

Dr Aldridge's book is better than *Depression: An Undiagnosed Illness* by the German psychologist Ursula Nuber. It's well-structured, informative and specialised without being dull and off-putting. Ursula Nuber's book was most likely first published in a series of articles, which explains why it's simplistic and shallow.

The German psychologist Sigmund Freud focuses strongly on our childhood experiences and recommends psychotherapy as the most efficacious treatment. British psychologists put less emphasis on the role that childhood plays in our psyche. Instead, they prefer to use medication, because they believe that long-term stress and pressure leads to a chemical imbalance in the brain, causing a drop in the level of serotonin. However, they also recognise the beneficial effects of cognitive therapy.

My personal remedy for depression: Faith + medication + cognitive therapy.

I am so impatient, the road to recovery is long.

When weakness and despondency take hold of me, I remind myself: "Whoever believes will not be in haste."[2] And: "They who wait for the Lord shall renew their strength; they shall mount up with wings like eagles."[3]

"God intended it for good to accomplish what is now being done."[4] God has His plans. We must put our trust in Him.

Pray, confide, give thanks. Serenity, patience, hope. Nurture joy and devotion in our hearts.

Notes

The weather is magnificent at this time of year. The temperature is between 20 and 30 degrees and humidity is at 50 percent. Sunshine and a fresh breeze. Beautiful and memorable days like these, you can count them on one hand.

Date: Morning of 23rd December 2002

Place: Consultation room in the Psychiatric Department of North Shenzhen Hospital

Characters: Professor Li, Li Lanni

Li Lanni poked her head through the half-opened door. The doctor seemed pleasant and gestured to her to come in. Happily surprised, she thought: "That's unusual. It's not often a doctor is free to see you right away. He's even smiling. Is it because I'm in a specialty department? Not necessarily. It's probably because they don't get a lot of patients here. Who wants to come here? Who wants to see a 'psychiatrist?' Even the name sounds peculiar. The consultation fees are expensive, 100 yuan. With my level two refund,[5] I only have to fork out 2.50 yuan for him to write me a prescription."

Standing in front of his desk, Li Lanni noticed his name plate said: "Professor." Anxious to inform him beforehand, she said: "I came to see you not because I'm ill, but because I'd like to have a prescription for sleeping pills. Would it be possible to prescribe me some for a few days?"

Professor Li: Please sit down.

Seeing that the doctor made no move to write out a prescription, she sat down.

Li Lanni: I often need to take sleeping pills, but some hospitals only prescribe them for three days, and I can't get them at the pharmacy. Could you prescribe me some?

Professor Li: I can only write you a prescription for seven days.

Li Lanni *(disappointed)*: Then...can you increase the dosage? Just a little. Normally I take two tablets of estazolam at one go, sometimes even four.

Startled, Professor Li shot her a disapproving glance.

Li Lanni: Well...yes...I overdid it a bit that time. I could hardly walk straight the next day. I kept bumping into walls, couldn't bend down and fell down a couple of times.

Professor Li: Tell me more about your sleeping problems.

Li Lanni was uneasy. Why was he asking her all these questions just for a couple of pills? Didn't he have any other patients to see to? Maybe he had to prove that he was worth every cent that his country had spent on his education.

Li Lanni: I have trouble going to sleep. With the sleeping pills, I manage to fall asleep around one or two in the morning, but I wake up around four and can't go back to sleep again. That's why I need a heavier dose.

Suddenly the doctor sat up on his chair, head bent slightly forward, a gleam in his eyes, like a police officer from the narcotics squad who had discovered a suspicious trail.

Professor Li: How long have you had these early morning awakenings?

Li Lanni: Er...about two months now. No, more than that. I've been having nightmares and sleep disturbances for over a year. I wake up in the morning feeling more tired than if I had stayed up all night.

Like a narcotics officer who had found a clue, he was absorbed in his own thoughts.

Professor Li: You don't suffer from ordinary insomnia. You should do a psychological test.

***Li Lanni thought to herself**: I don't believe you.*

Li Lanni: Er...no...it's alright. I'd like to have some sleeping pills, that's all.

Professor Li: Listen carefully. If for more than fifteen days you wake up in the early hours of the morning unable to go back to sleep, it's possible you might suffer from depression. Have you heard of depression?

Li Lanni: Depression? It's when you're so full of worries that you can't see a way out.

Professor Li: Not quite. It's a kind of mental illness. There are three clinical signs. One of them is waking up early in the morning unable to go back to sleep. Of course, there are also…

Li Lanni *(interrupts)*: I'm not depressed. I don't have to take care of my parents and I have no children. My working hours aren't fixed, so there's no pressure. I have loads of friends and my salary is enough for me to live on comfortably…My husband is a highly qualified professional and in good health. My brother is very caring and looks after our parents. So, you see, I've got no worries.

Professor Li: But…for an evaluation of…

Li Lanni: When I had my operation for my cancer, I didn't cry, even when I knew I had to have chemotherapy for metastatic cancer. Everyone I know says I'm cheerful and optimistic. How could I possibly suffer from depression?

Li Lanni didn't let the doctor get a word in edgeways. Being an insomniac didn't mean you're mentally weak or depressed. She needed to convince the doctor to prescribe her a heavy dose of sleeping pills.

Li Lanni: A friend said my cancer didn't seem to faze me at all. I was telling everyone about it, like I had won the lottery. Some people thought the hospital had made a mistake. How come she's in better shape than the rest of us?

Professor Li: Do you have a high level of self-control?

Li Lanni: Yes, since I was a child, I've always been independent and capable of excellent self-control. A lot of people like to confide in me, but I keep everything to myself. Once a school friend said: "Li Lanni, it's always me who comes crying on your shoulder. When are you going to have a good cry on mine? You'll feel much better afterwards." What she didn't understand was that I never cry.

Professor Li: That's not good. People who have a high level of self-control are like a bow that is drawn tighter, tighter and tighter and…Crack!…it snaps.

You can control yourself during the day, but at night your subconscious lets itself go, hence the nightmares.

Li Lanni was stunned. She remembered a dream she had not long after her operation. In her dream, she was crying in front of her friend: "Ququ, I have cancer!" Yes, that was the only time she cried, and it was in her dream. What the doctor said made sense, but to say that she was depressed was too far-fetched.

Professor Li: The two other symptoms for depression are: one, you lose interest in activities you previously enjoyed; and two... obsessive suicidal thoughts.

Li Lanni: Suicide has never even once crossed my mind! Cancer medications are now extremely efficacious, and the pain is not unbearable to the point of killing myself. I told my doctor that I'd never let cancer get the better of me. All the doctors say I have a healthy attitude towards life. I have nothing to be depressed about. If I'm depressed, then everyone in this province and half the world population would be depressed. (Laugh) Frankly, I'm the last person on earth who would be depressed.

———

I didn't sleep a wink last night. I was in the study until three in the morning, walking around in circles in the dark as if in a trance, a blanket thrown over my shoulders as I muttered these words in an effort to comfort myself: "Relax... Happiness... Tranquility... Beauty... Fresh flowers... Green grass... Blue skies." When I had finally worn myself out, I sat on the windowsill, watching the city sleeping beneath me. Then, leaning on the arm of the sofa, I said to myself: "Don't worry...no...don't worry. Don't be afraid...sleep...go to sleep." Even though I was exhausted today, I didn't want to take a nap. My head aches.

In her book *Depression Explained*, Gwendoline Smith[6] warns: "In remembering the wounds and unhappiness of the past, those who suffer from depression become prisoners of their past, plunging them deeper into despair. If they do not receive adequate counselling from a therapist, they will become further entrenched in their past."

Yes, I understand. But why do I refuse to remember the details of my operation? Why can't I talk about my depression in a meaningful way? I need to disperse the shadows surrounding me.

On the morning of 23rd December 2002, Professor Li of the Psychiatric

Department of North Shenzhen Hospital prescribed me seven days of alprazolam and seven days of paroxetine, an antidepressant. He told me to come back a week later for a follow-up. I took alprazolam, thinking it was the same as estazolam. I didn't take paroxetine and missed the follow-up consultation. As a joke, I told my friends about the Professor's diagnosis. They found it hilarious. Li Lanni depressed? Ha ha...who isn't? Even now, there are friends who don't believe it. A close friend once said: "What depression? If you're depressed, then we will be as well. You're the last person on earth who'd fall into depression. The doctor doesn't know what he's talking about."

In her book *Depression: An Undiagnosed Illness*, Ursula Nuber said that one common characteristic among those who suffer from depression is that they try to hide behind a mask that says: 'everything is alright.' The strength of their will and their self-control allows them to cope with the demands of daily life. But they keep their suffering to themselves, out of sight of everyone around them.[7]

A Taiwanese writer, San Mao,[8] hanged herself with a silk stocking in a hospital bathroom. People couldn't understand, saying: "We didn't know." Even the nurses on duty that night said: "But she seemed perfectly normal."

In 2002, the writer Yang Ganhua hanged himself with a belt in his dormitory room, leaving his colleagues in shock. "But we had no idea. He was at the meeting yesterday and there was nothing unusual about his behaviour."

Then there is Zhong Zishuo, editor of the review *Art in Guangzhou*. Half an hour before committing suicide, he was at work talking with colleagues and appeared calm and normal. He then went up to the rooftop of the building and jumped off.

And then there is...

There are people around us who are depressed, but they talk and laugh as if everything is going well in their lives. But in fact, they're planning their own suicide, going through it over and over again in their heads in cold blood, like a sniper taking aim at his target, ready to pull the trigger. Even when their bodies go into rigor mortis, all anyone can say is: "But we didn't know." Everyone is baffled and confused, because they have chosen to bury their heads in the sand, to say nothing, to play it down and forget.

When will we learn to reach out to those crying for help?

Who's next in line to be destroyed by depression?

22nd to 25th October 2005

Correlations

> **Excerpts from *"Seeing Red and Feeling Blue:***
> ***The New Understanding of Mood and Emotions"***

There are two main criteria in the diagnosis of depression.

Time: For at least two weeks and for the best part of the day, the patient is in a low mood and loses interest in life.

Physical and psychological symptoms: Below is a list of symptoms. If you experience five or more of the symptoms, it is likely that you suffer from depression:
- Continuous low mood
- Loss of interest in life
- Changes in appetite
- Sleep disturbances
- Feeling tired
- Unexplained feelings of guilt
- Trouble concentrating
- Suicidal thoughts

Susan Aldridge (England)

Complementary Notes

While copying the excerpt above, I became aware of how I, as a depression sufferer, am in conflict with the writer in me.

As a patient, I aim to transcribe the words of medical specialists and professionals so that I, as well as those who are in the same situation, can have a better understanding of our illness. However, as a writer, it bothers me to merely summarise what the specialists say instead of using words that express my individuality. I consider this to be professional negligence.

I am at once a depression sufferer and a writer. The two are incompatible and I am caught in the middle.

SEVEN

Diary
Wednesday, 25th June 2003 10:40 am

Last night, I dreamt I was sitting for an exam. Again.

It's been a recurrent theme in my dreams these last few years. I am always so anxious, either about not finishing the paper in time because I arrived late or that my writing is illegible. I know I have the ability to pass, but for some reason or another, I fail.

The first part of my dream last night was blurred. I only remember the last part where I was supposed to answer a simple maths question. Inside the division bracket was the number 12, but I couldn't read the number outside. I was stuck. Panic. Time was running out and I was about to give up when the teacher pointed to my paper and said: "It means you have to divide twelve by three." What a relief. It was that simple. I quickly wrote down "4", pleased that the exam was easier than I had expected. Woke up feeling pleased with myself. For the first time in years, I dreamt I had finished my exam.

Perhaps it's a sign that my health is improving. I'm making good progress. It's possible to change my negative mindset after all. "All things are possible for one who believes."[1] So happy.

Yesterday, Beijing was removed from WHO's list of "Infected Areas." Things are looking up. I must make a conscious effort to look on the bright side of life and nurture a positive frame of mind.

Notes

In June 2003, when the antidepressants began to take effect, I wanted to find out more about depression and the side effects of the medication. Why did I get sick? Who could teach me how to cope with depression?

I hadn't read any books on the subject. The first book I bought was at Learning & Excellence, a book shop near my home. The title was *Seeing Red and Feeling Blue: The New Understanding of Mood and Emotion*. The second book was *Depression: An Undiagnosed Illness*. They're both published by Sanlian Editions. The first one was printed for the first time in Beijing in October 2002; the second one was in January 2003. The SARS epidemic broke out in the spring of 2003. I wonder at which point during the SARS epidemic these books were transported from Beijing to Guangzhou and the conditions in which they were distributed. I'm grateful to those who translated these books, which aren't popular with the general public, and also to the book stores that sell them.

Writing my "Diary" stops me from falling into an abyss. But I often wonder why I added the section "Correlations." Maybe it's to reassure myself and others.

In reassuring myself, I take a step back from my bitter and painful experiences and reflect on how I can live with my depression and begin a new chapter in my life. In comforting others, I hope to reach out a helping hand and say: "Don't give up! Faith, love and hope will pull you through. Reach out for help and have faith that you shall be saved. Maybe your pain is greater than mine, and your path more arduous, but together we shall overcome the darkness. In saving ourselves, we save others in the process. Together we shall help doctors have a deeper understanding of depression. We shall help the families of depression sufferers provide the best possible care to their loved ones. Listen and you shall hear a faint voice crying for help. Look and you shall see a hand reaching out to you."

Dr Aldridge said: "Antidepressants need to be taken for one to four weeks before the beneficial effects are felt [...] For a patient desperately seeking help, it is devastating to find out that it takes several weeks for the medication to take effect. (Of course, it would be even more devastating not to be informed beforehand.)"[2]

Unable to carry on and with nowhere to turn, you have no other choice but to take medication. In despair, you find out the effects don't kick in immediately. You're like a fish from the Eastern Sea[3] that has landed on a cobbled road. You need water to stay alive. Those who promise to bring you water say: "Be patient. We'll fetch the water from the Western Sea." But before they reach the Western Sea, you are dried up by the sun.

27th November 2005

Correlations

Today, as I was tidying my study, I came across a yellowed piece of paper scribbled with notes. It's a checklist of things to write about when I started keeping a journal. But not knowing how to make it into an effective therapeutic tool, I stopped after the first entry.

The thing is, you can't plan your diary in advance. You jot down whatever comes to mind. Just tapping some words into the computer is a feat in itself. It's a spontaneous act, devoid of logic. My words are scattered and fragmented, like those of a patient who, in a state of delirium, rambles and babbles, spewing out all the pent-up chaos in him.

I thought I had thrown the checklist away, so it was a pleasant surprise to find it again. Here's a checklist of what I consider to be an ideal journal. I don't have what it takes to write such a journal, but perhaps my fellow depression sufferers will.

My ideal journal:

1. List out the things that make me happy, sad or worried.
2. Talk about the different schools of psychology, their theories and therapeutic methods.
3. Describe in detail my personal experience of therapy.
4. Sort out my thoughts, express myself without inhibition and conduct self-analysis.
5. Encourage myself, jot down the little things that make me feel good.
6. Make notes of the best passages I read in books on psychology.
7. Dispel all negative thoughts.
8. Give a thumbnail sketch of my health, energy level and mood.

Complementary Notes

The first month I was on antidepressants, I was in a bad way due to the secondary effects. Kneeling on the sofa, I watched the clock on the wall tick by, second by second. The words "fish of the Eastern Sea" kept going round in my head. I was like that fish in distress who thought: "I can't wait anymore! I'm dying!"

Like in the Chinese expression "fish stuck in a rut",[4] all of us have, at some point in our lives, found ourselves in a desperate situation screaming for help.

EIGHT

Diary
Friday, 27 June 2003 10:40 am

Saw a Chinese physician at the special consultation service, but still feel tired. Hope it won't be long before I regain my strength.

While flicking through the magazine *Good Health* in the waiting-room, I came across a question that many patients ask: How can you find the doctor most suitable for you? Answer: Patients suffering from a chronic illness should not automatically look for prominent doctors in senior positions with many years of experience behind them. Instead, they should look for specialist doctors who are responsible and sincere, and who have the time and patience to fully answer the patients' questions.

It's reassuring and encouraging.

I've been going regularly to the Psychiatric Department and the Traditional Chinese Medicine Department at this hospital. Although Professor Gong and Professor Chen aren't as well-known as the specialists in the other hospital, they're extremely patient and always take time to answer my numerous questions. Their therapeutic methods yield excellent results. This hospital is near the Sun Yat-Sen University. The staff is friendly, and the consultation fees are more than reasonable. Even though I have personal contacts at the other two hospitals, their location is far from home, the waiting-list is long, the consultation fees expensive, and the doctors and staff have little time for the patients.

Father God, full of mercy and worthy of my trust, You guide and protect me, and answer my prayers. Close the doors through which I am not meant to pass; open those through which I am destined to go; and allow me to move forward swiftly and steadily.

Lord, those who believe in You are blessed. Under Your guidance, all things are connected. Those who call upon the loving Spirit receive Your blessings. Facing hardships strengthens my faith. I feel more secure and will overcome the shadows of depression.

Notes

In 2003, on the eighth day of the first month of the lunar calendar, I dined with friends along the Pearl River. They were talking about how doctors were urging the public to stay vigilant during the influenza season and to watch out for any signs of coughing or fever. The following day, there were various updates on my mobile phone's newsfeed: what the different colours of sputum mean; people queuing up to buy white vinegar; lovers meeting up wearing surgical masks. For over 10 days the atmosphere in the city was tense, and then the situation calmed down. Thinking the SARS scare had blown over, I laughed about it with my friend, Wang Yun. I was in Guangzhou and she was in Beijing. We even talked about making a short comedy sketch, but it never occurred to us that a global tragedy was unfolding before our eyes.

During the SARS epidemic, many people stopped going into hospitals for consultations, but I continued as usual.

After the New Year, as I was packing for my trip to Shenzhen, I noticed that my brain had trouble coordinating with my movements. It was as if the connections between my body and my nervous system had broken down, like the communication cables in a robot's head gone haywire. My movements resembled those of a developmentally disabled person. Like a sleepwalker, my mind was absent. I had a host of physical and mental problems: exhaustion, insomnia, nightmares, despondency...The list goes on.

I returned to the Psychiatric Department of North Shenzhen Hospital for more sleeping pills. Although the consultation fees cost 100 yuan, the waiting-room was jam-packed. People were sitting on the sofa, listening carefully to the nurses giving out instructions. The person before me was taking ages, so I knocked on Professor Li's door and said to him:

"I'd just like to have some sleeping pills. It'll only take a minute, would it be possible to write me a prescription?"

"Wait for me outside," he said, looking at me sternly.

When a doctor has a lot of patients, time is precious.

Finally, it was my turn. After a few basic questions, he said: "You need to take antidepressants." I said I would think about it. I didn't for one second believe this nonsense about depression. All I wanted was my sleeping pills. However, I did notice that out of the three symptoms associated with depression, two of them had worsened. To prove that he was wrong, I had to find another illness I might possibly suffer from.

My first stop was at the Otolaryngology Department at the famous Oncology Hospital in Guangdong. Suspicious lymph nodes were found in my neck after my lymph node dissection in 2000. Towards the end of December 2001, at a national writer's meeting, I met the head physician of the Otolaryngology Department at the prestigious Oncology Hospital in Beijing. He advised me to stay in Beijing and, to avoid complications later, have both sides of my neck operated on immediately. Physically too frail for another operation, I opted to continue with chemotherapy. But what if the lymph nodes were malignant? Perhaps I should have a second operation. Should I have it in Guangzhou or in Beijing? Fortunately, after further tests, the specialist in Guangzhou said: "Don't worry. Everything is fine. Go home. Life goes on."

"But I'm always tired, even more than before my operation in 2000," I complained. "You warned me of an eventual brain or bone metastasis. Could I have a MRI scan, a radionuclide scan and a CT-scan?"

"These tests have harmful effects on the body. Go home. Your immune system is weakened, you should stay away from hospitals."

The doctor stood up (a hint that I should leave), patted me on the shoulder and said: "You're not depressed. How could you be? You're strong and optimistic. You're alright." Even the oncologist said I had nothing to worry about. I left the hospital feeling satisfied with myself, but doubts were niggling at me nonetheless. If my health problems had nothing to do with cancer, then what was the problem?

At the Gynaecology Department of another hospital:

Li Lanni was pacing up and down the corridor, glancing from time to time at the gynaecologist in the consultation room. She was the chief physician with over 20 years of experience. She was plump, heavily-built, had a broad face and a stern look. Had she been an obstetrician, wayward children would come into this world meekly and without a whimper. Doctors like her commanded respect. Li Lanni hoped that she would make a quick and succinct diagnosis. She was 99 percent sure she had some kind of menopause syndrome. It can happen anywhere between 30 and 60 years old, and taking hormones can regulate the body.

Li Lanni sat down as the doctor read through her medical file.

Li Lanni *(anxious but respectful)*: I think I'm going through menopause. I can't sleep, have nightmares and wake up tired. They say taking hormones can help, is that true?

Doctor *(glancing at her)*: Any hot flashes and night sweats?

Li Lanni: No.

Doctor *(calmly)*: Anxiety?

Li Lanni: No.

Doctor: Is your period regular?

Li Lanni: Yes.

Doctor: Mood swings? Are you more quarrelsome lately, flying easily into a temper?

Li Lanni *(surprised)*: I never quarrel with anyone, not even with my family, and I never lose my temper. Anyway, I'm too tired to get myself worked up.

The doctor was silent. After a routine examination, she put Li Lanni's medical record in front of her. She hadn't written a single word.

Doctor: Who said you were in menopause?

Li Lanni: I…I thought…

Doctor: You thought what? It's up to doctors to give a diagnosis based on science.

Li Lanni: But I have insomnia…

Doctor: Stop imagining things. Do some sports or housework. It'll do you good.

She made a hand gesture indicating that Li Lanni could leave. But Li Lanni refused to give up and opened the medical file.

Li Lanni: Could you prescribe some hormones? Shouldn't I be taking some medication?

Doctor: You don't mess around with hormones! You're not in menopause and you don't need them.

Li Lanni then went to two other hospitals, in the hope that a doctor would diagnose her as being in menopause and prescribe her some hormones. But it was in vain. She could read in the doctors' eyes: "You must be joking. You're out of your mind."

Li Lanni hated the word "depression." Depressed? Her? Ridiculous. Ludicrous. The doctors were so ignorant. Receiving a diagnosis like that was so humiliating. Li Lanni's strength lay in her fortitude and optimism. She never cried, even when the pain was deep. Since the age of 14, what hospitals hadn't she been to? Which doctors hadn't she seen? She was sick of hospitals: operating theatres, ambulances, body bags, mortuaries, coffins, funeral processions, botched operations, terminally ill patients, young girls with leukaemia, balding old women after they've been through chemotherapy or radiotherapy, pale waxen women suffering from uraemia and groaning in pain, women suffering from severe endocrine diseases whose faces were so bloated that they look like drowned corpses...The list goes on. She wouldn't go so far as to say she had come back from the grave, but she did come crawling out of numerous hospitals. She was used to sickness and death. So why should she be depressed?

Li Lanni went from one hospital to another. Exhausted and unable to sleep, she was hell-bent on finding a reason for her poor health so a doctor would prescribe her a treatment. Perhaps her chronic fatigue was due to stomach bleeding. She had a gastroscopy and a barium meal test. But the results were inconclusive: superficial gastritis or erosive gastritis. Maybe she could have a blood and urine glucose test. Diabetics usually lose a lot of weight. Don't they also suffer from chronic fatigue? But the blood tests were negative.

Next stop was at the otorhinolaryngologist's office. Sleep has something to do with the pharynx. You never know.

Li Lanni: Doctor, is it true that Guangzhou has a high rate of nasopharyngeal cancer?

Doctor: Are you from Guangzhou?

Li Lanni: My family is from Heilongjiang, but I was born in Guangzhou.

Doctor: You're fine. If you have phlegm, drink some salt water or eat preserved prunes or dried orange rinds. Women like them.

My brain was completely disconnected from the rest of my body, and it was getting worse by the day.

My head is floating in front of me. My limbs are trembling, as if dangling from the carcass of a headless frog. All my insides have been gutted out – my brain, blood, a shred of skin from my forehead, eyeballs... They're floating in mid-air. I never understood Picasso, but now I am one of his paintings. My body and soul are scattered, a bit here, a bit there, a lump here, a lump there: bruised veins, bits of bones smeared with pink flesh, fingers with brown wrinkled skin, scalp torn from my skull... They are just floating there, impossible to catch, impossible to put together again.

Eyes closed, I keep hitting my head with my hands. Pull yourself together.

Snap out of it. Stop! Stop, stop, stop. Control yourself. Immediately. At once. Now. You can't degenerate into this madness. You mustn't believe in such superstitious nonsense. Get a grip on yourself. I am normal. In front of doctors, I am polite and all smiles.

Next stop. Ophthalmologist.

My eyes hurt. My pupils are tired, as though they're hanging out of their sockets or have been churning in my stomach for a long time.

Maybe I have glaucoma. But the test results were negative. So why do my eyes hurt? Why have my dioptric measurements gone from 1.5 to 0.8? The ophthalmologist said: "Chemotherapy can have serious side effects. It can cause damage in your body: nervous, digestive, immune, blood and urinary systems. All that said, it appears your eyes have been spared."

Let's see, what other specialists do I have to see?

During the SARS epidemic, surgical masks were on sale at the reception desks in all the hospitals. Stocks were running out in the shops, so I bought four at one go. They were of good quality, like the ones you found in the 1970s. It had been a while since I had worn one and had forgotten how to put them on. Was I supposed to tie the strings behind my head or hook them around my ears? I managed the best I could. But it was too tight, and I couldn't breathe. All the windows in the hospitals were closed and people were taking the stairs instead of the lift. I walked up five storeys and the mask, humid from my breath, was sticking to my mouth. After that, I never wore masks in hospitals again and always took the lift.

I had tests for my lungs and heart, and two colour Dopplers for my liver, gall bladder and pancreas. I lost count of the number of blood tests I had. A neurologist palpated the small bump at the back of my head to see if it was the source of my woes. But none of the tests could explain my health problems.

I am not depressed. My life is free of worries. I don't work nine to five; I haven't been uprooted from my hometown to work elsewhere; and I have no children. As the famous song "Last Song" in *Dream of the Red Chamber*[1] says: "Know how to leave behind material possessions and worldly vanities." I am satisfied with my life; the country I live in is stable and peaceful; I have done nothing wrong and my conscience is clear. So I don't see why I should be depressed. But why have I lost interest in life? Why have I lost so much weight? Why am I slowly being eaten away by dissatisfaction?

My mental health deteriorated rapidly in the last two weeks of March. I dreamt that I was talking to the dead and even when I was awake, they were talking to me. Silently...continuously...they were asking me in their strangely soundless voices that came from nowhere: "Why are you still alive? Why? Are you afraid of death? Life has no meaning. You're better off dead. Do you know why others have chosen to die? Can you guess? Do you know the best and quickest way to die? Without suffering and in the least gruesome way?"

I was drained, physically and mentally. I made enormous efforts to shut these voices up and pull myself out of the bottomless pit. I was like a boat that had been sucked into the Bermuda Triangle.

A university hospital in Berlin conducted a survey of 130 patients who had consulted their family doctors for sleeping, digestive and sexual problems, as well as pain in the limbs. Ten percent were suffering from depression. Half of them received a diagnosis. And only one third entered therapy.

In her book, the psychologist Gwendoline Smith said that at first, she refused to accept that she had depression and doubted the effectiveness of drugs. She had been trying to find a "stable" state of mind for a long time. She had a two-hour session twice a week with a therapist. It was an attempt to sort herself out and learn how to cope with despair. But her condition was going downhill. Her therapist confirmed that she was suffering from depression and advised her to take medication, at which point she broke down in tears, holding her head in her hands, completely overwhelmed by a sense of failure. In her book, she talks about how many people refuse the diagnosis of depression. She regrets how mental illness is being stigmatised. If society is unable to dispel the fear and ignorance surrounding depression, then thousands and thousands of patients will never receive the appropriate treatment.

When I talk about Gwendoline Smith, this New Zealand psychologist, I can't help but compare the Chinese with the people in New Zealand, whose historical and cultural baggage are much lighter than ours. Since their system of social security is far superior to ours, the percentage of people suffering from depression should be lower. But even though the environment they are living in is more humane, their society is still fearful and ignorant. If that is the case in New Zealand, then the situation in China wouldn't bear thinking about. I am not optimistic about the future. It's my hope that people will someday have the courage and knowledge to deal with this problem.

For over a century, the Chinese people have lived through tragedies and immense social changes. Several generations have survived major social upheavals. As for my grandfather, great-grandfather, great-great grandfather and great-great-great grandfather, who among them lived in a strong, prosperous and peaceful China? Was there a generation not born into the tears and bloodshed of war? Buried deep in our collective subconscious are terrifying memories, feelings of vengeance and despair, and unhealed psychic wounds. Do memories of atrocities lay hidden in my father's subconscious, and that of the following generations? Are we healthy of mind? When will we take preventive measures against mental illnesses in the same way we do for SARS? If we don't, then in 20 years' time there will be an "epidemic" of mental illness and the death rate will supersede that of SARS and the Black Plague. It takes two generations to heal the scars of mental illness. There are two ways in which depression can manifest itself: inward movement which leads to suicide or self-mutilation; outward movement which leads to death or being attacked.

An affluent New China puts special emphasis on the notion of harmony. However, only the spiritual and mental well-being of its people can give rise to a harmonious society.

14th to 18th November 2005

Correlations

Excerpts from *"Never Retreat"*

We had moved into the city.

That year, we left the island of Haidao and settled in the city, where people were busy participating in the Cultural Revolution. Schools were closed. The older students had left for Beijing, leaving the younger ones at home with time on their hands, not knowing what to do with themselves.

Whenever my little brother and I entered the courtyard, eyes would be observing our every move. About a dozen children, the "gnats," would follow us and chase us out of the courtyard, throwing sand, stones and insults.

Every morning, I went to the canteen to fetch our breakfast and hot water. Before leaving home, I would be nervous, knowing the bullies would be waiting in the courtyard. They would throw handfuls of sand at me and I would shout in defiance: "You want to fight? Come on, if you've got the guts!"

Three months passed. One day at dusk, the children of the North and South Courts were playing the game "take the city by storm." But the North Court team was one player short.

"Come on, quick! Who wants to join us?" Those "inside the city" were waving their hands frantically. But no one in the cheering squad offered. Everyone knew that the South Court team was stronger, because it had the best fighter, a brawler called Ah Guang. I was standing beneath a tree some distance away. In spite of myself, I put up my hand and said: "Me!"

The battle began, and all were plunged into confusion. It reminded me of the Japanese invasion and the battle of Triangle Hill during the Korean War. Dripping with sweat and covered in dust, I fought the enemy, shouting: "It's your life or mine!" I had lost track of time when suddenly there was a deafening silence. I looked up. There were only two fighters left in the courtyard: me and Ah Guang. I knew I was done for. We were standing in front of our "cities," staring each other down. I must have looked as desperate as a rabbit who found itself staring into the face of a big grey wolf. Looking at me with disdain, a smile on his lips, he gestured with his hands and said casually: "Surrender. You're finished." The enemy was about to storm the gates of the city. I saw red, and without a second thought, rushed headlong into him. If I were to die, then I was going to bring him down with me. Ah Guang dodged to one side and my head hit the ground. I felt an exploding pain, and everything went black. I had knocked myself out.

The next day, head down, hand over my nose, I scuttled across the courtyard to fetch breakfast and hot water. My nose was scratched, red, and swollen, and had smudges of gentian violet on it. I looked ghastly. But none of the children laughed at me that day. And they never threw sand or stones at me again.

Summer of 1991

Complementary Notes

The excerpt above, taken from a short story of mine, provides a glimpse into my childhood. As a military child, I was brought up with the notion that "life is like a battlefield." In other words, never be afraid of death. My upbringing made it difficult for me to accept that I had fallen into depression. The very notion that I was suffering from a mental illness shook me to the core, ripping my dignity to shreds. I was in denial, filled with anger and frustration.

If only I had had some basic knowledge about depression, I wouldn't have suffered the way I did. That image of myself is coming back again. I "broke my nose," so to speak. In a big way.

NINE

Diary
Saturday, 28th June 2003 10:20 am

I am happy, but in a cautious way. Since I got up this morning, I've been in high spirits. Unlike other days, I haven't felt the usual aches and pains: headache, weak limbs, stomach ache, bloated tummy, chest pressure, shortness of breath, slow pulse, nausea, dizziness, sore throat and eyes, anxiety and difficult urination.

Such joie de vivre is so rare for me. I am happy. Before, the word "happiness" was devoid of meaning. It was something beyond the grasp of my imagination even. But this past year, I've been given a taste of what it's like to be healthy (albeit temporarily) and to lead a normal life (again temporarily). It's what I call happiness. Why cautiously happy? Because such moments are few and far between, and life is unpredictable. I am grateful for my blessings and cherish this fleeting happiness.

These last couple of days, I've been forcing myself to read, do sports or write in my diary. My problem is that once I start reading, my brain works non-stop, taking the enjoyment out of it. It becomes an exercise, an effort to cram in knowledge that I have to memorise in case I need it at a later date. It puts me under pressure, makes me tired and nervous, and my mind quickly reaches its saturation point. As soon as I begin to read, I feel sick, my eyes are sore and my head aches. What's more, I forget what I just read.

It's the same when it comes to sports. I'm always pushing myself to do more, for a longer time, and it ends up being an ordeal. A few days ago, my Chinese physician said I suffered from Deficiency of Energy. Because I lack physical strength, I should avoid doing too many sports. I had bought a jump rope, but he advised me against it. It could aggravate my condition.

Rereading the entries from a few days ago, I realise I tend to push myself to the limit. My aim is to do a psychological self-analysis and write up the different therapeutic methods for depression. But it puts me under a lot of pressure. So it's hardly surprising that I am stressed and irritable whenever I think of my diary.

There has been so much pressure these last few years that I am not even conscious of it anymore. But this must change, otherwise I'll never be free from depression. These past two days, I've been going with the flow, not forcing myself to read, do sports or write in my journal. Just doing my best to live simply and naturally.

Notes

Sitting in front of the computer in a state of exasperation, I had my chin in my hands or my head thrown backwards, eyes closed. I am supposed to write about what happened between the end of March and beginning of April 2003, but my mind is on strike. Not feeling up to it.

Last night, I dreamt I was sitting for an exam again. I had no pen and the other candidates were scribbling away on their test sheets. I had to manage with a ballpoint pen refill held between two bamboo strips and loosely tied together with a red string. It kept falling apart and I kept having to tie it back up again. Panic. Whenever I started to write, the pen refill would disappear in between the bamboo strips. I wanted to walk out of the exam, saying to myself: "Why get yourself into such a state? You don't have to sit for this exam. Don't bother, just walk out." But I hesitated. Walking out was against the rules. I stayed in my seat, struggling like an idiot with the make-do pen and telling myself: "Relax...don't be scared. Since you don't have a pen, the teacher will understand. You can abstain from writing your exam papers, but you can't just walk out." Just then, the teacher announced that the exam was cancelled, and we were to gather outside. I was so happy and relieved.

Dream continues. There was a party at school and my classmates were putting on their costumes backstage, but I couldn't find mine. The reputation of our class was on the line and our teacher and class monitor were pressuring me. They told me to choose something from a pile of velvet costumes and they picked a pair of tight-fitting ballet trousers which were too small for me. Then they picked a low-cut dress which was too big. I tried on several costumes, but none fitted. By now, my teacher was angry, telling me I must remember where I had put my costume. The harder I thought about it, the more confused I became. The stage manager came over to complain about upsetting the order of the programs. I felt so ashamed that I wanted to disappear and hide. But I was accountable to my class and therefore had no choice but to stand there backstage and take a scolding from the stage manager. The class monitor ordered me to go back to the dormitory to find something that would fit me. I ran back to the dormitory and knocked on every door. Out of breath, I thought desperately to myself: "You're running out of time. You can't make it. Don't let your teacher and classmates down. Don't get them in trouble. Do something. Make up for what you've done." I woke up before I could find my costume.

I am reluctant to relive in my mind the period between the end of March and beginning of April. Words can't find the right communication channel. My subconscious refuses to talk.

About one week before 1st April 2003, Li Lanni had asked just about every friend who was a doctor but not a psychiatrist this question: "A professor said I was suffering from depression, do you think it's likely?" Everyone said no.

Li Lanni sent a SMS to a friend to briefly explain her situation and ask for help. The friend replied straightaway and put her in touch with a specialist.

It was the morning of 1st April 2003. He was a prominent psychiatric specialist and the department's head physician. In truth, Li Lanni wasn't expecting a diagnosis, just the confirmation that she wasn't depressed.

SARS patients were treated at that hospital, which was at the forefront of the fight against the epidemic. There were horror stories about SARS on Hong Kong television every day and people were extremely cautious, so Li Lanni thought there wouldn't be many people at the hospital. But to her surprise, she discovered that Guangzhou folk were tough and resilient. The consultation department was full, and few people wore masks or took the stairs. All the seats in the waiting room were taken. The head physician had given authorisation for Li Lanni to register at reception and told her to wait patiently for her turn. If the Psychiatric Department was crowded during the SARS epidemic, then wouldn't it be swamped in normal times? Li Lanni observed the faces but couldn't see anything unusual about them. None showed any signs of insanity. Most of them were watching television while waiting for their turn; some, looking pale, had their eyes closed. But then, the people of Guangzhou have a naturally pallid look, which has nothing to do with the quality of their sleep.

At 10 past midday, a nurse called Li Lanni into a small room to fill in a questionnaire on the computer. There were 90 questions, which had to be answered within three minutes. The nurse said not to answer the questions any old how just to finish them on time. Li Lanni thought to herself: "A questionnaire like this? A piece of cake." She finished the questionnaire, skilfully dodging the "traps." She had no intention of cheating, it was just that her subconscious was desperate to rule out every single possibility of depression, and she knew exactly the "right" answers that would keep her out of trouble. The nurse was surprised she managed to finish in just over a minute. When Li Lanni was on a creative writing course at Nanjing University, she and her fellow students often played around with these kinds of psychological tests. She was into palmistry and the study of physiognomy and could read someone's future and their past, especially when it came to their misfortunes. When she was reading someone's fortune, her hands and body would go cold as ice, even on a hot summer's day. Having played at this game for several years, she was an expert at it. Now she knew how to fill in the questionnaire and what to say in front of the specialist in psychiatry.

Li Lanni: It's half past midday. You're tired and overloaded with work, with no time to rest. How do you manage this every day?

Head Physician: It's okay. There's not a lot of people today.

Li Lanni wasn't just trying to be pleasant, she really did think that doctors in China were over-burdened with responsibilities and overtime. The doctor read wearily through her questionnaire. She could tell from the expression on his face that her answers didn't raise any suspicions. Looking at the stack of medical files on his desk, she knew he had to sacrifice part of his lunch hour to see to his patients. Feeling slightly guilty, she told herself not to go into too much detail about her illness and to carefully choose her words so the consultation wouldn't last for more than 10 minutes.

Li Lanni: In cases like mine, you don't need to take antidepressants, right?

Head Physician: Apart from insomnia, what other symptoms do you have?

Li Lanni: There aren't any! Everybody who knows me says I'm not depressed. A lot of people have warned me against antidepressants and told me about their harmful effects.

Head Physician: New drugs have fewer side effects. Do you... sometimes have suicidal thoughts or the feeling that life isn't worth living?

Li Lanni: No, never. I'm a very cheerful and optimistic person and have lots of friends. Maybe my insomnia is work-related and my fatigue is due to the high dosage of chemotherapy. I was going to have five cycles, but my cardiac...

The doctor nodded and carried on reading, trying to come up with a diagnosis.

Li Lanni *(eagerly)*: Oh, and another thing... I don't like eating out. Every time I'm invited out, I get nervous. Sometimes I accept hoping it'll be cancelled.

Head Physician *(smiling)*: I don't like going out to eat either. But that doesn't mean anything. It seems unlikely to me that you suffer from depression.

The doctor wrote a prescription. Ah yes, alprazolam, she thought...I know it. One tablet at bedtime can improve sleep and reduce anxiety. Relieved, as if she had received a grand pardon, she picked up the prescription, murmured a "thank you" and scampered out of the door. The pharmacy downstairs was closed, so she went to the emergency service and bought the medication for two yuan. Then she called her friend to tell her the good news: "I'm not suffering from depression! I don't need to take antidepressants!"

On the evening news that night, two Hong Kong television channels announced that the singer Zhang Guorong had committed suicide. He had jumped off a building.

Zhang Guorong, who suffered from depression, had just killed himself!

It was sensational. His face was everywhere. Everyone was talking about him: journalists, eye-witnesses, music fans, movie fans, television presenters, friends. We heard his songs, saw clips from his concerts and films...

Zhang Guorong, his face... eternal, youthful...is staring at me from the television screen, his eyes wrinkled at the corners, a smile playing on his lips, the look in his eyes – mischievous, anxious and weary. It says: "It's April Fool's Day, won't you come and play a game of death with me? Who wants to play? Come on!"

I shuddered. It was just as well that the doctor had told me that morning that I didn't suffer from depression. Otherwise, would Li Lanni have lost her mind at the shocking news of Zhang Guorong's suicide?

19th to 20th November 2005

Correlations

Excerpts from *"Glimpses of Childhood"*

The Cultural Revolution began when I was 10 years old. I was a boarder at a school that was part of an important military base. On the first day of the school holidays, the teacher said to me: "Your parents have left the military base. Your father's friend, Mr Jia, will come to fetch you, you can leave with him."

Stunned, I wondered where my parents were. How could they have disappeared like that? How long was I to stay with Mr Jia? Was I now an orphan?

Mr Jia lived in a courtyard belonging to the political department. Both of his daughters had their hair cut like a boy's. When they saw me, they said:

"Another snotty kid. Hey, we're the big sisters around here." The elder one looked me up and down and said: "Can you sing President Mao's songs? There's a rule in this house. You have to sing a song before every meal, if you can't, then you get nothing to eat."

The dinner bell rang. A bowl in my hand, I followed the two girls meekly into the canteen. I rinsed the elder sister's bowl and chopsticks and chopped the spring onions for Mr Jia. They had soya sauce, sesame oil and spring onions at home. I didn't like raw garlic or spring onions, but beggars couldn't be choosers, I could no longer be picky.

One day, I overheard the younger one say: "Snotty Nose has manners, haven't you noticed? She never goes through our stuff and never sits on our bed." The older one replied: "I don't like her. She seems so old, there's nothing innocent about her." I thought to myself: "Old? I'm not even ten years old." I wondered what "innocent" meant. It upset me so much that when the older sister told me to fetch the stool at dinner, I brought her the chamber pot instead.

One evening after our bath, the three of us were playing together. The older sister suddenly wrinkled up her nose, sniffed and said:

"You've been using my sandalwood soap again!"

"Oh rubbish!" the younger one retorted.

There was only one year difference between the girls, but the younger one was taller. They were both in their second year of secondary school and bickered all the time.

"You know very well you did. Lying fiend!" said the older one, throwing herself on her sister.

"Lying fiend? Come on, smell me!"

Suddenly, I felt a gaping hole crack open in my chest. Black cold air came rushing out and the pupils in my eyes froze. I could smell wafts of sandalwood scent on me. Usually only the older sister used sandalwood soap. The younger one used soap with an ordinary scent, and mine, which was given to me by my teacher, had no scent. But I loved sandalwood soap. Mother used it, and it reminded me of the warm fragrance of her body. The sisters were bickering away, and their words were stabbing into my flesh.

"I'm sorry, it was me... I took it by mistake..." I opened my mouth and wailed. Before I could finish, I broke into sobs and cried myself sick.

Early the next morning, I left a farewell note and returned to school. I became used to being alone after one semester. As a boarder, the school provided me with food and lodgings, as well as stationery, toothpaste and soap. I didn't have one cent on me, but I didn't go hungry. In the summer, I wore my winter clothes with the sleeves cut off; in the winter, I sewed the sleeves back on.

Time passed, and it would soon be my tenth birthday. I squeezed all the toothpaste into a seashell and sold the tube.[1] I sold other things in my possession: a pair of leather sandals, the handle of my toothbrush,[2] unused notebooks and scraps of fabric that I had cut from my pillowcase. With my one cent, two cent, and five cent coins in my pocket, I went to the military base's photographer and said to him: "I'd like to have a birthday photo."

"Smile," he said. "Why do you look like an old maid? You don't look at all innocent."

His words made me think of the two sisters. Suddenly, I missed the family who had taken me in.

Many years later, the birthday photograph still holds the unspeakable sadness of that day.

Complementary Notes

At the time when I was writing this story, it's likely that I already had depressive tendencies. Every morning, I would wake up in low spirits. The apartment was filled with a strange kind of sadness. I saw glimpses of my childhood, as if my brain had been soaked in photograph developing solution, bringing out images of the past. My mind and body were bathing, drowning even, in this chemical solution. My friend, Li Mei, once said to me: "Why do you insist on opening up old wounds? They've already healed, but you keep on wanting to prod them open again. It's like you're addicted to your pain."

She said these words casually, but they shook me up.

After that, every morning upon waking, I would try not to think of things that made me sad. But it felt odd, as if without these sad thoughts and images, I didn't know who I was, nor where I was. All day long I felt lost, like a walking corpse searching desperately for its missing soul. The feelings of bewilderment and fear distressed me even more than my previous sadness. So I let myself sink back into the chemical solution, waiting for Li Lanni to resurface again.

TEN

Diary
Monday, 30th June 2003 10:40 am

I make an effort not to push myself to the limit these days. When I am outside doing my exercises and fatigue sets in, I stop. I don't set myself a time limit. In most of my activities, I am careful not to deplete my energy, but, as people would normally say, "nourish and build up my energy resources" instead.

Although the garden where I take my daily walk is dull and uninteresting, there are always lots of children playing there. It's calm and peaceful. There I feel the presence of God. He is saying: Look at those children and learn from them.

Yesterday, I read *On the Sense of Anger*[1] by the Swiss psychologist Verena Kast. She says that anxiety is a normal part of life and that we should learn how to face up to it, deal with it and overcome it. You can't run away from it forever. The longer you hide, the bigger the impact will be when it hits you. If you can successfully overcome it once, you'll have acquired the experience to overcome it again.

Mother called me this morning, worried that she might have tuberculosis. I told her she should stop going to that so-called prestigious hospital, and instead of imagining all sorts of things, come to Guangzhou earlier for a check-up and seek a diagnosis. I try not to be affected by her unnecessary worrying. She's the perfect example of a neurotic depressive personality. My relationship with her is like this: Someone who can't swim tries to save someone who can barely swim. Her arms are hanging around your neck, and not only can you not save her, you risk being drowned in the process.

I wish she'd get help. I used to worry excessively about her, but now I know God has His plans and all I can do is pray, have faith, be grateful and wait in patience.

"If you believe, you will receive whatever you ask for in prayer."[2]

Notes

In my "Diary," I talk about how Mother gets on my nerves.

In recent years, I wrote a novella called *Courtyard of My Childhood Years*, in which I talk about my childhood wounds. When Mother read it, she called me and accused me of selling her out for a few pennies of writing fees and threatened to jump off a building. My brother also accused me of lacking in filial piety and humiliating Mother and demanded that I delete all the relevant passages.

I analyse the negative thought tendencies that have become part of my life: fear, resentment, suspicion and confused thinking. Unable to run away anymore, I must face up to myself and free myself from the burden of the past. In doing so, I touch upon sensitive family matters and personal issues. Keeping a journal is a form of therapy, much like emptying the mental waste stored up inside.

I'd like my journal to be as spontaneous as possible. These are words that come from deep inside of a survivor and not some literary work filled with trivialities. It's a medical file that could be of interest to psychiatrists and psychologists. It also documents my observations on society and could be useful to sociologists. It could also speak for those who suffer from mental illness and end their lives in silence and anonymity. And lastly, it could serve to encourage those who are trapped by depression, anger, and anxiety without understanding why to actively go out and seek help.

This isn't merely a record of my own fight against depression, but that of a whole generation. I'll try not to digress, but as I comb through my negative thoughts, I might at times repeat myself like a broken record and even say the same things every day.

In today's entry, three times I touched upon issues about my private life. Since they could be prejudicial to someone's reputation, I decided to delete the relevant passages. After much hesitation, I kept those about my parents. The anger and resentment some children feel towards their parents is a taboo subject in the Chinese tradition.

Ever since I can remember, I've never been a devoted daughter.

Ever since I can remember, I've never felt close to my parents.

When I was 22 years old, I stayed in the endocrinology service at the Zhongshan University Hospital in Guangzhou. The services for both nephrology and orphan diseases were on the same floor. I often saw corpses being wheeled out on stretchers. I shared a small room with a young woman around 27 years old. Her bed was by the window and her parents, who lived in Hong Kong, came to visit her every weekend. I never received any calls, nor letters from my parents, who lived in the western part of Guangzhou.

When I was operated on for an angioma at the age of 14, I took a military bus and admitted myself into hospital alone. Afterwards, with the stiches still in place, I returned home, which was several hundred kilometres away. At the age of 17, I spent six months at the First Military Hospital. Between National Day and the Chinese New Year, I didn't receive a single word from my parents, who were in the northern part of Guangzhou at the time. I didn't cry. I was used to it. At the age of nine, I was already independent.

At Zhongshan Hospital, several patients died a few days in a row in the room next door. On the first night, someone was weeping mournfully. Twice I heard the young woman toss and turn in her bed. It was bright and sunny the next morning. She sat in front of the window combing her favourite oil into her hair. She was pretty, but unable to take in solid food, so she relied on parenteral nutrition. As a result, she had become thin, pale and frail. That morning, she had dark circles under her eyes. I thought maybe she was annoyed at being kept awake by the crying the night before, but she called me over to show me how shiny her hair was. The following night, we heard weeping again. It sounded like parents crying for the death of their child. I heard a nurse say that someone had cried so much that she had fainted. In the darkness, I saw the young woman get out of bed. She stood, arms across her chest, hands holding onto her shoulders, listening to what was happening outside the room. Through the mosquito net, I could barely make out the expression on her face.

"Are you afraid?" I asked her softly.

"They're crying for the dead," she said suddenly, after a moment of silence. "Who's going to cry for me?"

"But you have your parents," I said naively. "Me, I don't have anyone."

Without a word, she went back under the mosquito net. I stared at the pale white moon outside the window. Suddenly, an immense sadness welled up inside me. If I were to die tonight, who would cry for me? Where were my parents? Were they thinking of me?

My nose was prickling, and tears filled my eyes. It was unlike me to be so emotional. I wiped away my tears. That night, I needed to cry, but tears refused to flow. They stayed stuck at the corner of my eyes. I thought of a child crying for her mother, her face streaked with tears. I called out silently: "Mother, Mother." But it felt strange, as if there was a lump inside. Then I called out silently: "Father, Father," but it felt unnatural. I felt so wretched, but tears still wouldn't come. Who could I think of? Who could I call? Who could I count on to comfort me and give me courage? In the darkness of the night, when the angel of death was roaming from room to room, who could I call to protect me?

The children of any given generation can harbour resentment toward their parents. Times change, the reasons for their resentment change, but the bitterness remains buried deep inside.

I came back from the dead. I climbed out of a mass grave, where the skeletons did not speak. They dared not speak, because no one would listen.

Today, I can truly say that I no longer resent my parents. Because I have finally dug out the stone lodged inside me.

I've read books by psychologists and psychiatrists of different nationalities: American, German, British, Swiss, Canadian, New Zealand, Iranian. They all say that childhood wounds are related to depression. I must admit that having read all these books, I still don't understand why I suffer from depression. Many factors come into play: childhood, genes, severe illness, daily stress, work stress, a dysfunction of our neurotransmitters... However, among those who have had a difficult childhood, painful family history, deep wounds, or those under extreme stress, perhaps one out of 10 become depressed. Why is it that nine come away unscathed and one falls into depression?

Some time ago, I was talking to my friends about the unhappy memories of my childhood. Before I could finish, they all jumped onto to me, saying: Do you think you're the only one who lacked security as a child? Have you ever seen a mother die in front of her child? Do you know what it's like for a child to lose her mother? Do you know what it feels like when your parents hate you for no reason?

I had known my friends for many years, but it wasn't until that day that I realised that they too had suffered as children.

22nd to 23rd November 2005

Correlations

Excerpts from *"A Hundred Dumplings"*

As a child, I never understood the meaning of the word "family." Military children become used to living in a community very early in life. Boarding school begins in kindergarten. It was the 1960s and the ambience of the times can be summed up in these verses: "Raging seas, tempestuous skies raining down fury/Five continents tremble, lashing wind and roaring thunder."[3] As military children, we were very conscious of our role as the torchbearers of communism. We went home once every school term. If during the summer or winter holidays our parents were on deployment, we would stay at school.

Our teachers told us how we would probably be the last generation who still had ties to our families. Following the Cultural Revolution, the family unit would eventually disappear. A child would be given over to the state at birth. The nation would be our family. Encouraged by this idea, we were nonetheless slightly troubled: Would our parents be taken away from us? Would we have to call every man and woman we came across "Mother" and "Father?"

We lived a carefree life at school. Meals were at the canteen, and the school provided us with everyday items: uniforms, textbooks, pencils, pencil sharpeners, notebooks, biscuits, sweets, fruits, towels, soap and a wash basin. The school took care of our medical expenses and we watched movies in the big playground.

However, one day, the Great Proletarian Cultural Revolution came along. Teachers were humiliated, then driven from schools or sent back to their villages. We felt both afraid and excited at the same time. Freedom! But our portions at the canteen grew smaller and we began to go hungry. Our uniforms became worn out, but the school no longer replaced them with new ones. At the weekend, there were no more sweets and biscuits, nor fruits. The movie sessions were cancelled. We no longer celebrated People's Liberation Army Day, nor National Day, nor Chinese New Year. Electricity was cut off at night. Our dormitory had become as bleak and desolate as an abandoned cemetery. We only had one thought on our minds: Where were our families? We had had no news from our parents for a long, long time.

One day at midday, a jeep took away a second-year boy with curly hair. The following week, another student was lucky enough to be taken away. The hope of going home began to spread like cholera among the students. But under the orders of the "left wing" of the Party, army officers were not allowed time to take care of their children. Nor did they know the Revolution had reached the schools, and the schools were closed.

The summer of that year, I felt the poignant absence of my family. I didn't know where my parents were, nor did I understand why they hadn't come to fetch me. Distraught and hurt, I asked myself: "Has the Revolution abolished the family unit? Has my family abandoned me?" I even stopped dreaming about them at night. The harder I tried to remember their faces, the blurrier they became.

Having no summer clothes to wear, all the students developed heat rash. The girls made sleeveless tops out of old handkerchiefs. We sewed the handkerchiefs together to make a big piece of cloth. Then we cut a hole in it and slipped it over our heads. The simple top sat neatly on our shoulders. One day, as I was sewing my top, an army officer I had never seen before appeared at the door. He called out my name and said: "Your father sent me to take you home." Hearing the word "family" was like being hit on the head with a football. I felt numb and confused, as if I suffered from a head injury. Without a word and empty-handed, I followed the officer outside. During the ride on the bus and boat, I didn't ask where my family was. Troops often changed garrisons, and military families moved from place to place. We arrived in a town with a strange name, Foshan, meaning "Buddha's Mountain." But there were no Buddhas, nor mountains in sight.

I saw my father. I had forgotten how long it had been since I'd last seen him. I was indifferent. No tears, no smiles. I was still numb from the "head injury." Or maybe I had missed my family so much that my heart, tired and empty, had become old and crumpled up, like the handkerchiefs we sewed into shirts.

Father smiled, tapped me playfully on my shoulders and said: "Hey, how come you look like a street urchin?" He looked at me the way a company commander would look at a soldier who, having lost his way, had finally joined the ranks again.

Not knowing what to say, I sat in my father's office, dunce-like, withdrawn and unresponsive. Father kneeled down in front of me, studied my face and asked:

"What's the matter?"

"When are we going home?" I asked, looking up.

"Mother and your little brother are with Grandma in Jiangsu…"

Before he could finish, I wailed: "I want to go back to school…"

I stood up, ready to run outside, but Father held me back.

"Don't you miss your family?"

"No!" Blinded with hatred for my parents, I wanted to shout: It's you who destroyed my family. You didn't want me, and I don't care.

Many years have gone by and I still don't know what it means to have a family. Whenever I think about it, I become confused and distressed. I feel fear and pain, but, strangely enough, there is also hope. The hope is vast like a cliff and deep as a valley. From afar, I see a bright and never-ending light, but close up…I can't see anything. For I have never even come close to experiencing hope — endless, boundless hope.

June 1994

Complementary Notes

The notion of "family" I just talked about has various connotations: a sense of security, parental love, family ties, moral support, the source of life, the foundation stone of childhood and adulthood. My childhood experience has taught me to keep a certain distance from my family. For many years, instead of a safe haven where I could heal from my wounds, my family was a place of stress and obligation. Tired of drifting, I wanted to go home. But after several days at home, I wanted to leave and be alone again. Isolate myself in a capsule so I could mentally let go. When it came to my family, I was incapable of giving and receiving. From an early age, I was used to taking care of myself. I trusted no one.

ELEVEN

Diary
Tuesday, 1st July 2003 11 am

I called Ya Li and Liu Lei to ask them to make an appointment with a specialist for Mother. I don't see these friends very often, but whenever I need a favour, I can always count on them to do their best to help without asking for anything in return. I am so grateful to have such friends, especially in times like these when human relationships are reduced to mere commercial exchanges.

As I was out strolling yesterday afternoon, it occurred to me that my health has improved significantly. Sometimes I forget that I am in a much better state of health.

"Be free of anxieties." "Don't look back, go forward." Psychologically I am in a bit of an odd spot: Mentally I find it hard to adjust to the fact that my health is improving daily. It's like having a fish bone stuck in my throat. Although the doctor has removed it and my life is now back to normal, I still feel the pain and discomfort of having a foreign object lodged in my throat. Anxious and worried, I dare not move or breathe.

Just got off the phone with Chen Zhihong. We talked about how it's so important to take care of ourselves.

Notes

Are you ready to go back to what happened between 2nd and 12th April 2003? You managed to trick the psychiatrist into thinking you didn't need antidepressants. On the morning of 12th April, you saw four different specialists in two different hospitals in the Pearl River Delta area. Then what? You can't hide anymore. Talk.

It's painful between my eyebrows, my abdomen is hard and bloated and I feel sick. I want to run outside, lie down on the grass in the sun. I have nothing to say. Fatigue is taking hold of me again. I don't want to see anyone, talk or answer the phone. I didn't say a word all morning. Don't make me.

Don't be scared. Do you need some help? On the morning of 1st April, the psychiatrist prescribed you alprazolam. It's an anxiolytic and a sleeping pill. You took one tablet half an hour before bedtime and you felt better, didn't you? Talk. Can't sit still in your chair? You already drank a cup coffee to perk you up and ate a banana and some chocolate to put you in the right state of mind. Then you waltzed madly around the apartment, doing a Tibetan dance. "Tra la la ba ta di...Receive my thanks...La la la... Peasants have become masters... Forever grateful...Tra la ba... Red mountains and rivers... La ti ta..." But what do the lyrics mean? They don't make any sense. Even your dog snuck back into his cage, too embarrassed to watch. You're like someone walking alone in the dark who is so afraid of her own shadow that she starts to desperately sing and dance to muster up her courage. But it's daytime and the sun is out. The temperature is between 14 and 24 degrees, humidity is at 70 percent with a light wind from the north. Go on, talk. Afterwards you can go up to the rooftop on the 16th floor and do your light therapy. The sun is at its strongest around 1 o'clock in the afternoon. The rooftop is close to the sky. You can turn your face to the sun, hands outstretched, back slightly arched, and let your body soak in the light, dissolving all the shadows lurking in your memories.

I dreamt that my maternal grandfather came back from the dead to ask me to save him.

    He got up from the stainless steel trolley at the mortuary. I was wearing a hospital gown and a nurse told me my grandfather wished to see me. I thought: "But he died at the age of 87, didn't he? That was ages ago. At the time, my little brother and I were in Pingxiang in Jiangsu Province. We saw his body being carried out of the ice-cold mortuary and then taken to the crematorium. Is my memory playing tricks on me? Lord, maybe the doctors made a mistake? Maybe Grandfather isn't dead. Did someone forget him at the hospital?"

    The man lying on the floor was indeed my grandfather. He looked so wretched. The nurse didn't give him a hospital gown. He was lying curled up on the floor, in the freezing cold, naked, his back curved like a bow, and you could see the bony notches of his spine. He grabbed my hand and begged me to help him: "The doctors told me to go, because I've only got one day to live. They said I must leave the hospital. You've got to help me." His hand was icy-cold. I was kneeling on the floor and didn't want to let go of his hand. I couldn't cry or go into a panic. I had to be brave for Grandfather, give him the courage to stay alive, channel my life force to him and save his life. I kept on talking, telling him to hold on for one more day, so he could prove the doctors wrong. I told him not to worry, promised him that I would never let go of his hand and never let him die. Then his head fell onto his knees, as if he had fainted. No one came over to help. I was frozen to the bone. If I stayed like that any longer, I would freeze to death. I was afraid of passing out and letting go of Grandfather's hand. His life was literally in my hands. "Even if I do of cold or exhaustion, I must never let go," I thought. But my strength was ebbing away. Panic, fear, guilt and anger came over me... In my distress, I wondered why no one came over to save Grandfather. I wished someone would take my place. I would then be free to die.

I was numb with cold... Then I woke up, chilled to the bone.

I had similar dreams three nights in a row and felt exhausted in my sleep. The recurrent themes of these dreams: I was watching other people die; others were watching me die; I was at my own funeral; I found myself in a strange town with people from my village who were dead.

Another dream.
    I was in an arid mountain region with a group of tourists. Those in front shouted to say there were corpses lying in the bushes. Not daring to look, I squinted as I went past. Then we were on a Jiefang[1] truck, watching the landscape roll by. Parts of the mountains were bare. There was a canal that looked like the Red Flag Canal. It was only a couple of inches deep and the water current was slow, perhaps due to a water shortage in the region. As the truck was going uphill, it stalled, and all the passengers got off. Look over there! There's blood and dismembered bodies of dead school children in the water... elbows, feet, heads, school satchels, shoes. Don't look! Why were there so many dead children in the canal? Why was not a single body intact? Then more bodies gushed out of the canal opening. Two were slumped on top of each other, blocking the mouth of the canal. Unable to take this anymore, I shouted hysterically: "They're children, school children! Why are so many of them dead? How did they die?"
    I woke up. Dismembered limbs... an elbow here, a thigh there... were floating in my mind's eye... a child's head stuck in the canal opening... a primary school pupil lying face down...

During the period when I had these kind of dreams, every time I closed my eyes, I would see dead bodies. And when my eyes were open, the dead would talk to me, especially those who had committed suicide. They would explain to me why they had killed themselves, whispering in my ear: "Come on, let's go. Let's leave this world together."
    Stop. My stomach hurts, and I feel sick. There is someone in my brain who is on the verge of a nervous breakdown. I try to stop her, tame her, but we're both tired from the struggle.
    Spare me for today. Please. I must go out into the sun, take my dog, Lele, for a walk at the Sun Yat-Sen University campus. I need to switch off my memories.

24th November 2005

Correlations

Excerpts from *"Grandfather's Smile"*

My maternal grandfather had aged. The frightened, hesitant and wary look in his eyes betrayed his feelings of impotence and hopelessness. The mocking smile at the corner of his thin lips was tinged with something odd and unfathomable.

"When you sit on a chair, what kind of energy does it entail?"

After some hesitation, I stood up and looked dejectedly at the teacher... my grandfather. He wore a stern look on his long thin face. He patted the physics book to dust off the chalk. Standing in front of me, he repeated the question several times, as if he were reciting a magic spell.

"Answer the question, please. When you sit on a chair, what kind of energy does it entail?"

I racked my brain for an answer and suddenly it struck me:

"I know...Friction!"

Ha ha ha...the whole class burst out laughing.

"And what else?" Grandfather asked, the expression on his face silencing the peals of laughter.

"I don't know," I answered, playing with the cracks of the wooden desk.

Annoyed, he let out a long drawn-out sigh.

Winter came. One day, at the end of the first lesson, we heard a funeral procession passing near the school. All the pupils rushed outside to watch. Sixteen large strong men were carrying a coffin covered with a red silk cloth embroidered with phoenixes and dragons. At the front of the procession, people were carrying flags and lighting firecrackers. Those at the back were weeping, playing the flute or drumming on a tambourine. It was a major event. I had lost track of time when suddenly I remembered that school was not over. I rushed back to school, but the classroom was empty. Grandfather was standing by himself on the teaching platform, a blank look on his face.

Grandfather had retired. He led a drab and lonely existence in the teachers' accommodation that was once an abandoned temple. He no longer talked about his life as a teacher. Whenever the school bell rang, he would become agitated and pace up and down, or stand at the doorway, a strange smile on his lips.

July 1981

Complementary Notes

For some reason, during my depression relapse, I often dreamt of my dead maternal grandfather.

He was my school teacher for two years. In high school, he gave me tutorials in maths, physics and chemistry every day. Having only studied for one year in a state school, I didn't even have a basic grasp of combining like terms. As I was quite slow, teachers were often frustrated with me. And Grandfather was often at his wit's end with his granddaughter. Working in the fields would make me feel faint. I would eat my meals alone, sitting on a wooden stool in the doorway because Grandfather worried that I might choke on chilli peppers. He asked the class delegate to keep an eye on me. Unable to vent his frustration on pupils who couldn't keep up, I bore the brunt of his anger. It didn't matter that I was the head of the Communist Youth League, or that I was a radio show host at the school's radio station. By venting his annoyance at me, he regained some of his dignity as a teacher.

Grandfather and I loved to eat candies when Grandmother wasn't watching. She kept the New Year candy treats in a ceramic jar: dried sweet potatoes, rice fried with sugar, strips made from sugar cane that were bought with food ration tickets, packets of white sugar Mother had sent us. It was our little secret. We would steal them while Grandmother was cooking. First, I would check to make sure she was in the kitchen and wouldn't come back into the house. Most of the time, Grandfather would be preparing his lessons and I would be doing my homework. The lid of the jar was heavy, and we were careful not to let Grandmother hear the clinking sound of the lid as it opened and closed. The sugar spilled easily. Grandfather took a pinch of sugar, letting it slowly dissolve in his mouth. I copied him. I was a quick learner. With sugar in our mouths, we both looked at each other and giggled. It was a moment of tender complicity between a teacher and his pupil.

TWELVE

Diary
Wednesday, 2nd July 2003

After my telephone call with Chen Zhihong yesterday, my computer overheated. So I stopped writing. It's just as well. Since I don't force myself to do anything these days, I am not stressed, restless or despondent.

29th June was a Sunday. I was at home watching *Hour of Power* on a Hong Kong international television channel. In his sermon, the Reverend Robert A. Schuller of Crystal Cathedral quoted verses from Psalm 37, written by King David:

> *Do not fret because of those who are evil*
> *or be envious of those who do wrong;*
> *for like the grass they will soon wither,*
> *like green plants they will soon die away.*
>
> *Trust in the Lord and do good;*
> *dwell in the land and enjoy safe pasture.*
> *Take delight in the Lord,*
> *and he will give you the desires of your heart.*
>
> *Commit your way to the Lord;*
> *trust in him and he will do this:*
> *He will make your righteous reward shine like the dawn, your*
> *vindication like the noonday sun.*
>
> *Be still before the Lord*
> *and wait patiently for him, [...]*[1]

"Do not fret because of those who are evil" means one shouldn't worry. "Take delight in the Lord" means one should always stay positive. The verses remind me of these four things:

1. Don't worry.
2. Stay positive.
3. Trust in God.
4. Be patient.

Each minute of our lives is a gift from God. He who created us has plans and knows how we can serve Him. We must learn to be patient. The Reverend said today that people are impatient. They need instant gratification, and to satisfy their desires, they resort to all kinds of illegal or immoral ways, shortcuts, unfair competition etc. This causes chaos, prejudice, fear and anxiety. A truer word has never been said. I must reflect more on my shortcomings, learn how to bide my time in gladness and to live my life in hope. Every day, I remind myself that God has gifted me with health, and that I should free myself from worry, fear and doubts. God is with me. He has bestowed his blessings on me and helps me to succeed in my endeavours.

Sometimes I wake up depressed and, as if out of habit, start brooding over the unhappy things, which, most of the time, have nothing to do with me. But over the years, my thoughts have tended to drift towards the negative. So I usually wake up depressed, and as the psychological can influence the physical, I feel weak and suffer from all sorts of aches and pains. It drives me further into a depressed state. A vicious cycle.

Under the guidance of the Holy Spirit, I begin each day with the blessings of God. Each minute of my life is a blessing from Him.

Notes

My maternal grandfather passed away one morning in early spring. He had cancer. Maybe an old man of 87 years dying from cancer wouldn't have suffered much. He was hospitalised in Pingxiang in Jiangsu Province. On the first night, he ate a fried egg. He was still conscious at 6 o'clock the following morning, then at 8 o'clock he passed away.

Elders say that, at birth, we come into this world on a boat and at death we leave in a car. Fate decides the time and place of our departure and the passengers who will travel with us. That morning, Grandfather left on the 8:30 car. He didn't have time to say goodbye to us.

When he died, my brother and I were on the train. We arrived at the station at 10 o'clock and decided to go straight to the hospital. Since I've been in and out of hospitals for much of my life, my brother, who was worried that it might upset me, suggested I should leave earlier and offered to stay on for a few more days.

We learned of his death when we arrived at the station.

One night, I dreamt of Grandfather standing in front of me. He was wearing a dark blue Sun Yat-Sen jacket[2] with black buttons. He looked well. He had a smile on his long thin face and looked 10 years younger. Happily surprised, I looked at him and asked: "Grandfather! Where have you been?" He pointed to the floor to say that he had been in the ground. Puzzled, I wondered how it could have been possible. Was there an underground city? Did he leave in a car via a tunnel?

"What were you doing down there?" I asked.

"I'm a teacher there," he replied, laughing.

"But you're already retired."

"They asked me to take up teaching again," he said, pleased with himself.

Alarmed, I said to myself that Grandfather was already dead. Then I woke up.

In my dream, Grandfather wanted me to tell Grandmother not to worry, that he was teaching again and was well.

In April 2003, around the Qingming Festival,[3] every time I dreamt of Grandfather, he was always in trouble.

Between the 2nd and 12th April, every dream I had was related to death. A mysterious force from the kingdom of death was exerting its power over me, trying to take me away.

There is a popular expression in Cantonese-speaking regions: "To be in the grip of a malevolent force." After Zhang Guorong's suicide, some said his soul was trapped in the ghost movies he had starred in; others said he was "in the grip of a malevolent force." There were numerous cases of suicide during the four days following his death. According to the media, they were people who wanted to imitate Zhang Guorong, and it was a chain reaction set off by a series of bad news.

The truth is, every year around the same period, there are people suffering from severe depression who commit suicide. But the death of these ordinary people doesn't make the headlines. They are tears that evaporate silently, without leaving a trace. The death of Zhang Guorong turned society's attention toward depression. The image of him jumping off a building will always be etched into our minds. The sensational nature of his death shocked us out of our ignorance.

Be on your guard.

The month of April 2003 was dedicated to Zhang Guorong. He was on television everywhere. Radio stations played his songs non-stop. Some newspapers said he had killed himself because of relationship problems, others thought he had AIDS. I avoided watching television but heard everything I didn't want to hear when others were watching. The more I tried to stay away from the bad news, the more it was shoved in my face. A portrait of Zhang Guorong appeared on the television screen. It was a perfect photo, because Zhang Guorong sought perfection. It had obviously been carefully chosen, and all the fans who loved and respected him recognised it instantly. It was the embodiment of all that was charming and fascinating in him. Suddenly, I caught his eye. He said: "Do you know why I left this world? Jumping into the void is the best way to go. You can see how happy I am now, can't you? Why dilly-dally? I know what I'm talking about. Listen…"

No, no, no… I don't want to listen. Lord, help me. Give me strength and courage. Guide me onto the right path.

On my bad days, I dreaded seeing his films or any documentaries about him. Even hearing his name made me cringe. I hid the DVD of his film *The Life of Ah Q*. I loathed seeing the DVD cover of his comedy drama *East Meets West*, which showed him surrounded by other actors.

He was ushering me into the car that would take me to my death.

Go on, hurry up. It's time to go.

On the morning of 12th April, I consulted a doctor at the otolaryngology department of the Oncology Hospital. The doctor said the size of my lymph nodes hadn't increased. I left the hospital feeling confused, not knowing where to go. As I was crossing the Haiyin Bridge in a taxi, I decided to go to another hospital.

When I arrived at the specialists' department, I made appointments with three different doctors. The head physician in gynaecology said: "You don't show any symptoms of menopause. There's no need to take hormones." The chief physician of Traditional Chinese Medicine said: "You suffer from a Deficiency in *yin* and *yang*." She prescribed three doses of "Decoction of the Four Noblemen"[4] and "Decoction of Suanzaoren-Ziziphus."[5] She stressed that time is needed for the *yin* and the *yang* to find their balance. Then the nurse at the reception called out: "Li Lanni. Psychiatry! Li Lanni. Where is Li Lanni?"

When I left the hospital, I had two bags of antidepressants, enough to last me for seven days. Face the truth, Li Lanni. Two of the three psychiatrists you have consulted said you are suffering from depression. As for the third one, you didn't even want to listen to him. They said you were crazy and you didn't like it. You've got some nerve, lying to the doctors.

25th to 26th *November 2005*

Correlations

Excerpts from my medical file at the psychiatric department
(External consultation)

12th April 2003

Poor quality sleep, depression, loss of interest in life, irritability (more than 3 months).

For the past 3 months, the patient has been waking up early in the morning for no reason. Reports of depressed mood, loss of interest in life, slow reaction, diminished concentration, poor memory, irritability, nervousness, mental and physical agitation, heaviness in chest. She has received treatment in this region.

Hypothyroidism. She underwent surgery for thyroid cancer in 1998, followed by several surgical procedures and chemotherapy.

Her mother has a history of depression.

Before her illness, she was outgoing, and moods were stable.

Depressed mood and loss of interest in life. During consultation, the patient answered all the questions correctly. Absence of any negative thoughts.

Further tests for depression are recommended.

Complementary Notes

Spring of this year, I found my old medical files again. I copied down parts which are related to this book. I never read the medical report following a consultation. I don't care what the doctors say. In any case, medical reports are just a formality. As I was reading the reports, blurred images came floating out of my memory, as if the lens of a camera were badly adjusted. Maybe this is how a doctor perceives a patient suffering from depression.

THIRTEEN

Diary
Monday, 7th July 2003 10:45 am

Feeling better. I was extremely tired a few days ago and never thought I'd be back on my feet again so soon.

It's rare I feel so calm, relaxed, light-hearted, energetic and carefree. If only every day could be like this. Hope tomorrow will be even better.

Like it says in a song of praise: "I give thanks to God for giving me hope, I thank Him always."

Just now, I managed to overcome a psychological block related to my depression. I answered the phone. From now on, I must make an effort to reinforce my social network.

When I fall into a state of depression, I'm incapable of dealing with my social life. I can't answer the phone or go out. I dread people coming over to see me or hearing the phone ring. I am scared of all sorts of things. I am even scared of myself.

I still can't bring myself to relive the dark period between the end of March and beginning of May when my illness took hold of me. I am incapable of analysing the progression of my illness in a rational way.

Don't force yourself. Take it easy.

Self-therapy: dispel my fears, strengthen my social ties, don't be afraid of answering the telephone or seeing other people, go out more often with friends, have regular social activities. This therapy is to cure social anxiety.

The Lord said: "My grace is sufficient for you."[1] Amen.

Since last Friday, I've been doing an exercise that enables me to overcome my fear of the telephone. At first, anxious and afraid, I wanted to give up. Then I scolded myself for being a coward. It was a struggle between me and myself, and I finally convinced myself to do it.

It was a small step forward. I dialled a number and, to my great relief, no one answered. I could go back to hiding in my world, temporarily, at least.

Today, I accomplished this exercise under the guidance of God.

Remember this: When faced with difficulties, never be afraid. Trust in God and wait for Him to come to your aid.

Notes

Exhausted. Restless. Something isn't right.

I refuse to believe that I am that weak. Pluck up your courage and scratch a tiny corner of your memory…I don't want to see anyone, I don't want to talk on the phone, I don't want to answer the phone. I can't concentrate.

My heart is like a stove burning on low-quality charcoal. The fire, sometimes blazing, sometimes dying, gives off clumps of dirty ash. At times, my primitive soul jumps out of my body, leaps into the air, mouthing soundless cries. It screams at me in a freakish voice: "Let yourself go! Let yourself sink into insanity!"

No, don't die, don't give into madness…I can't… I can't take this anymore.

I am worn out during the day. All of my energy is spent on controlling my mind and body, just to maintain a semblance of normality. But at night, dark malevolent spirits come into my sleep and dreams, dancing and laughing.

I dreamt that…. my teeth were broken. Mouth closed and clenching my teeth, I could hear them grinding against each other. Feeling that the upper and lower teeth were about to come loose, I dared not clench my jaws too tightly. A third of the teeth touching the side of my tongue and inner cheeks were all broken, their pointed edge driving into my tongue. I consulted several doctors in different dental hospitals. One of them said: "I can't help you. All your teeth are broken. There's no point in seeking treatment in a hospital. All your teeth will fall out when you open your mouth."

I left the hospital in a state of distress. Not knowing what to do or where to go, I kept walking along the main road. I couldn't open my mouth or relax my jaw without my teeth falling out. Unable to drink, I would die of thirst. I felt pain in my head, cheeks, chin and temples. Relaxing my jaw a little, I immediately felt my teeth coming loose. There was nothing I could do except keep my mouth shut. Not knowing how long I could go on like this, I became increasingly distraught. What was I to do?

I dreamt that… some sort of cultural activities were being held at a holiday resort. I didn't know any of the people who were signing up in the main hall. After registration, I went into a room with my suitcase. As I was putting my clothes in the wardrobe, there was a knock on the door. I opened the door to a woman who I think was an editor of a magazine. She smiled and said: "What took you so long? Ms Liang is looking everywhere for you. She wants to know if you've arrived."

"Where is she?" I asked. "It's been years since I last saw her. I'll go and see her later."

Suddenly, my heart stopped. Ms Liang… Wasn't she dead? A fellow student at the Lu Xun Institute told me a few years ago that she had died from cancer.

An invisible weapon shot through the air. Where am I?

At times, the boundary between life and death fades out. And some are doomed to forever wander between the two worlds.

I dreamt that... I was in an alleyway. People were sticking pieces of black paper on the planks of wood that covered the ground. The tension and sadness in the air stopped me from going towards them. Then someone said there was a corpse somewhere ahead. I tried to turn back, but the alleyway had no side street allowing me to escape.

A crowd of people dressed in black were coming towards me. Those in front were carrying a woman who had just hanged herself. They were walking hurriedly, as if trying to find a doctor to save her.

Not wanting to look, I stood against a wall, but saw that the woman had a thick hemp rope around her n. eck. I wondered why they hadn't taken it off, because left like this, she'd be dead even before they arrived at the hospital.

I wanted to tell the people, but fear prevented me from speaking. Not wanting to look at the woman's face, I looked up and saw enormous letters forged in red metal: Yuanhai Theatre Company. I wondered what a theatre troupe was doing here. The crowd was coming closer and closer. Where could I go? Why didn't the alleyway branch off, providing me with an escape?

It's been a month since I stopped writing in my diary. I've been having nightmares again. A lot of them. I had the dream about the alleyway last night. I'm going through a rough patch and should stop rummaging through my memories.

I need to regain my strength. I'm not going to give up talking about my feeling just because it might set off another bout of depression.

I hope that someday someone feeling lonely and helpless will find this book. You aren't alone in your plight. You aren't alone in your fear. To carry on living isn't easy, but perhaps your destiny is to keep on fighting. We will strive to be beacons in the world.

28th December 2005

Correlations

Excerpts from *"Spring"*

I had turned 21 that year. In early spring, I was staying in a prestigious regional hospital. I had been in and out of different hospitals since the age of

17. At first, I was in rooms large enough for ten people. Then I stayed in medium-sized rooms for six.

When I was 21, I was put in small rooms for three. When a patient's condition began to deteriorate, she was moved into a single room. Those who were in single rooms usually had no more than three days to live. After that, they were taken to the mortuary.

I had been in the small room for two days when the woman in bed number three was moved into a single room. Sitting in a wheelchair, weak and frail, her head hanging to one side, she muttered that she didn't want to change rooms, nor put on an oxygen mask. Twenty minutes after she was moved into the single room, she stopped breathing.

Bed number three was now empty.

For several days, the patient in bed number one and I kept staring at the empty bed. The mattress was thick and lumpy with patches of dirt stains. It looked like a grotesque and puffy face. At night, I often had the impression that someone was sleeping in the bed and wanted to scream. The next morning, I would go out onto the balcony and look at the sky and trees to dispel images of the mortuary from my mind.

The single room was located on the third floor. Opposite was the balcony, which was accessible through a set of swinging doors. Two tall magnolia trees stood on the side of the balcony.

It was early spring, and the buds had not yet appeared. Instead of being a light green, the leaves were dark, as if they were in pain. I couldn't feel the spring that was in the air.

On a Monday, at midday, clean sheets were put on bed number three. It was for a young peasant girl from the Guangzhou region. She had an oval face and beautiful lively eyes that were typical of the women of the province.

I showed her the magnolia trees. She picked a small purple flower and a few blades of grass that were growing in a corner of the balcony.

I said to her: "Careful. You'll get your hands dirty."

She smiled. It was a smile of innocence.

I took a small empty medicine bottle, filled it with water and put the flower in it. Suddenly, the atmosphere of the room was infused with a sense of spring.

A week later, I heard that she had leukaemia and the doctors said she had only two months left to live.

Her mother wept uncontrollably. Her three brothers, all farm workers, had faces streaked with tears and took turns to give her blood.

A month later, she could neither get out of bed nor walk. But her dark eyes were still bright and alert.

Impatient to see the magnolia trees come into bloom, every day she would ask me to go out onto the balcony to pick a few magnolia leaves for her to use as bookmarks.

It was only then that I learned for the first time that trees also shed their leaves in the summer. The leaves that fell were green. I no longer wanted to see the magnolia trees blossom. I wanted time to stop, because by the end of spring, the young girl would be lying in a mortuary, swept away like a small green leaf blown by the wind.

One day, seeing that her mother had left the room, she sat up in bed and said to the woman in bed number one and me: "The doctors say I'm going to die."

Startled, the woman and I looked at each other.

"Don't be silly," the woman chided her. "How can you die? You're so young."

The girl looked at me, an innocent and trusting expression on her face.

"I don't want to die. I want to live, live, live. I want to, I want to, I want to!" she said, her voice filled with determination. She was like a school pupil who kept on insisting: "I want full marks in my exam. I must, I must, I must!"

Time passed. Her health deteriorated day after day until she no longer had the strength to take even semi-solid food. But her eyes were still bright and alert.

Soon she could no longer eat. One day, during one of his rounds, the doctor gave instructions for her to be moved into the single room that evening.

She didn't protest and only said: "Don't forget to tell me when the magnolias blossom."

For me, spring of that year came to an end in the darkness of that very night.

March 1993

Complementary Notes

I saw the many faces of death in my youth: ugly, evil, tormented, hellish, decaying.

On the other hand, I also saw people die in beautiful and moving circumstances, like magnolia buds falling silently to the ground.

Before dying, some people intentionally do harm to others. Filled with hatred, they act under the power of an evil force. Others hurt their family and loved ones, their bitterness filling the hospital room like poisonous gas.

Then there are others who, like the young girl, don't want to die, but aren't afraid of death. For them, the process of dying is transformed into drops of rain that fall from a starry sky and are carried away by the wind, leaving a fragrance that penetrates into our hearts.

Sometimes, I wake up from a nightmare puzzling over why the faces and behaviour of the people in my dream seemed so real. I don't know them and have never seen them before in my life. Where did they come from?

Maybe I met them many years ago in a hospital, and their images imprinted themselves into my subconscious. Perhaps the negatives of these images, buried in me for a long time, are now being "developed" by my subconscious.

FOURTEEN

Diary
Wednesday, 9th July 2003 11 am

My parents are arriving in Guangzhou on Sunday. Anxiety crept in after our phone call yesterday afternoon. I kept telling myself to stay calm and not to worry.

Conflicting feelings towards my parents are eating me up. I'd like them to come to Guangzhou so we could spend some family time together, but I dread it because Mother makes us all so tense and nervous. Ever since I can remember, life revolves around her. The family atmosphere changes depending on her moods, which are as fickle as the weather. Since she stopped working and became a homemaker, she is psychologically unstable and pesters the whole family with all her aches and pains.

She doesn't mean to hurt her children, but could it be a sign that she is suffering from depression? She has no self-control whatsoever. It's more likely that she suffers from phobic disorders. According to one medical book, one characteristic among depression sufferers is that they put on a mask which says 'everything is normal.' Extremely aware that something is wrong, they still manage to cope with daily life through their strong willpower and great self-control. They keep their pain inside, never letting those close to them know how they feel. Specialists call this Perfectly Hidden Depression (or concealed depression).

They say depression is hereditary. I wonder if that's true for me. But my symptoms are different from my mother's. Instead of pestering everyone else with my problems, I prefer to keep them to myself and put on a normal, happy face. This kind of depression where you isolate yourself from others is dangerous. Because if you go over the edge and commit suicide, those around you would never know the reason why. I must stop this.

Currently in therapy for severe depression, my moods are unstable. It's not a good idea to see Mother too often. Most of the time, she just talks about her own worries and negative things and it might affect my therapy. But I can't run away. She thinks she has tuberculosis but can't get a diagnosis in Maoming. My parents are natural worriers. It's my duty as a daughter to find them a good doctor who can put their mind at ease, even if nine times out of ten she isn't sick.

I am confident that with the help of God, I will be shielded from harm.

Can you think of anything these last few days that has made you happy?

1. I seem to have fewer nightmares, and even when I do, the anxiety is less intense.
2. Go on, think, you'll find something. Yes... I wasn't tired after my doctor's appointment yesterday morning. I kept thinking how I should live out the rhythm of my life - physical, mental and spiritual – in accordance to that of God's. Felt much better after that.
3. Is there anything else? Surely there must be. Why do moments of happiness pass by so quickly? Why is it so difficult to remember them afterwards? And why do painful memories never stop tormenting us? It's so discouraging. Oh yes...yesterday I bought a few comedy DVDs and went to the hair dresser. Feel much lighter.
4. Go on, there must be one more thing. Got it. My computer was working perfectly today. It didn't freeze once. Compared to a few days ago, I am less tense when working on it. That's right, a smile is coming back to my face. My mood is improving.
5. The timing of my days off this month suits me. Pleased about that.
6. The summer heat is unbearable, but I am in better health than in spring.

A verse from the Bible comes to mind, bringing me comfort. I repeat silently to myself: "God intended it for good to accomplish what is now being done."[1]

Notes

The Chinese New Year holidays are over, but my health is still poor.

I want to write about what happened after 12th April 2003, but as soon as I delve into my memories, I am overwhelmed by sadness and various other sensations: darkness, nausea and feelings of being cold and broken. My heartbeat slows down so much that I can't feel it anymore; my pulse seems non-existent; my head aches like hell, as if an explosion has blown a hole in the middle of my skull that is pumping out white smoke; and my soul, shattered into thousands of tiny pieces, is scattered in the wind. Crouched in the bottomless pit of my hysteria, I keep praying: "Shut the door! Shut the door!" A high-pitched voice inside me is screaming: "Ah... ah... ah... I'm going insane... ah... ah... ah!"

My heart is in bad shape. Went to the hospital. Same old problem: my heart rate is too slow. Nothing unusual there. Maybe the sudden surge of bad memories is weighing on my heart.

Some passages of my diary talk about my daily life. They're like a screen of vegetation behind which I can take refuge, and I am like a wounded soldier of the rear guard in view of enemy forces. I need to hide behind the bushes to recover from my wounds and change the dressings. The enemy is approaching. Stuck in the process of reviving my memories, bogged down by depression and desperate, I dig an underground passage.

Depression is a deeply distressing illness, because there are no outward signs, no open wounds, no scars, no tumours. But inside the heart is bleeding and burning to death. Rahel Berglinger, a Swiss patient wrote: "They keep telling me that it'll get better, that light is at the end of the tunnel. Most of the time, I shut up and say nothing." As I read this, I so wanted to shake the hand of my spiritual brother. It's exactly that. You must shut up.

Someone who has influenza and is coughing sits next to someone who suffers from severe depression. Others sympathise with the person who is coughing, concerned that she might cough up blood, while the one who has depression is bleeding inside… No, her mental state is even more horrible than bleeding, but she doesn't complain. When someone pats her shoulder and says: "It'll get better. Pull yourself together," it's like telling a diabetic that her body is going to produce more insulin by itself. It's absurd. It makes no sense to tell them to relax or "snap out of it." In *Depression: An Undiagnosed Illness*, the German psychologist Ursula Nuber says: "It is like asking someone to put her finger on her wound when that is exactly what that person is unable to do, because she lacked the strength."

A doctor who has depression, said he would have preferred to be sick with cancer, because at least he could have talked about it. With depression, you can't see it, you can't smell it, there's nothing.

So far, I haven't come across any books written by someone who suffers from depression, has cancer and has been through chemotherapy. Even if such a person does exist, she might not have survived. Those who are willing to write about such an experience are few and far between.

In a way, I am pleased that the surgical procedure has left a scar on my neck. It shows I have a deep wound. I am equally pleased that I have had chemotherapy, because it helps me cope with the side effects of the antidepressants.

People misunderstand the word "depression." As soon as they know that you suffer from it, they say: "You must look on the positive side of things. Be strong." Others, without being asked, say: "Look on the bright side. Life isn't perfect. Depression, you've inflicted it on yourself. Be optimistic."

People try to "comfort" you without having the faintest notion of what depression is. What can I say? It's one of the reasons why some patients end up taking their own lives.

Unfortunately, this type of misunderstanding is quite common. That's why in psychiatric wards you often see written on a board: "Depression has nothing to do with your willpower or moral character." It reassures those who consult a doctor for the first time, and I am grateful for it.

If my depression is due to a chemical imbalance of the neurotransmitter serotonin, then it follows that I should take medication for it. Consulting a doctor wouldn't help me in the least bit.

The New-Zealand psychologist, Gwendoline Smith, suffered from depression. In her book, *A Complete Guide to Depression,* she wrote: "As a clinical psychologist, I often see the suffering on the faces of my patients. However, in the past, I never understood the depth of their despair, nor how mentally fragile they are." Every time I read "in the past, I never understood," I can't help but think that the doctors who themselves have suffered from depression are the ones who understand the patients the most. Medical skills and personal experience are two different things. Throughout the history of China, renowned physicians have attached great importance to the role personal experience plays in medicine. They tested medicinal herbs on themselves and some, infected by the plague while tending to the patients, found the remedy that cured the epidemic.

Of course, I don't want doctors to fall ill just to become better doctors. But I do believe that medical health care professionals today lack sincerity, compassion and respect. They say when western medical hospitals were first built in China, 80 percent were built by religious organisations and 70 percent of the nurses were nuns. The doctors worked selflessly and lived by the religious principle: "Love thy neighbour as thyself." In the Chinese tradition, physicians were either Buddhists or Taoists, who lived by the principles of compassion and humanity. To them, "Saving a life rises beyond the pagoda of seven storeys."[2] Medical professionals today attach greater importance to technical skills than the moral aspects of medicine. No matter how competent and brilliant a doctor may be, without humanity, he or she can never excel in his or her vocation.

Today, urban citizens like to consult doctors and take pills. This is especially true for heavy drinkers and smokers who rely on doctors and medications. Hospitals are now livelier hubs than marketplaces in the countryside. Exhausted and overworked, with no religious beliefs to fall back on and unable to help themselves, where can doctors find the necessary strength to understand compassion? According to some books, prison guards' mental health is the lowest on the scale. Medical professionals' mental health is probably somewhere similar.

It's extremely difficult to be an outstanding physician these days. Achieving high educational qualifications is a relatively easy feat, but it's far more difficult to put into practice the principle of loving thy neighbour as thyself. Moreover, you need stamina and an iron constitution to become a medical professional. All these factors come into play when you aspire to be a great physician.

Other countries make the distinction between a psychiatrist and a psychologist.

Psychiatrists receive special training in medicine. As doctors, they focus on the patient's symptoms before giving a diagnosis and then decide if medication is necessary. They are able to prescribe whatever medication they decide is necessary.

Psychologists, on the other hand, focus on the psychological and emotional state of the patient resulting from family conflicts, financial difficulties and other situations that cause stress. Psychotherapists and psychologists are not qualified to prescribe medication.

One must always try to find out if depression originates from physiological or psychological problems.

In every hospital I've visited in China, the department of psychiatry and the department of psychology are one and the same. Psychiatrists and psychologists are both qualified to prescribe medication. That is why patients often consult the wrong doctors. For some, a chemical imbalance is at the root of their depression. But instead of seeking treatment that addresses the physiological causes, they are treated by a psychologist, which naturally has no effect whatsoever on their illness. These last two years, I've been paying close attention to information on different methods of tackling depression. I can't help but think of those who end up committing suicide because they were unable to find help. If only they knew where to look, they wouldn't have ended their lives.

Stop. Am I digging an underground tunnel for myself? No, it's the ear canal of a cat. The wound is still bleeding.

I dreamt I was at an exhibition. Seeing there was a mummy inside a case, I backed away, but I could still see parts of its chest and abdomen. Its skin was like wind-dried beef. The glass case was dirty and covered in grey spider webs. Next to the mummy was the dead body of a yellow mummified cat. It was extremely life-like. I remembered an old taboo against putting a cat next to a corpse, because the corpse would then rise and grab whatever is in front of it, and it would be impossible to make it let go. I think it's called a zombie. I was scared. How could someone put a cat next to a corpse? If it got up, would I be able to run fast enough? The people next to me were saying how the yellow cat was there to protect its dead master. A gust of cold wind blew through the dark exhibition hall. I wanted to leave. I didn't know what the theme of the exhibition was and didn't want to know. I looked for the exit but couldn't find it. The mummified body of the cat was haunting me. Although I am not fond of cats, I felt sorry for it. I was scared of the mummy, and its black dried-up skin made me sick.

Like me, many people who suffer from depression are in pain. One image often comes to mind: with one hand, I'm hanging onto the edge of the rooftop of a skyscraper; dangling in mid-air, I am about to fall. I don't know how long I can last, nor when I can climb back up onto the roof. The weight of my body is hinged upon the three fingers of one hand. I just want to let go.

A country with bright mountains and pure crystal clear water. Does it exist?

One week in my ideal world: early in the morning, I sign up with other patients also suffering from depression. The doctor patiently explains to us: "Don't force yourselves to control your reactions. If you feel the urge to sink into insanity, do it."

After being hypnotised by a specialist, Li Lanni, who, until that moment, was curled up at the bottom of her subconscious, jumps outside. She was in some sort of online virtual reality. She runs around and cries like a madwoman, bashes her head against the wall, jumps into the void, slits her wrists, stuffs herself with sleeping pills, shoots herself in the head... She does everything she wants to do.

This enables patients of an introverted nature to give free rein to their suicide wish, just as Da Yu was able to drain the flood waters.[3] It also allows patients of an extroverted nature to indulge in violence, like a volcano that erupts, spewing out molten lava. Sixth day: tranquillizers, waking up, convalescence, primitive energy restored. Evening of the seventh day: back to reality.

15th to 17th February 2006

Correlations

Excerpts from *"Autumn Melancholy"*

"She must be operated on immediately," the doctor said.
The girl had a tumour on her neck... Biopsy... Malignant... Hospitalisation... the sooner the better.

Hospital...a word she was only too familiar with. In her memory, all she could see were silhouettes of the hospitals she had stayed in.

When I was 14 years old, on an island lost at the far end of earth, a military doctor said to my father: "It's an angioma. She must undergo surgery in a hospital."

My father was young. The red badge on his cap made his black hair stand out, and his red scarf enhanced his shiny square face. He had a way of walking with his head tilted slightly upwards, and his splayed feet did not undermine his military gait in any way.

"Did you hear that? You're going to have an operation. Father must attend a meeting very far away. You have to go home by yourself."

Before the doctor could take me to my room, Father had driven off. All I knew was the number code for the military hospital and that we had spent the whole morning driving in a Beijing[4] jeep.

"How old are you? You're very brave," said the head surgeon, appealing to my pride. "Will you join the army when you grow up? You'll make a very brave soldier."

Feeling flattered, I let them poke around inside me in the operating theatre for two hours. The tumour was next to a vein. Tired, legs aching, dripping with sweat, fingers working clumsily, two junior military women doctors were struggling. Finally, it was the head surgeon who saved the day. Head slightly to one side, my hand on the surgical wound, I left the operating theatre and ran to the canteen. I knew there would be no one waiting for me with warm milk and fried eggs.

A few days later, I hitch-hiked back home.

"You've still got your stitches," Mother said. "Didn't the doctors and nurses take care of you?"

Grabbing a pair of scissors, I stood in front of the mirror and cut the black and bloody suture threads with bits of flesh still stuck to them.

I was only 17 years old. It was in a military hospital in Guangzhou.

I spent six months in hospital and felt annoyed every time someone asked me: "Why don't your parents come to see you?" My family wasn't used to showing their affection. In any case, there were a bunch of inept doctors looking after me.

Hey, love, we have to do a second gastric fluid analysis. Last time, we forgot to do a fasting gastric juice pH measurement.

Alright.

Hey, love, we have to a duodenal biliary drainage.

Alright.

It was in the heart of winter. A tube was passed through my nostril, down the back of my throat, through my stomach and into my duodenum. The metallic tip at the end of the tube came off and, like a martyr, I was rushed into the X-ray room.

Hey, love, we'll do a pneumogastrogram, shall we?

Alright.

The doctors put into practice what they had learnt in class. And there I was, my abdominal cavity filled with air. For two weeks, there was a small red flag at the head of my bed.

"Why didn't you say 'no?' Why...?" Five, six years later, Mother kept asking me.

I was 21 years old. I was seriously ill and needed to go to a prestigious regional hospital.

Father took out his phonebook, in which he had written down all the telephone calls he had previously made. The pages were well-thumbed, and the edges ragged from use. He went through the list, trying to find a hierarchical superior or a subordinate who could help us. He wrote them letters, but none of them replied. Then, one day, a letter arrived. This person had never benefitted from any favours from my father and had little contact with my family. Going by the standards of today where relations are based on mutual interest, this person was in no way obligated to go through the trouble of using his network to help us. I was admitted into hospital. This incident opened my eyes to life: good and evil; sincerity and hypocrisy.

What I want to talk about, I've already done so in my novella. And what I don't want to talk about, I've already forgotten. I hope one day I can help someone who is in a similar desperate situation.

The last time I was in hospital was last year.

It was the first time I found myself in such a bright and spacious room. Every day, light would fall through the curtains, spilling red and green petals on my hospital gown. Someone came in to clean the floor, bring me meals and hot water, but blank-faced, as if I weren't there.

It was the first time I had seen such a beautiful woman doctor. She had short, thick black hair and wore a bright red skirt that was slightly longer than her white coat. Looking relaxed and at ease, with the weight of her body shifted onto her right leg, she casually rested her elbow on her narrow waist. She spent about 20 minutes at each bed.

On the day of my operation, Red Skirt, in her usual stylish manner, and an absent-minded young junior doctor came to fetch me. I was anxious. On the operating tables next to me were two young women from Hong Kong. They had come to mainland China for an abortion. Three-fifths of the patients in the operating theatre were there for abortions, and half of them were from Hong Kong. This hospital came to the assistance of our compatriots, filling their coffers at the same time.

When they were sewing me up, the anaesthetics began to wear off and I felt nauseous. Looking up at the beautiful woman doctor, I imagined her holding out a warm and comforting hand. I got up and said to her: "I feel dizzy. I'm going to faint!" She looked at me coldly… No, it can't be… before she could finish her sentence, I lost consciousness. When I came to, I found myself curled up in a corner of the operating theatre.

"You gave us a fright there," Red Skirt said. "Go back to your room. I'm finished for the day." She walked off, swaying her hips.

"The operating theatre is closed. You must leave now. Steady yourself against the wall."

A couple of podgy nurses were counting wads of cash while mouthing advice.

"I'm going to faint…"

"Want some milk? Fifty cents a cup."

Cold tears ran down my cheeks. It was bitterly cold.

Last year, the frost of spring froze in my heart. This time, I'm going to a different hospital and will pay for the medical expenses out of my own pocket. My parents offered to pay for me. "Let us make it up to you."

The look in Father's eyes often made me think of the Ma Zhiyuan's song: "Tianjingsha Autumn Melancholy."[5]

In my novella, I wrote about the resentment those of my generation feel towards their parents. We needed their love and protection but suffered from their absence.

It must be fate.

The people of my generation have never experienced a happy family life, nor parental love. They don't know how to give or receive love. No, that's not entirely true. They do know what love is, otherwise how could they feel resentment?

"You must undergo surgery as soon as possible," my brother said. "If you don't want to do it for yourself, then do it for Mother and Father."

In September, as soon as I received the letter of admission for a creative writing course at a university, I immediately left for the southern region of Jiangnan.

Leave, leave. As quickly as possible.

Ungrateful daughters only know how to say goodbye.

What about Mother and Father? They were sad. Heartbroken, even.

October 1987

Complementary Notes

After I finished the autobiographical narrative above, the following year (that is, in October 1988), I underwent surgery. However, it wasn't until the spring of 2000 that I knew it was a total thyroidectomy of the right lobe. Worried that I might not withstand the shock, the doctor and my parents hid the truth from me and my family.

My parents and my cancer aside, many parents and children hide the truth from their loved ones. They all say it's done out of love, but ultimately it has unintended and unfortunate consequences. Tradition dictates that we only talk about the good news, never the bad. We're secretive about major and minor things alike, which inevitably makes life complicated. At the root of this habit is human fragility, as well as a lack of mental strength. Human relationships become dysfunctional, because the communication, trust, complicity and mutual support, which underlies all interpersonal relationships, are not sufficiently developed.

During the course of the last century, our fatherland, weakened and frail, suffered spiritual wounds and its primitive energy was depleted. We have lost faith. If we have no faith, then from where do we draw our strength? How can we survive on this earth? Without faith, how can we live in peace, harmony and in good health?

FIFTEEN

Diary
Monday, 14th July 2003 10:50 am

Tired these days. Although I had no intention of writing in my diary today, since I have some time on my hands, I'm going to jot down a few thoughts.

On *Hour of Power* this morning, the special guest was a pretty woman by the name of Xueli. She is a television presenter at *The 700 Club*, a musician and a writer. She fell into a depression 10 years ago and stayed in a psychiatric hospital. During therapy, the doctor would ask her: "Who are you?" She would always give the same answer: "I'm a television presenter at *The 700 Club*." It wasn't until many years later that she understood this: Being a television presenter was her job and not a part of herself. Her answer then changed, and she would say: "My name is Wei Xueli. I am a daughter of God." When she was first admitted into hospital, she refused to take medication, believing that prayers and reading the Bible would cure her. Then she asked herself: "How do you know which method God has chosen to save you?" She then began to participate fully in her therapy and achieved excellent results. However, since being discharged from hospital 10 years ago, she hasn't stopped taking antidepressants. Recently she published a book entitled *The Most Essential Things* in which she says that our greatest sin is not believing in God. She says that the will of God is not difficult to fathom and that we don't need to learn by rote all the rules and commandments. We just need to remember this: "Love God, love thy neighbour." The will of God is as simple as that. She even told her six-year-old son that he didn't need to achieve good grades at school or learn complex theories. He only needed to remember this: "Love God, love thy neighbour." When she finished her speech, she sang a hymn and was applauded by the congregation.

In his sermon, the Reverend Robert A. Schuller quoted from *Epistle to the Philippians*, Chapter 4, verses 4 to 7. A summary in three points:

1. "Rejoice in the Lord always."
2. "Do not be anxious about anything."
3. "[...] by prayer and petition, with thanksgiving [...]."

He then sang a hymn: "Rejoice in the Lord always. I say, rejoice, rejoice, rejoice, rejoice... I say, rejoice. Rejoice in the Lord always..." This is the chorus. It's fun and easy to remember.

The Reverend Schuller says that prayers and giving thanks to the Lord is a way of life. Under the guidance of the Holy Spirit, we breathe, walk, think, work... God is with us, always. And thus, we obtain "[...] the peace of God, which transcends all understanding [...]."

I love these words: "The peace of God" and, "Still, my soul be still."

Yesterday afternoon, I went to fetch my parents at Guangzhou station. All is well. God is guiding and watching over me.

Notes

Three days after Li Lanni started taking antidepressants, her suicidal tendencies took a turn for the worse.

The warning on the package leaflet for paroxetine says:

Possible side effects include worsening of symptoms for those who suffer from mental illnesses or are at risk of suicide.

For patients who suffer from depression, whether they are on antidepressants or not, symptoms can worsen and/or suicidal thoughts or behaviour can occur. Such risks exist until there is an improvement in the patient's condition.

Bad luck. Li Lanni only read the warning this morning.

Normally, hospitals in China don't advise patients with mental illnesses to read the package leaflets for medications. This in order to avoid mistrust and prejudice. In China, psychiatrists and psychologists cannot prescribe medication for more than seven days at a time. But 99.99 percent of medical specialists have never experienced depression. They only know about the effects of the medication from theories and patients' experiences. They don't necessarily understand what a patient suffering from severe depression would go through during the first seven days of treatment, nor the devastating effects it can have.

Before her treatment, Li Lanni had heard about the side effects of antidepressants and that different medication had different effects on different people. Since she had been through chemotherapy, she has a higher tolerance for side effects than most people.

However, during the first seven days of her treatment, she felt even worse than being in chemotherapy.

She was in a bad way: burning sensations on the face, neck, and scalp; severe nausea; spasms from the oesophagus down to the stomach; icy-cold limbs; cramps in the arms and legs; blurry vision; burning and watery eyes;

dizziness; uncontrollable trembling; sensations of hot and cold; unquenchable thirst; dryness on the tip of her tongue; painful urinary hesitancy (sitting on the toilet for hours on end without being able to urinate); and cold sweats. She had the sensation that her blood was burning hot. It was pumping around in the blood vessels of her limbs, head and neck, as if her insides were being burnt by smoke coming from a furnace. Sometimes she felt like her head was so bloated that she couldn't feel it anymore; other times, she felt her apartment was shaking like a drunken monster swaying from side to side, and the sky was about to crash down on her head.

After taking her medication in the morning, she remained slumped on the couch with a plastic basin next to her, hugging two cushions against her chest to stop the pain. Sometimes she would kneel on the couch and throw up into the basin; sometimes, with her feet hanging onto the back of the couch, she would bang her head on the floor to dull the pain. At other times, she would be in such a state of agitation that she didn't know whether to sit, stand, walk or lie down. Li Lanni stared at the clock, watching the minutes crawl by. The doctor said the side effects would decrease after one month, along with the depressive symptoms. 10 minutes... another 10 minutes... how many "10 minutes" are there in the space of one morning? There are 30 days in a month. How many "10 minutes" are there within a 30-day period?

Among those who have committed suicide, some were on antidepressants but stopped their treatment, unable to cope with the side effects.

During this long and torturous process, the graceful silhouette of the angel of death came to me, like Prince Charming coming to take Cinderella away.

Go on, jump. The balcony railings are low enough for you to just hop over them. Come, follow me. Together we will fly high up into the sky. You are a butterfly. Come, take flight.

His voice was soft and clear. He was so patient and attentive.

No! Suicide is a shameful act.

No, there's no shame in it. People with incurable diseases have the right to choose euthanasia. It's not selfish. Those who accuse you of being selfish are themselves selfish and cold-hearted. Go on, jump! There are only 12 storeys. It'll be all over in a minute.

In her head, Li Lanni started to write a simple will and testament for her family. Then she wrote a letter to a close friend. A few dozen words. Words of thanks. Her last words.

In his will of about 100 words, Yang Ganhua said that his death was no one's fault. He told his family where he had left his personal belongings, and that they were to return the things he had borrowed from other people. Not one superfluous word. Zhang Guorong's suicide note was short, written on a paper napkin. She understood. Suicide notes, she knew how to write them by heart.

The terrace was surrounded by a safety railing. Li Lanni found the key to the door that led out to the terrace. Don't bother with putting on new clothes. Just put on something loose and a pair of lace-up trainers, so passers-by won't be disgusted at the sight of a pair of purplish-red feet. You must stay clean and well-dressed. That's the least you can do. To jump, you must choose a time of day when there are few passers-by. Her last act will be done on a sunny day.

Lord, forgive me. I can't go on like this. I lack the strength. Help me, I beg you. Take me back into your arms.

Merciful God, answer my prayers. You say there is a time for everything. There is a time to live and a time to die, a time to kill and a time to heal. I can't wait any longer. But without Your consent, I do not have the courage to take my own life, so afraid am I of not being received into heaven. Before You only, suicide becomes a sin. Lord, show me Your intention. If You would allow me to return to You, I beg You, let me die. If You should forbid it, then save me, I beg this of You.

People are crowding around me and whispering in my ear. I know some of them while others I have never seen before. They're all babbling away.

San Mao said: "Do you know why I hung myself with a silk stocking? The windows of the hospital room were closed, so I couldn't jump outside. People don't understand why I took my own life. I couldn't not die. You understand?"

Yang Ganhua said: "I chose to do it with a belt, because it's strong. I told people I was sick, but no one understands that dying is easier than living. Now do you know?"

Virginia Woolf said: "My friends and my husband were so good and kind to me. It made me feel even more guilty. I was afraid of my domestic servants, of today's problems, of tomorrow's problems. I had no other choice but to seek refuge in the water. Do you understand?"

Li Lanni's father-in-law committed suicide in August 1966. At the time, he was the deputy head of the Department of Culture of the military region of Guangzhou. When he came back from the symposium on art and literature that comrade Jiang Qing had organised at the behest of comrade Lin Biao, his mood changed abruptly. One evening, he jumped off the top of a building without anyone understanding why. Li Lanni only saw the photograph of the deceased. His superior said to her: "For decades, no one understood why he committed such an act, but you guessed the reason behind it. It was depression."

Zhong Zishuo said to Li Lanni: "People thought there was an obscure reason behind my suicide. But there wasn't. It was depression. I ended my discussion with my colleagues and then jumped off the roof. It was as simple as that. The building was very high."

Zhang Guorong stayed silent. He stared at me with his laughing eyes, as if to say: "Don't you want to leave as well? We're waiting for you."

She was in a daze.

Head thrown backwards, back facing the terrace, Li Lanni shouted: "Lord, help me! Help me resist this temptation!"

She saw, as if through a fog, crowds of faces and mouths, gathering and jostling in front of her, pushing her to leave. She couldn't stand it anymore. Everywhere on the terrace she saw hands like spiders pulling her into their webs, but a force in her body was resisting and stopping her.

All of a sudden, there was nothing, as if an electric current had been cut off. She didn't know how long the power cut lasted. A few minutes. Maybe a few seconds.

When Li Lanni came to, she started hitting her head violently with her hands. She just kept on hitting, hitting and hitting. A voice was screaming: "I don't want to die! I don't want to die! No, no, no…" This strange voice echoed throughout the apartment. Li Lanni was terrified, and her body was shaking. Suddenly, drained of all her energy, she collapsed on the floor. Was she going to lose consciousness? What could she hit her head with? A club on the head and she'd be in a coma for a whole month.

She was confused.

She nearly jumped. Why didn't she? Li Lanni screamed that she didn't want to die and then there was nothing. Did she lose her memory? Her brain didn't register what happened afterwards. Her memory had failed her.

Did she have hallucinations?

Did she go into a trance while in the throes of a schizophrenic reaction?

Did she lose her mind due to a severe bout of depression, or due to the adverse effects of her medication?

Wipe out all traces of this incident.

There are some experiences you must delete from your memory. Other people must never know about them. The universe holds secrets that we would never have imagined in our wildest dreams. If we are to remember, then just pretend. Our memory is subjective and imperfect. Our knowledge of the universe is limited. My heart is filled with respect and gratitude.

24th February 2006

Correlations

Excerpts from *"Ordinary Days"*

[...] I sealed the cracks of the windows and door with scotch tape. Then I made an incision in the gas pipe of the kitchen stove and, listening carefully, I heard a soft whistling. I took a blanket and a pillow from the bedroom and put them on the kitchen floor. I closed the door and lay down serenely on the floor, waiting for the angel of death [...]. But 10 minutes later, I was still conscious. I jumped up and turned the gas tap on. Suddenly, I heard a loud bang. The explosion had blown up the window and extractor fan [...]. Keeping my nerve, I called the firemen and rushed outside to wait for help to arrive.

[...] I bought some poison commonly known as *hongshanai*. Its chemical name is thallus cyanide. Just a small spoonful is enough to kill you [...] I poured half the bottle into a glass of water. The water turned a bright red-orange and looked rather inviting. I sat on the bed and took a large gulp. A cold sensation immediately spread through my body. A second later, I felt nauseous. Another second passed, and I threw up all the liquid I had just ingested...

Li Yuying (Mrs Li Oufan)

Complementary Notes

Mrs Li describes her pain so succinctly. This is because the feelings inside her are impossible to express. As a fellow depression sufferer, I admire her. As one of her readers, I thank her

As Mr Li Oufan, her husband, said: "Chinese society lacks a deep understanding of depression, leading to many misconceptions. I sincerely hope that those who have suffered greatly from depression can talk about their experience."

SIXTEEN

Diary
Thursday, 17th July 2003 11 am

Around 10:30 am my computer froze. Not having anything better to do, I cooked some spare ribs with bitter cucumber. The computer restarted after that.

My friends say I should hire someone to do the cooking, but I prefer to do it myself. I've read in books that physical activities help reduce stress.

I almost never used to cook. As a child, I ate at military base canteens. Later, when I was studying or working in different cities, I still took my meals in canteens. My hectic lifestyle and numerous writing assignments meant I mostly ate either fast food or in restaurants to maintain my social relations. Now I am making up for it.

This makes me think of how the people of my generation have weathered drastic changes: Some have reached the top and are now on the decline. Some, like me, have survived a serious illness and want to retire from active working life; others became civil servants and experienced a dramatic reversal of their fortune. Then there're others who have been demoted... When faced with such a grim reality, it's easy to be disheartened.

While reading the Bible two years ago, I felt God had sent me this message: "Come with me by yourselves to a quiet place."[1] But I didn't follow His advice. In my ignorance, I wanted to leave my mark on society by writing an outstanding literary work. I thought it would allow me to become an instrument of God. Also, I was afraid of withdrawing into the desert. I lacked willpower, intelligence, strength and patience. I thank the Lord for teaching me, forging me, saving me and healing my wounds. Thus, I come to a better understanding of His intentions.

Lord, grant me strength and courage, and with the help of the Holy Ghost, guide me to that "quiet place."

Notes

One February morning after my surgical operation in 2000, I was looking out of the hospital room window, head slightly tilted to one side and a dressing on my wound. The 10 coldest days of the year in Guangzhou are around the Chinese New Year. It was a dark and cloudy day. Outside it was raining and a cold wind blew. People were hurrying to work. Buses were crammed full of passengers crushed together like sardines. Soaked to the bone, cyclists were struggling to keep their rain caps on their head. Pedestrians looked glum and wretched, hunched under their umbrellas. I remembered how miserable I was too, when I went to work in such foul weather. But that day, I envied those people struggling in the rain. Little did they know, there in an old building a stranger was watching them with envy, longing for the day when she could be among them again. I thought that if I were to survive and to go back to work again, I would never ever complain of bad weather again.

There were four beds in the room. A woman in her 50s had the bed closest to the window. She had advanced breast cancer and was in hospital for radiotherapy. She hardly looked out the window, sitting up in bed instead, head down and deep in thought. Her husband and children rarely visited her. My bed was next to hers. I liked looking out the window. The view was uninspiring, but it was better than the sad and dreary room. An old woman in her 70s was in the bed next to mine. She had a malignant brain tumour but was too old to undergo surgery. She was bald, and her hair follicles were dead. I heard she didn't have long to live, that she was going blind and would soon become unconscious and die. The nurses said she no longer needed to be in hospital, but her sons felt that as long as she was there, it gave them hope and comfort. Since she couldn't walk, she was either in her wheelchair or lying in bed. Her three sons took turns at her bedside. She was mostly silent, looking proudly at her sons from time to time. And they looked at their mother, eyes filled with love. Mother and sons shared many moments of such tender complicity.

A young woman, no more than 30 years old, had the bed closest to the door. She underwent surgery for metastatic cancer of the upper jaw. Her face, nose and mouth were disfigured by scars and I was afraid to look at her. At night, she often stood in front of the dimly-lit toilets, like some hideous and malevolent ghost. This ghastly image stuck in my mind long after I left hospital. Her parents brought her soup every day. Her husband, a good-looking man who was the same age as her, came to the hospital every day to feed her. Every time she swallowed a spoonful of soup, she would cough and splutter. It made me want to throw up. Sometimes, I would hide under the blanket and cover my ears. No matter how painful it was for her, no matter how long it would take, she would always try to swallow the food. She had a two-year-old daughter and was fighting to live. Of all the patients in the room, she was the one who had the most challenging problems to face. But it was she who held onto life with hope and optimism.

Only my mother and my husband visited me. My father had severe hypertension with systolic pressure at over 230, and my brother was in another hospital with a high fever of 40 degrees. My mother took care of both my brother and me. My husband didn't take any days off and carried on with his teaching duties. Of all my friends, I only told Ququ that I was in hospital. She wanted to come, but I wouldn't let her. I didn't want my friends to see me in such bleak and dreary surroundings and feel sorry for me. And too tired to talk, I would end up feeling guilty and blaming myself.

The number of patients who live a normal life during the first year following surgery is increasing. Oncologists told me that some patients who had the same type of cancer that I did, and even in less severe cases, died 20 days after surgery. Often, they're weak psychologically; in other words, they were "scared to death." There are others who go back to work during the first year and resume a normal life. Some have a relapse one or two years later, their cancer cells spreading at an uncontrollable rate. Like me, numerous cancer patients have witnessed far too many sad and tragic stories in hospital wards. Surrounded by death, we don't have the luxury of thinking about when we'd go back to work. The only question we ask ourselves is: "How much longer do I have to live?"

When I learned that my cancer had spread, my first thought was: "It's lucky I don't have children. Just give me some powerful painkillers, so I don't die in terrible pain."

I examined my conscience and asked: "Li Lanni, do you have a clear conscience?" I was afraid of giving myself a straight answer. Lying in my hospital bed, eyes closed, I reviewed my entire life beginning with my first memories. A few days later, I found my answer: "Yes, my conscience is clear. Definitely." A sense of relief came over me. I was free to leave this world. I would never forget that wonderful feeling of being able to die, free of worries and with a clear conscience.

The year following my operation went by smoothly. Proud of myself, I said: "Li Lanni, I'm satisfied with you. Cancer didn't kill you. They say if you survive a critical illness, good things will come your way. Let's wait and see."

That was the second Chinese New Year after my operation. I was gushing with confidence, like a child holding a coloured balloon that had just been inflated. On the second day of the New Year, wearing a padded jacket, woollen trousers and ankle boots, and with a smile on my lips, I was walking briskly towards a shopping centre. Suddenly, I felt my body flying through the air, then my mind went blank for a few seconds. When I came to, I found myself lying on my back at the entrance of the shopping mall. What happened? Did I fall? Really? How embarrassing. I sat up, head in a daze. My trousers were ripped through to the lining at the knees, where there was a gaping wound.

It was a bad omen. Falling flat on your face at the start of the New Year is enough to spook even those who aren't in the least bit superstitious.

After the New Year, I bought a magnolia bonsai for my balcony. It was the prettiest tree among the seven or eight that were at the florist's. It had begun to grow leaves of a delicate spring green that were very soothing to the eyes. Soon I would smell their fragrance. Excited by this thought, I made a wish: to recover my health and strength, like this tree in bloom. But the next day, when I went out on the balcony in the afternoon, the magnolia had been sliced in half. A metal pole I used to dry clothes had fallen, cutting through the trunk, leaving a stump in the earth. I had made a wish the day before and it made me nervous. No, no, it doesn't matter. It's nothing at all. I tried to save the magnolia, hoping it would bud and flower. But it had succumbed to its injuries.

Was it a bad omen or a warning?

Cancer patients have this one thing in common: often before the onset of their illness, they've reached a high point in their lives. They have a flourishing career, many doors are open to them, their morale is high, and they are in the best physical shape of their lives.

This was the case for one woman who had advanced breast cancer: The year before she learnt she had cancer, life was smiling on her. Many of her colleagues lost their jobs, while she kept hers. Her personal finances were strong; she had gained the trust of the factory directors and her prospects of promotion were excellent. Her sister said to her: "You've never looked so beautiful in your life!"

It's the principle of the "waxing and waning of the moon."

The year 1999 was the busiest I had ever been in my whole life. I had numerous writing assignments: television series, film scripts, short stories and essays. I worked on the pre- and post-production of several documentaries, attended a premiere in Macau and evening galas at the Great Hall of the People in Beijing, was appointed to an important position, won awards, etc. I spent the New Year in Beijing and returned to Guangzhou for the Chinese New Year. It was a busy and productive year. Over the Chinese New Year of 2000, I worked on a television series with the director He Jun. When the first manuscript was finished and before undergoing surgery for cancer, I told the director to find someone else to complete the project.

All cancer patients, whether they are university lecturers, white-collar workers, entrepreneurs, journalists, editors, television hosts, civil servants, writers, directors, actors, etc, seem to have one experience in common: They fall from the top of the mountain into a precipice. Take my magnolia tree for example. Before being sliced in half, it was healthy and blooming, which makes its death all the more unfortunate. I held onto the hope that it might come back to life and start blossoming again.

Those who are at the bottom of the precipice are like me at the start of the New Year: Sitting on the ground, wondering how I could have fallen flat on my face. Luckily nothing was broken. Too much time has been wasted, we must now make up for lost time. Come on, get up and climb that hill. Show what you're capable of. We cheated death and a happy, healthy life lies ahead of us.

What's happiness? Having high social standing? Being productive at work? Creating artistic works? Being famous? Making profits and more profits? Having a squeaky clean reputation? Living up to your family name? Having a happy ending?

I don't know what happiness is. And I don't want to know. It's something nice, that's all.

Hurry up. In your public and private life, you must move forward as part of a team. In this way, you'll climb even higher.

In public life, it's the bonds of comradeship and friendship that matter most. A decent person is always grateful to those who have helped him: family, nation, parents, friends, hierarchical superiors, those who were by his side during troubled times, those who helped him in times of need. In turn, he too must come to their aid.

If you've run 9,900 kilometres in a 10,000-kilometre race, it would be a shame to give up.

Life is unpredictable. The wheel of fortune is turning constantly. "Carpe diem": "Seize the day."

A teacher can never give up on his students, a bank director on his employees, an actor on his audience, a writer on his readers, a public official on his Party.

Private life is simpler. To live and to recover from an illness, you need money. To treat cancer, you need money and social relations. To earn enough money, you need a certain social standing. The higher your social status, the more chance you have to obtain things. This principle is true for everyone, whether he or she is sick or not.

To feed your family, you need a job. In order not to be eliminated from the job market, those who are sick must fare better than those who are well.

To live is to cope with problems.

Cancer patients are twice as busy as those who are in good health. Except for retirees.

Keeping yourself busy helps give you courage, hide your fear, obtain benefits and favours, protect your family interests, keep your place in society, do... do many, many things.

A year after my operation, I announced that I was returning to an active life. I began reading extensively, wrote essays and short scripts, conducted interviews.

During the summer of 2001, I was feeling very restless. While on the balcony taking in the evening air, I often had this thought: What if I jumped into the void?

The first time it happened, I found it rather amusing. Li Lanni, you're funny. However, after several times, a sense of unease came over me. My reason tried to intervene: This is ridiculous. Don't be silly. Even though I was unaware at the time that it was a type of pathological thinking, I tried to control myself and stop these thoughts. When my mind was still, this thought came to me: Retreat into a quiet place. When I felt a light wind touching my face, I murmured: "Retreat... into a quiet place... Go... Go to... that... quiet place..."

On 17th December 2001, I was plunged into despair when the otolaryngologist advised me to undergo surgery immediately after the Writer Representative Conference. It meant my cancer cells were active again, taking me back to where I was in February 2000.

To have peace of mind, I searched in the *Cihai*[2] for a definition of the common expression: "Retreat from the world to nourish your energy." I reread the principle of "emptiness" in Buddhism, as well as an annotated edition of the *Dao De Jing*.[3] As I was reading these texts, I thought I understood them. But once the books were finished, I was plagued by doubts again.

I attempted to find rest in remaining still.

I could retreat into the wilderness, but what if my mind kept on thinking about the material world? I tried to turn my thoughts on other things, but they kept galloping around in my head like wild horses. What was I to do?

Today people have the misconception that "finding rest" means not going to work and that "remaining still" means mediating for half an hour every day. We want everything, and we want it now. If we rest for half an hour, it's for the purpose of storing up enough energy to either indulge ourselves for 10 hours afterwards or throw ourselves into all sorts of activities with increased fervour. Like the barely perceptible movement of a hound before it pounces on its prey.

Between the end of 2002 and the beginning of spring in 2003, mankind, which is so disrespectful of nature, received a warning in the form of the SARS epidemic. And punishment was inflicted on me for not having retreated into the "quiet place." If you missed the warning signs God gave you through cancer, then He'll give you a lesson through depression.

Throughout my punishment, I had no choice but to retreat into the "quiet place." I was incapable of doing anything other than listening to music and watching television. I was forced to cut myself off from the outside world and give up my professional activities. Lying alone on the couch, I could do nothing but pray. It was then that I finally understood the phrase: "Retreat into the wilderness, where there is no man, but only spirits dwell."

During the time when I was cast out into the spiritual wilderness, I learnt to rest, gather strength and immerse myself in spiritual essence. I discovered that my illness and my sufferings had a positive effect on me. It helped me find rest and gather strength, like laying my body down by still waters that soothed my thirsty, fearful heart. I also understood the meaning of this verse: "In repentance and rest is your salvation, in quietness and trust is your strength."[4] So true. When you're at rest, you understand the meaning and purpose of your life.

But I was still weak and blind. I "retreated into the wilderness" by force of circumstance. Once the punishment came to an end, I went back to my old habits. But I had confidence and hope that I would be saved.

15th March 2006

Correlations

Excerpts from *The Power of Positive Thinking*

This, believe it or not, was the prescription. His patient was to take two hours off every working day and go off for a long walk. Then he was to take a half-day off a week and spend that half-day in a cemetery.

In astonishment the patient demanded: "Why should I spend that half-day in a cemetery?"

"Because," answered the doctor, "I want you to wander around and look at the gravestones of men who are there permanently. I want you to meditate on the fact that many of them are there because they thought even as you do, that the whole world rested on their shoulders. Meditate on the solemn fact that when you get there permanently the world will go on just the same and, as important as you are, others will be able to do the work you are now doing. I suggest that you sit on one of those tombstones and repeat this statement: 'A thousand years in Thy sight are but as yesterday when it is past, and as a watch in the night.'"

The patient got the idea. He slowed his pace. He learned to delegate authority. He achieved a proper sense of his own importance.

Norman Vincent Peale (United States)

Complementary Notes

An increasing number of people are incapable of letting themselves go. If all the elites in China were to spend half a day in a cemetery, they would probably throw themselves back to work at an even more frenzied pace and hang on harder to power. Each minute of our lives must be exploited to the fullest.

SEVENTEEN

Diary
Friday, 18th July 2003 10:10 am

Made an appointment with a specialist for Mother.

A few days ago at dinner, she was complaining again about how she was coughing blood. It's becoming obsessive. She's already had a sputum cytology test, blood test and a chest X-ray. Everything is normal. She's even had a CT-scan. One doctor thinks she might have excessive production of mucus but didn't eliminate the possibility of pulmonary tuberculosis. The head physician at the hospital told her she was fine, and she was discharged four days later. But she is still convinced she has tuberculosis or some other serious illness and is going to die.

Fed up with hearing the same complaint all the time, I snapped at her: "Even if it *is* tuberculosis, it's no big deal. If you had cancer like me, you'd be dead by now."

Mother gave up her job when she was quite young because of a stomach disease (the real reason being that she was afraid her family background would get her into trouble). She was a homemaker for many years during the Cultural Revolution. Although she went back to work again after that, she was no longer entitled to claim her pension rights. She refuses to face up to her mistakes and inadequacies by hiding behind her "illness." My brother and I got used to her mood swings at a very early age. Our family life revolves around her. Because she is "sick," she must come first. What she doesn't realise is that unconsciously she is willing herself to be sick. Then she'll be the centre of attention, allowing her to run away from the resentment and dissatisfaction she feels inside.

If I understand why she behaves like she does, why do I let myself be affected? Maybe it's because my childhood wounds are still open.

Somewhere in my subconscious, I don't consider her my mother. Everything she says and does gets on my nerves and makes me feel insecure. Talking to her depletes my energy. Sometimes she triggers all sorts of aches and pains in my body: headache, heaviness in the chest, stomach ache, restlessness.

Stop making yourself unhappy with these unpleasant thoughts. She is also a victim of her times. I am in therapy to alleviate my anxieties and overcome the shadows of my childhood. Since Mother likes to wallow in her role as a sick person, it's up to me to keep a certain psychological distance from her and stay a simple observer. I refuse to fall into the trap of playing the role of her "emergency nurse." I won't lose my nerve, won't contradict her and won't answer back.

Lord, support me with Your mighty hand. I beg of You, drive away Satan.

Lord, shine Your divine light on me and dispel the darkness from my heart. May Your eternal light shine in me and warm my heart forever. Amen.

Notes

In my diary I wrote about the worries that have plagued me all these years. Since depression can be hereditary, in this "Notes" section I will go back several generations in an attempt to explore possible hereditary links.

From the point of view of character, experience and family environment, my grandmother should be the one most prone to depression and I the least out of the four generations of women in my family – my great-grandmother, grandmother, mother and I. But as it turned out, my grandmother is the strongest of us all. Today, at 95 years of age, she is clear-headed, her handwriting is legible, and she always wins at mah-jong.

I'm going to explore the lives of these four generations of women spanning an entire century, as well as the hereditary nature of depression in this ordinary Chinese family.

Rather I should say five generations, if I were to count the one after mine, but I've made the choice not to have children.

Ten years ago, Zhang Mei, Ququ and I made the conscious choice to not have children. Our colleagues named us the "three ladies without heirs."

It was a decision I made before I was married. After my marriage, I had three abortions. People of the older generation tried to make me change my mind. They said that from the point of view of my destiny and marriage, having children would be beneficial to my future, health, family life and old age. Others said my choice was tied to the fact that I had faced many setbacks in life. Although not obstinate by nature, I stood my ground.

Not having children of my own doesn't mean I don't like them. Being a mother is a great responsibility and I don't have what it takes.

When I was 20 years old, I realised that I lacked a positive maternal figure in my life. In my mind, there were only negative images. I've never met the kind of mother figure that Bing Xin's[1] teacher writes about in her book. When I was growing up, I remember seeing slogans that conveyed images of the "ideal mother figure." But I never had a kind-hearted and optimistic mother who was healthy in body and mind, capable of giving a sense of security to her children. Women who grew up in situations similar to mine tend to have emotional problems, are emotionally insecure and easily fall prey to despair.

Faith, hope and love are the psychological building blocks of a person. But due to my hereditary factors and family circumstances, I lack these spiritual tools. If a woman like me were to have children, she would be incapable of providing a healthy and balanced family environment. The conditions would be far from ideal to raise children in.

History mustn't repeat itself. And taking into account the rapid demographic growth, I decided not to have children. From that moment on, criticisms like "not having descendants is a filial impiety" and "but you will die without heirs" no longer bother me.

I never knew my great-grandmother. They say she lacked the beauty and talent of her daughters. The rest of the family likes to make fun of my grandmother, mother, and me by saying: "It goes downhill from one generation to the next." From the first day I was born, people have been finding faults with my appearance. Both men and women alike in the army used to say: "This child is not as good-looking as her parents." Later, when I visited my maternal grandmother, the family used to say to my face and behind my back: "She's not as pretty as her mother or her grandmother. Look at her eyes, nose, mouth, ears and skin. She's going to be taller than her grandmother. Times have changed. Children feed on cow's milk now."

My great-grandmother's nickname was Xigu. My grandmother's nickname is Xiaotao, and my mother's is Lanlan. These three women of different generations have their own stories to tell and have their parts to play in the history of depression in my family.

As a young woman, Xiaotao was as beautiful and graceful as a peach blossom. Her eyes, full of charm, were like petals moist with dew. Her face was round. Her teeth, slightly protruding and white and smooth as white jade, made you think of the yesteryear actress Shangguan Yunzhu, as well as the Hong Kong actress Zhou Huimin, who has a faint smile on her lips even when she isn't truly smiling.

Lanlan joined the Artistic Regiment of the army as a young woman. A young war hero fell in love with her and sent her love letters through the internal organisation of the Party. Even my father says she isn't as beautiful as her mother. The first time he saw Xiaotao, my grandmother, she already had eight children, four of whom were dead. She was a woman in her 40s who had lived through many hardships.

Xiaotao's mother was Xigu. Her father was a poor scholar of the provincial examinations of the Qing dynasty. When his granddaughter was a child, he betrothed her to a boy born in the same year. Xiaotao was a few months older than her future husband. She was born at the dawn of a new era, in January

1911, and was the first generation of young girls to receive a western education. In secondary school, she was one year ahead of her fiancé. But she didn't like him, finding his face too long and his academic performance too mediocre, unlike herself. She was a good student. Her best subjects were Chinese and English. Her grandfather praised her essays, which the teachers marked with a red pen. The school uniform was plain: white shirt, black skirt, white socks and black shoes. Xiaotao, a brilliant and ambitious pupil, wanted to study in the best universities in China. But life is unpredictable. The day before she was to receive her secondary school diploma, her father died suddenly due to sickness. Xiaotao's life was changed overnight. Her only source of income was gone, destroying her dream of going to university. Her mother, now a widow, had to feed the family, and her brother needed to go to school. At 17 years old, she was faced with only one choice: marriage.

Why do I think that, out of the four generations of women, Xiaotao should be the one most vulnerable to depression? Because she was beautiful and talented. Having grown up during the period of the May Fourth Movement, she wanted to pursue her freedom: emancipate herself from feudal values, study at university, be free to choose her husband and determine her marital relationship, be part of the new generation of youth, and build a stronger and more prosperous country. All of her cousins were successful. Some were studying abroad, while others studied at the Universities of Beijing and Shanghai and became women of the new generation. Even though Xiaotao was the one with the most promising future, she spent her entire life at home. She never knew what happiness was, had no social status, and endured many hardships and humiliations. No one understood her, and no one could help her change her circumstances. Her life before and after her marriage were two diametrically opposite worlds.

I lived with my grandmother for two years during secondary school. The image of her, frail and always troubled by dizzy spells, is deeply etched into my memory. She didn't have money to buy medication or food supplements. When she felt faint, her face would turn pale, and with a trembling hand, she would open the ceramic jar where she kept the white sugar Mother had sent her from Guangzhou. She would take out a small packet, carefully undo the string, take a pinch of sugar and put it in the palm of her hand. With a guilty look on her face, she would let out a small sigh as if to chide herself for being wasteful, lower her head slightly and put her hand against her mouth. Then, reluctantly, she would throw her head backwards, and the sugar would fall into her mouth. She would then lean against the headboard of the bed for a while before getting up to resume her tasks.

I wondered if her dizzy spells were due to low blood sugar, anaemia or a lack of adequate nutrition.

When I visited her a few years ago, I heard Mother scold her: "You don't have money to buy tofu that costs only a few cents. And even when you want to eat it, you can't afford it." It broke my heart. Entirely dependent on others, she never had an income. She had to be accountable for every single cent that was spent. At 90 years old, she didn't have a house to her name. I was upset and wanted to cry out at the injustice of it all. But Grandmother never let this get her down and never felt sorry for herself. Earlier this year, I received a letter from her just before the Chinese New Year. She wrote: "My greatest regret is not having joined the workforce after the Liberation." She told Lanlan and Nizi: "As long as I'm alive, I'll continue to share with you the blessings I have received. The secret to my longevity is to be content with what you have."

For Lanlan, her 16th year proved to be the turning point in her life. She was in secondary school. One day, after class, she joined the People's Liberation Army with her classmates. She didn't go home to fetch her belongings and left without telling her family. She believed it was her first step on the road to communism. That day, her father was in the middle of a mathematics lesson when the high school students shouted: "Mr Zhang, your daughter has left with the People's Liberation Army!" If Lanlan hadn't left that day, she would never have become a soldier. She would have become a primary school teacher and would never have suffered from depression.

For Li Lanni, her ninth year was the turning point in her life. She had, until then, enjoyed good health, physically and mentally. But from her ninth year onwards, many things happened that eventually led her into a state of chronic depression. Even the smallest and most insignificant of things contributed to her decline.

We have all experienced events that have changed our destiny and our mental states. Once we are diagnosed with depression, we should try to remain level-headed and go through our mental life with a fine-toothed comb. At which stage of our lives did problems begin to surface? In which part of ourselves are the hidden wounds? Where are the blockages? How deep are the fissures?

Have you ever tried to analyse yourself in this way?

6th April 2006

Correlations

Excerpts from *Courtyard of My Childhood Years*

1

The courtyard had no door. An old longan tree stood at the entrance.

Every year, the longan tree bore fruits which, barely bigger than a small pea, would dry up and die. A few days later, they would fall silently onto the sand and shrivel up, one by one, like a still-born foetus. The trunk leant to one side, its branches hanging low. From afar, it looked like an old woman bent over in pain, her back hunched-up, hands out-stretched, reaching out to her dead children.

There were a few yellow one-storey houses in the courtyard. My family lived in the one that stood in the east but faced west.

Mother locked the door, closed the curtains and told my brother and me to sit on her bed. Then she said in a quiet voice:

"We've moved into this new place, and there are going to be two new rules. One: You're the big sister, and you're going to look after your little brother. If he's naughty, both of you will be punished. Two: You must never talk about your maternal grandmother's family."

"I know why. Grandmother's family are landowners!"

"Nonsense!" said Mother, giving me a small tap with her fan made of palm leaves. "Grandfather is a teacher of the people. Never forget that. I became a soldier when I was a teenager and we're against all landowners. Nizi, be a good girl. You must help Mother."

My brother nodded eagerly, but I was left speechless.

"Another thing... don't ever say that your mother can read," Mother continued. "If... something ever happens to me, Father will marry another woman. If you have a step-mother, then there'll be a step-father..."

Mother had resigned from her job the previous year. She said she was sick.

2

Xiao Yuzi's family lived in the house opposite ours. Xiao Yuzi was eight years old and didn't go to school. The women in the courtyard said she had a heart disease and that she was going to die before reaching adulthood. They said the hospital where she was born had strange practices and should never have let her come into this world, because she brought nothing but trouble. But it would have been too cruel to end her life and, what's more, it was illegal. She was a burden to her family and was a waste of money, ration tickets, and tofu.

Xiao Yuzi brought bad luck. Her mother lost a lot of blood during her delivery, which left her suffering from facial paralysis.

At one time, when Xiao Yuzi's mother took the quilts out of the trunks to air them in the sun, she found a nest of mice inside. The suckling mice were half the size of a thumb and their eyes were still closed. They had soft round bellies and translucent skin, and their flesh was pink and tender.

As if she had discovered a treasure, Xiao Yuzi's mother rushed out to buy a bottle of Shiwan rice wine. She put the mice in the wine, sealed the bottle and left them to soak in the wine like dumplings. Then when the wine reached maturity, she drank a small cupful every day.

Xiao Yuzi's mother liked to eat meat and she always managed to find some.

She never threw away the black mice she caught at home. Following a Cantonese custom, she would skin them, split open their bellies, rip out their innards and sprinkle the abdominal cavity with salt. She kept their bellies pried open with a small stick and put the mice out in the sun to dry until they turned red and stiff. She would cut a piece off when she was cooking, put it in a casserole to stew with fermented soya beans, ginger and garlic.

3

Mother pursed her lips, her eyes making quick nervous movements. The wrinkle between her eyebrows was as hard and sharp as a knife.

She had resigned from her job when she was in her 30s due to her cardiac and stomach illnesses. She was anxious all the time. She was probably thinking of her parents.

Her father had been denounced and sent to the countryside. My grandparents ate what they managed to grow. Mother was worried about her parents, but couldn't talk about it, so she took it out on us.

I kept myself busy. I folded the quilt on my bed and climbed up to the upper bunk to see if my brother had folded his. I picked up a strand of red wool that was lying on the floor.

4

The sparrow was still moving, but its wings were smeared with blood. The feathers on its tiny head were bright and glossy. Its eyes were closed, and its body was trembling violently either out of fear or pain.

Zhang Xiaoxia pressed down hard on the sparrow with the palm of her hand. It stopped moving.

"It's fainted," I said, feeling sorry for the bird.

"Let's eat it," said Zhang Xiaoxia.

Putting the slingshot into her belt, she started plucking the sparrow with clean quick gestures. It moved, desperately clawing the air. Unable to cry out in pain, it could only move its head.

Suddenly, I thought of Xiao Yuzi. She lay on the floor, moving her head in the same way after her mother had hit her with a stool.

"Do we have to eat it?" I asked quietly.

Zhang Xiaoxia glared at me, her eyes bulging.

"Go and fetch some dried leaves."

The sparrow was no more than a lump of red flesh with wrinkled skin. Its belly was trembling and, except for around the neck, all its feathers had been plucked out.

Sitting on the stone steps in front of the meeting room, Zhang Xiaoxia lit a fire with the dried leaves. She pierced a stick into the anus of the sparrow and started grilling it over the fire. I carried on collecting the dried leaves. The bird turned black and was shrivelling up.

"It smells good, doesn't it?" Zhang Xiaoxia asked, pulling off a wing and putting it into her mouth.

The sparrow's neck was twisted, and its eyes were half open slits. As if it refusing to resign itself to its fate, it was smiling in mockery of its missing wing. Its cadaverous eyes stared at me, watching to see if I liked the taste of its flesh.

"Go on, eat up," said Zhang Xiaoxia, giving me the other wing. "If you don't eat it, I won't play with you."

I licked the charred wing with the tip of my tongue. Then I took a small bite, chewing slowly just to show Zhang Xiaoxia that I was eating.

I didn't want to eat the little sparrow but was afraid that Zhang Xiaoxia wouldn't play with me anymore.

"It's tasty, isn't it?" she asked, pulling off the head.

She was chewing on the neck and the corners of her mouth were moving up and down. Now and then, she spat out bits of pink flesh.

"The meat tastes a bit rotten. You just have to get used to it," she said, ripping apart the bird's body. Blood slowly dripped out.

Zhang Xiaoxia's lips were black and her teeth were smeared with red.

Complementary Notes

The manuscript of this novella was refused a few times. Since the story has little literary value, I've included it in this book as part of my medical records intended for psychiatrists.

It's one of my favourite novellas. The characters and events are real, and I changed the names by replacing one Chinese character with another. The courtyard in the story is part of a military base located in Foshan.

One day, my parents left without a word. The family was reunited two years later.

We moved from the island of Haidao, a military outpost, to a busy and lively town. I changed from a school for military children to a regional one and found it difficult to adapt to my new environment.

Also, Mother had changed. She seemed strangely distant and I felt uneasy around her. From that time on, I learnt to be psychologically independent of my parents and of other people whenever I was in a new environment. I became rebellious towards my family. From being introverted, I became an extrovert.

The courtyard holds the thoughts and impressions of a 12-year-old child.

I long to return there to reconnect with my memories, and to relive the sights, sounds and smells of my yester-years.

EIGHTEEN

Diary
Saturday, 19th July 2003 11:20am

Slept badly these last two nights. It takes me longer to fall asleep and I wake up dizzy with a headache. It's probably because I've reduced my medication. Two days ago, I started taking half a tablet less of alprazolam at midday and in the evening. But last night, feelings of anxiety were again present in my dreams.

Dreamt I was sitting for an exam. The notification took me by surprise and I rushed into the examination hall in a state of panic, but the session was nearly over. The teachers scolded me for arriving late and said there would be consequences. It was so unfair, but I didn't know whose fault it was and couldn't justify myself. To save time, I took a copy of the examination paper, knowing full well I wouldn't have time to finish. But to my dismay, the teachers couldn't find my name on the list of candidates. I didn't know where to sit, nor what the examination subject was. One of the teachers said it would be a waste of time to keep on looking and that I should sit for the exam. At that moment, a senior teacher came in. He looked like a retiree and commanded respect. He said: "We can't find her name on the list. Just say she isn't registered for today's session." I had no idea what he was talking about. The other teachers said an observer was always more lucid. Then, one of them said: "They got it mixed up. I've already finished my session. Today's session has nothing to do with me." Overcome with relief, I thought: "Great. I don't have to sit for the exam today." A weight had been lifted off my shoulders, I felt light and cheerful, and began chatting to the exam invigilators. Smiling to myself, I thought: "Phew! Just a storm in a teacup. It turns out I've already finished my exam."

This dream provides an insight into my mental state.

Now that I've lessened my intake of medication, I should take more care of myself and not get myself worked up. Regression is a normal part of the process. Anxiety and depression behave like criminals. Seeing that the number of sentinels guarding the entrance has been reduced, they rush through the breach, wreaking havoc on the other side. To guard against the enemy, I must be positive and stay alert.

When I can't sleep, I pray. When I wake up with a headache, I pray. I firmly believe this: "If God is for us, who can be against us?"[1]

Notes

Exams are a recurrent theme in my dreams. It symbolises stress, but I also wonder if it's in any way related to my family history. My great-grandmother's father was a provincial examinations scholar. Does my fear of exams come from him? Before he passed the examinations at the provincial level, he must have sat for many others: end of the year exams, local exams, etc., all of which were extremely intellectually demanding. Stories of how difficult the imperial examinations were are only too well known. The criteria for selection was much stricter then and must have wreaked havoc on the nerves.

I never knew my great-grandmother. And I never made the effort to find out more about her and her mental world. I would hear fragments of information here and there: She was kind and good-natured, and had lived through the rise of a New China.

I'll call Mother to ask her if Great-Grandmother knew how to read and write. What was education like in a family of scholars? But then, Mother's information is never 100 percent accurate. Since I'm not doing a historical study, I'll let my imagination do the work. What were my generation's great-grandmothers' psychological journeys like?

Xigu was born in the 1880s. I don't have much of any idea of what a young girl's life in that time would have been like. However, the following events will give us a glimpse into Xigu's life.

In the same year that Xigu's father passed the provincial exams, two events took place, one happy and one sad. The unhappy event: The family didn't have enough money to pay for the journey to the capital city, where Xigu's father was to take the court exams. He gave up hope of ever becoming a public official. At that time, the ambition of every scholar was to become an official in the imperial civil service. Otherwise, what was the point of pursuing academic excellence? How could you put your talents to good use, help the people, and become a pillar of society? Li Bai, Du Fu, Su Shi and Xin Qiji,[2] all these immensely gifted men were imperial officials. Tao Yuanming[3] was a civil servant in the imperial court before returning home in the countryside to "pick chrysanthemums growing on a wooden palisade facing east."[4]

Without money, Xigu's father could not travel from the mountains of Wubei in the province of Jiangsu to the Forbidden City in the capital. Her family was unable to raise enough money for his journey. I wonder if it was because they couldn't collect sufficient funds from the villagers, or if it was because they were unwilling to beg the wealthy and cold-hearted. Was he a noble scholar or did he have a weak and bland personality? He never took that journey to the capital and remained a poor provincial examinations scholar all his life. He taught and composed texts for a living: beautiful parallel sentences written in fine calligraphy, inscriptions for wooden tablets and steles, texts and letters for villagers. His house was big and spacious, which suggests that a provincial examinations scholar was able to make a good living from writing.

He was the equivalent of today's freelance writer.

Such a coincidence. My brother called me this evening to tell me that Grandmother has been admitted into hospital for a heart problem and that her condition was worrying. Morbid thoughts surfaced in my mind and a superstitious fear took hold of me: Did I violate a taboo by talking about my great-grandmother? Stop. No more. Wait until Grandmother is better.

There's nothing I can do except pray, over and over again. I believe God's intentions are good. Don't be afraid, have faith.

10th April 2006 at 11 pm on the dot

Correlations

Excerpts from *Courtyard of My Childhood Years*

9

"Nizi is actually quite pretty," said Mrs Gong, looking at me. She was sitting at the foot of a tree, combing Xiao Chun's hair. "At first I thought she was very plain, but with time, I began to find her rather pretty."

My heart leapt with joy. I picked up Xiao Chun's red ribbon that had fallen on the ground and gave it to Mrs Gong.

"Nizi, when did your mother stop working?" she asked, frowning.

"When she was seventeen. Her stomach was sick."

Mother joined the army when she was 16 years old. She followed the troops to hunt down bandits. The armed forces marched night and day from Jiangsu Province to the province of Guangdong. As part of the Artistic Regiment, she played the Chinese castanets, sang and acted in shows to raise the troops' morale.

"Girls today are too sassy," said Mother Hu, taking a bamboo stool to sit down with us. "Around that time, I left with my eldest daughter Yi Hong to look for her father. We went from village to village asking people for food."

Mother Hu was holding a sewing basket on her knees. It held scraps of rectangular cloth with which she made patchwork pillowcases.

"Her father had left, and we had no news from him for several years. I said to myself, if he had gotten himself killed, I'll stay a widow and not remarry for the rest of my life. But if he had become a civil servant and had abandoned me and my girls, then I'll kill myself, jump into a well and take him with me!"

Si Hong, Mother Hu's fourth daughter, was the same age as my little brother. But she looked old, just like Xiao Yuzi's grandmother. Her face was wrinkled, two of her teeth were missing and her front teeth were long and elongated. They say that the older you grow, the longer your teeth become. But Mr Hu was only in his 40s. He had coal black hair, a square face and eyebrows shaped like swords. He was a striking man.

"Nizi, did your mother teach you to sing?" Mother Hu asked me all of a sudden.

"Yes, she knows a lot of songs."

"You see," Mother Hu said to Mrs Gong. "She's no ordinary woman. And she says she can't read."

10

"Nizi, is your mother home?"

It was Mother Hu's voice. Mother rushed outside the house to stop Mother Hu from coming in. She never let anyone inside.

In the camphor wood trunk was a silk pouch embroidered with a pair of mandarin ducks. Inside the pouch were a pair of gold earrings and a silver bracelet that was broken in half. At the bottom of the trunk were two small boxes of books. It was strictly forbidden for us to touch these boxes. You would think there were land mines hidden inside.

"Did you hear? Last night, Xiao Chun's mother..." said Mother Hu, lowering her voice. "She threw a fit again."

I climbed onto the bed without making a sound and stood tip-toed on two big pillows, peering out of the small window. Mother and Mother Hu were standing huddled together.

Mother was speaking in hushed tones and I could barely make out what she was saying.

"Why did she do that? She should consider herself lucky her husband didn't ask for a divorce."

Mother Hu rolled her eyes and pouted, as if Mrs Gong had scored a point over her.

Even Mrs Gong had secrets! All the families in the courtyard had their own dirty little secrets then. If it was true, Mother's secret wouldn't be so awful after all.

"If it's your sister's child, then there would be a family likeness, wouldn't there?" said Mother Hu, stifling a laugh. "You'd better watch out...men can never be trusted. Mark my words."

Mother Hu lowered her voice even further and I heard Mother say: "Nizi's father... he... he wouldn't..."

"Xiao Chun's father wasn't faithful... they're all the same."

"No, it can't be... but if it's true... then it's awful," said Mother, frowning.

"What would you do?"

"I'd leave with my children."

"Think again! Or you could have another son," Mother Hu chuckled.

11

When Mother brushed her teeth, she would cough and splutter, and her veins would stand out on her temples. Mrs Commander in Chief would tease her and say: "You're not pregnant, are you?" Her mouth full of toothpaste, Mother replied: "I'm always like this when I brush my teeth."

Every morning, I would watch my mother brush her teeth. I didn't like to see her cough and splutter. It frightened me.

"Mother, are you pregnant with a little brother?"

"No," she replied with a smile, surprised. "Don't be silly."

If Mother were pregnant with a little brother, I would want him to die in her belly. I didn't want any more brothers or sisters.

I confided my thoughts to Zhang Xiaoxia and she swore she would never tell anyone:

"I swear on Chairman Mao's life. If you don't believe me, then I'll tell you a secret." Brushing a strand of hair from my ear, she whispered: "My mother's father is a capitalist."

Zhang Xiaoxia's kindness touched me deeply.

Calm was restored on the streets and Father came home more often.

At night, Mother had nightmares and cried. Awake and staring at the mosquito net, I would hear Father talking softly to her. They would talk in hushed voices. Their words were raindrops dripping slowly from the rooftop.

My eyes were heavy with sleep, but their whisperings would keep me awake.

"I want to send Mother something... life is hard in the country..."

"You must be careful... send the parcel from another village..."

"Do you think... they'll receive it?"

"People... must... never know... about... this..."

I put my fingers in my ears. My heart was pounding.

Complementary Notes

The small courtyard where my family lived holds a special place in my life. It's where I made my psychological journey from childhood to adolescence.

Every family in the courtyard had their own secrets and neuroses. It was a time in history when sickness prevailed: families were sick, parents and children were sick, neighbours were sick. Sometimes I think life in that small courtyard could be the basis for a television script with neurosis as the central theme. It could, for example, be a Chinese version of the film *Spellbound*.

Mrs Commander in Chief was probably the sanest person out of all the residents of the courtyard. In the eyes of a child about to enter adolescence, she was a deeply maternal woman. She knew how to protect her own children, as well as those of other people. She didn't have emotional highs and lows, didn't harass others with constant blame and didn't flare up in bouts of hysteria. A child of 12 needs to be able to identify with a parental figure who is healthy in body and mind.

NINETEEN

Diary
Tuesday, 22nd July 2003 10:20 am

Feel awful. Since the day before yesterday, I've been helping Mother prepare for her medical consultation.

Two nights ago, I went over to Junya Residence to explain to my parents how to get to the First Guangzhou Hospital by taxi and how to deal with the administrative formalities. Got up at 7 am yesterday to get ready. But just as I was about to leave, I was told that Dr Xiao, the head physician, would be absent that morning, and it wouldn't be until 2:30 in the afternoon that we'd know if he'd be working that day.

Dr Wang kept me updated on the situation. I went to Junya Residence at midday to wait for further news. Then my parents and I took the underground to the hospital. Once we arrived and were told that Dr Xiao wouldn't be working, we immediately made an appointment with another doctor.

It wasn't all for nothing. Good news: Mother doesn't have tuberculosis. To her relief, she doesn't have anything infectious, and life can go back to normal. Bad news: The doctor can't rule out a problem with the pulmonary vessels. Further tests are needed. Meanwhile, she must watch out for blood in her sputum.

Afterwards, I took my parents home and talked to Fanding about Mother's follow-up medical tests and consultations.

I was shattered when I got home at 8:30 pm. Only then did I realise I had forgotten to take my alprazolam, Euthyrox etc.

My state of health being as it is, having to deal with these kind of problems leaves me drained. But what can I do?

What irritates me most is Mother's endless neurotic complaints. She always thinks the worst, broods over everything, and is suspicious, disparaging and full of blame. I am in therapy for my depression and she pushes me back down into my hole. But God is by my side. I often ask Him for help, otherwise I would have had a nervous breakdown ages ago.

Before I left Junya Residence, Mother was complaining that she had lost a lot of weight and was worried sick that people were saying she looked like a matchstick.

All I could say was: "You think you're thinner than me? You're one metre sixty-one tall and weigh just over fifty kilos. You've always been like this. Me, I'm one metre sixty-five and weigh fifty kilos. A couple of months ago, I was even down to forty-eight kilos. But I don't care. People also say I'm thin. Hu Ququ even teased me and said I looked like a toothpick. But I don't think I'm thin. I'm perfectly happy with my weight."

She stopped after this.

I maybe unstable, but I rarely complain to others about my problems: operations for my cancer, chemotherapies, severe depression.

Everyone is struggling to make a living and has their own problems to solve. Who doesn't get sick? Who doesn't have problems? If I complain to others about mine, it just adds to theirs. There are lots of things in life we must face alone. Other people can't help you. Why drag them down with you?

Only the Lord can help me. The Almighty Lord is my Saviour. He saves my life and my soul. He helps me always.

Notes

Every year in March and April, the number of people suffering from depression explodes. Suicide rates increase dramatically, and we often hear about them in the news. Recently there were four cases of suicide in a university in Guangzhou. I always take extra care of myself this time of the year.

I was born and brought up in the province of Guangdong, where the four seasons of the year aren't clear-cut. So I am not particularly sensitive to the transition from winter to spring. What's odd is that I always get sick in spring.

My coughing fits used to be so bad in spring that they'd make my insides ache. When I lay down at night, I would cough until tears welled up in my eyes. I would leak urine, and all the blood vessels and meridians in my body felt as though they would explode. I had penicillin shots twice a day and I lost count of the number I had. The puncture site, covered with bruises, was as big as the palm of my hand. The skin was so hardened that the needle couldn't penetrate the skin. I was coughing all the same, and it wasn't until the end of spring that it gradually stopped. The decrease in my thyroid function, my low heart rate and depression get worse every spring.

It's normal for me to be sick and abnormal to be healthy. I "qualify" to be admitted to hospital at any given moment. A few years ago, Mother underwent surgery in a military hospital to have her gallbladder removed and was worried sick about it afterwards. The head surgeon, a family friend of ours, said to her: "Actually you're in better health than your daughter. She can cope because mentally she hangs on. It isn't easy for her."

Ever since my operation for an angioma at the age of 14, I have often been sick and needed to be hospitalised. At the age of 22, I had an endocrine function test at Guangzhou Hospital. The doctors were puzzled by the results. People who have hypothyroidism or severe dysfunction of the endocrine system usually suffer from stunted growth, physically and intellectually. They're usually diagnosed with impaired cognitive development or pituitary dwarfism, but there I was, 22 years old and still growing. I was already one metre sixty-five and my intelligence was relatively normal. How was it possible?

I became a medical case study for this hospital. Specialists in Chinese and western medicine, local and overseas medical students all pored over my case and used me as part of their clinical studies.

After three months, they were still unable to find the cause of my hypothyroidism. The doctors advised me to go on long-term sick leave. The head of my unit came to Guangzhou specially to inform me of my status. He said: "In compliance with the regulations, you're entitled to sick leave benefits longer than six months. When you're discharged from hospital, go to the national health insurance offices and file the application papers."

Due to my hypothyroidism diagnosed during my teens, I never had acne and never went through any adolescent crisis. You can say I never had an adolescence. I never knew what it was like to be young.

In my life, youth, sickness and death are closely intertwined. In my subconscious, my conscious mind, and within the intricate web of my neurotransmitters, the "seeds" of youth had barely begun to germinate when they died for no reason at all. I've never strived to live a perfect life, because absolute perfection doesn't exist. Some say a childless woman is unfulfilled. But I never wanted to have children, nor be a perfect woman.

I came to know imperfection at a young age through illness and death. Imperfection can't be made whole or transformed into perfection. It's an intrinsic part of life beneficial to mankind. I accept imperfection. Its beauty is unique. Without knowing what imperfection is, how can you recognise perfection?

Went to North Shenzhen Hospital for my antidepressants this morning. I had made an appointment with a specialist, Professor Li, and we were talking about this book that I am currently writing. Recently I keep hearing about suicide cases related to depression. Among the recent victims were university and high school students, teachers, civil servants, entrepreneurs, journalists and even psychologists.

How can you identify those who are at a high risk of suicide in China? Some say children these days are too psychologically vulnerable. When they come up against the slightest difficulty, they choose to end their lives. But I think it's more like the straw that broke the camel's back. In my book, I want to compare the changes in the psyche of different generations in a given family.

Take myself, for example: I am one metre sixty-five tall; my mother is one metre sixty-one; my maternal grandmother one metre fifty-six; and my maternal great-grandmother just under one metre fifty-five. In our family, one generation is physically taller than the last, but psychological resilience diminishes from one generation to the next. Why is that?

Professor Li told me that he had also suffered from depression. No wonder he could diagnose my depression so quickly. He said I had the full support of all the specialists in psychiatry for my book. He had suffered from depression for six years. There were no obvious symptoms for the first three years. At the time, he was studying for a doctorate. All he felt was that something wasn't quite right with himself.

It wasn't until he was transferred to Shenzhen that his condition began to deteriorate. When he experienced early morning awakenings, which is a somatic symptom of depression, he finally understood what was happening to him.

He took antidepressants and recovered his health a year later. Having lived through his depression, he was particularly aware of the symptoms and asked me a host of questions about my insomnia.

Fanding called me to say that the hospital had contacted him. Grandmother keeps saying: "It's too late. It's too late."

She's thinking of us. Fanding is catching the 9 o'clock train tomorrow morning. I so badly want to go, but Fanding is worried it might trigger a depression relapse and strongly advised me against it. We wondered if we should tell Mother but decided not to say anything. We're in the middle of a high-risk period for depression and must do our best to protect her.

11th April 2006

Correlations

**Excerpts from the chapter "Depression"
in *A Family Guide to Health Care*[1]**

The notion of depression belongs to that of *yuzheng*.[2]

The strict definition of *yuzheng* is emotional, mental and energy blockages resulting in the following symptoms: depressed mood, tearfulness, heaviness in the chest, irritability, anxiety, distrustfulness, mood swings, fear, insomnia, the sensation that something is stuck in the throat, etc.

Spiritual Axis:[3] Sickness of the Mind:[4] "Melancholia causes stagnation and depletion of vital energy."

Spiritual Axis: Verbal Questions:[5] "[...] When someone is sad, anxious or fearful, the heart beats quickly and hinders the function of the internal Organs."

Hua Xiuyun[6] said: "*Yu* is the stasis of *qi*.[7] If it lasts for any length of time, it then transforms into Heat, which consumes the Organic Liquids and impedes circulation. Consequently, the body will lose its capacity to regulate its ascending and descending movements. At first, there is a deficiency of *qi* and Blood, which then transforms into *yu*."

In the chapter "Yuzheng" of his book *Ordering of Patterns and Deciding Treatments,* Lin Peiqin[8] wrote: "Most illness is caused by *yu,*" and that: "All illness originates from *yu*. This is the reason why in treating an illness, one must consider the element of *yu*."

Medications that are used to treat the syndrome of *yu* must not be too strong.

One must avoid destroying the stagnation of *qi*; wasting the *qi*; causing any dysfunction of the Stomach; causing any syndrome of dryness; and consuming food that contains too much oil.

As it is indicated in the chapter "Yu" of *Case Histories That Act as Clinical Compasses:*[9] in order to treat illness that is related to *yu*, "it is essential not to administer medications which have a purgative or tonifying effect. Food with a bitter taste expels Heat without causing any dysfunction of the Stomach. Spicy food regulates the circulation of *qi*, but one must be careful not to cause any deficiency of *qi*. Use medications which are of a Humid nature to reduce dryness and increase astringency without overly lubricating the body. One must activate the circulation without causing any dysfunction."

Complementary Notes

Psychiatrists in the west believe that physicians in Ancient Greece had an understanding of depression.

In the Bible, King Saul suffered from depression. David played the harp to soothe his headaches and ease his irritations and agitation. It's the equivalent of today's medical therapy.

I am curious to know under which dynasty depression was mentioned for the first time in China. Not being knowledgeable on this matter, I didn't know where to look. As a last resort, I did some research into Chinese medicine and gathered some information here and there. It's better than nothing.

In my experience, Chinese medication takes too long to be effective when I am in the bottomless pit of my depression. It's more efficacious in preventing depression and during convalescence.

I believe Chinese drugs can cure depression. Chinese medicine was in the world spotlight for its role in the SARS epidemic. However, have Traditional

Chinese Medicine research organisations listed the prevention of depression as an essential part of their programmes?

New generations of antidepressants are regularly introduced into the market. Can Chinese medicine produce new generations of the "Carefree Formula?"[10] Can it modify and improve on an ancient formula to cure depression?

While reading these medical texts, I was overwhelmed with respect for the physicians of ancient China. I hope more doctors of today will continue the work of their predecessors and open up new therapeutic possibilities to be of service to society.

TWENTY

Diary
Friday, 25th July 2003 10:40 am

I can't stop thinking of this proverb: "Illness hits you as suddenly as a mountain that collapses and recedes as slowly as the reeling of silk cocoons."

The words "reeling of silk cocoons" weigh heavily on me when I'm doing my exercises, consulting a doctor or lying on the couch exhausted.

As for the "mountain," we're often too distracted to see that a mountain is building up in front of us. In fact, we don't even see it until it collapses, burying us under the rubble. It's only then that we realise the kind of mess we're in.

We wait painfully for the "reeling of the silk cocoon" to finish. One day is like 10 years and we ask ourselves over and over again: "Why is it taking so long?"

I must learn to wait: "Wait for the Lord."[1]

I am like a pile of earth. God took a handful of earth next to me and with it made a work of art, which is then exhibited in the best museums in the world. He took some more earth and made some very pretty toys. Then He picked me up and made an ocarina out of me. I was softened, kneaded, rolled, cut, sliced, stretched, pinched and left to dry. I was fired in a kiln for several days, taken out and rigorously inspected. I was immersed in water, then shaken up and down, left and right. I became a plain and ordinary ocarina. God created me, forged me, put me through hardships. With His blessings and the help of the Holy Spirit, I will produce sounds and music and become the angel that brings comfort.

Maybe this is my mission in life.

Lord, may all that I accomplish be in accordance with Your will and plans.

Notes

Grandmother has also fallen into a depression.

Fanding called me from the hospital in Pingxiang. He arrived at 7 o'clock in the evening and went straight to the hospital. Grandmother was still up.

The doctor said she had heart problems.

She refuses to have injections, take medication or wear an oxygen mask. She asked only to be euthanised.

When she knew that Fanding was arriving, she asked for an oxygen mask, because she had things to say to him. When he arrived, she was so overwhelmed with emotion that she immediately blurted out three things: 1. He mustn't tell our parents she was in hospital. 2. When Grandfather was alive, he never owed anyone money. She would reimburse Mother for the money she had lent her to pay for Grandfather's cemetery plot; she would reimburse me for the money I had lent her for an air conditioner. 3. We mustn't cut our ties with the rest of the family.

After that, she tore off her oxygen mask and stubbornly refused to take her medications. Fanding said he had never seen a 95-year-old woman with so much energy. He couldn't stop her from ripping off her mask. And she only had this to say to the doctor: "Get me euthanised."

Fanding stayed at Grandmother's bedside. In the middle of the night, she touched his hand and asked him, the grandson she had brought up so lovingly: "Fanding, are you hungry? You must be tired. Do you want something to eat?"

My grandmother has a heart of gold. Even when she is ill, she is still thinking of others.

It breaks my heart.

The truth is, Grandmother's illness has less to do with her cardiac problems than with the sorrow that weighs in her heart. She is kind, compassionate and loving.

She has suffered injustices all her life and her heart is bursting with sorrow. For her, it's harder to live than to die. She has reached a breaking point.

The incident with the air conditioner still upsets me. In Pingxiang, the temperature soars over 40 degrees in the summer. She lives in a horrible little hut of four square metres built on a terrace. In the summer, it's a furnace inside. In winter, the temperature drops below -10 degrees and it's an ice cave inside. I sent her money for an air conditioner, but her son's family complained: "No, electricity is too expensive." I said: "But I'll pay the electricity bills. Can you install the cables?" Naturally, it was too much to ask.

The third thing that Grandmother said: Don't cut your ties with the family. Maybe she was referring to that incident.

Grandmother, you're always thinking of others, of your children and grandchildren. Why do you never think of yourself? Since you were 17 years old, you have lived for others, suffered insults and humiliations in silence, kept your dignity, swallowed your pride and buried your resentments.

What can I say? What can I do? It breaks my heart.

12th April 2006

Correlations

Excerpts from "Grandmother and International Women's Day"

The first time I heard of International Women's Day was when I was in secondary school. At the time, I was living with my grandmother in the province of Jiangsu.

My school was holding a symposium on 8th March. I was surprised to receive an invitation and said to myself: "What's that got to do with me?" I told my grandmother about it after school and, to my surprise, she took an interest in it.

She kept saying: "It's a good thing. Many people who want to go aren't invited. Why don't you want to go?"

I was 17 years old and full of myself. I will always remember the look of disappointment and also of affection in her eyes.

She said: "If my father had lived a year longer, I would have gone to university. But it wasn't my destiny."

She had given birth to a daughter. In the first month, her mother-in-law never gave her so much as an egg to eat. She cooked for the whole family and mended their shoes. The neighbours felt sorry for her and gave her six eggs, which kept her nourished.

Her daughter died a few months later. The letters from Beijing were becoming few and far between, the reason being that Grandfather was spending his weekends strolling in Beihai Garden with the daughter of a public official.

For four years, my poor grandmother cried herself to sleep at night. But she had no hate in her heart. She blamed herself for the misfortune of having been born a woman.

Fifty years later, Grandfather said to her, jokingly:

"Count yourself lucky that I'm a decent person. I didn't abandon you. I came home."

"You know what?" said Grandmother with an ironic smile. "If you hadn't come back, I would have left and started a new life."

Later, Grandmother told me: "If I had divorced at the time, it wouldn't have been such a bad thing. I was young and educated, I could have become a teacher and done as I please."

After the Liberation, she wanted to join the workforce, but Grandfather was used to having his wife take care of him. She stayed a homemaker all her life. "If you feel deeply for someone, how can you stop those feeling at will?"

Grandmother will be 80 this year. It is her wish to celebrate International Women's Day.

If only she had gone to university...
But there are no ifs.
She is still going strong, like a 100-year-old plum tree: beautiful, but its fragrance nuanced with bitterness.

21st February 2001 at Kangle Residence

Complementary Notes

This year, just before International Women's Day, the chief editor of the Arts and Literature section of *Southern Daily* asked me to submit an article. I sent him this story about my grandmother. After Mother had shown her my story, she said to me on the phone: "Lanni, I read your story. It's very well written. Thank you. Thank you very much." I felt ashamed of myself. It's not well written. What Grandmother couldn't express, someone else said for her. It was just a few sentences here and there amongst all that was pent up in her heart. But it brought her some comfort.

TWENTY-ONE

Diary
Saturday, 26th July 2003 12:10 pm

Reducing the dosage of my medication is having adverse effects on me. Had anxiety dreams several nights in a row.

Last night's dream:

I was visiting a city with Hu Ququ, Zhang Mei and Cheng Zhihong. The hotel we were staying in was average. The three of them shared a large room with several other women and they were talking and laughing together. I was alone in a miserable little room opposite theirs and heard them talking about where they were going to shop for clothes. Ququ came over to say they were going to the night market and asked me to join them. After some hesitation, I said I couldn't go, because the sole of one of my shoes had come off and I couldn't walk properly. At first, I enjoyed the peace and quiet of being alone in my room, but boredom soon set in. Then Fanding arrived. I was glad I hadn't gone out, otherwise how could he have found me? He said he was going away on a business trip to a hydroelectric station for five days and asked me to return to Guangzhou to look after our parents and his family. Assuming my responsibilities, I said I would leave right away. I walked Fanding to the hotel entrance and told him not to worry. When I returned to the hotel, Ququ, Zhang Mei and the others were already back. They said they were leaving on the next minibus for Guangzhou and were in the middle of packing. While mending my shoe in my room, I kept an ear out for what was happening in theirs. Then, hearing rapid footsteps, I hurriedly gathered my belongings, which were strewn all over the floor. It was so quiet in the room opposite mine that you could hear a pin drop. Grabbing my suitcase, I ran out, disappointed that Ququ and Zhang Mei didn't come to fetch me. I could have done with some help packing. My friends were nowhere to be seen outside the hotel. I returned the key to the reception, and as I was walking past my room I noticed that I had left the key to my suitcase on the tea tray. As I was picking up the key, I saw my raincoat hanging on the back of the door. I panicked, thinking the minibus might leave without me. A few of my belongings were still in the room, but I didn't want to take them. Head spinning and in a state of utter panic, I rushed outside into the courtyard thinking: Are they going to notice that I'm missing? Are they going to check the minibus before they leave? The suitcase was heavy, and I could barely see in the dark. I was exhausted and sick with worry.

When I woke up in the morning, I was completely drained. This dream is indicative of my emotional state. Why do I get myself so worked up?

I am disappointed with myself. Instead of taking two-thirds of a tablet, I took a quarter. Reduce the dosage just by a fraction and I go to pieces. Why am I so weak?

Notes

Today is 13th April. Fanding sent me a text: Grandmother's condition is deteriorating.

Holding her hand, he said to her: "My heart is with you. We'll always be one family." She understood. Reassured by Fanding's words, she didn't want to talk anymore.

Fanding was crying on the phone, not because Grandmother is sick, but because she had a sad life.

Lord, Grandmother has done so much good in her life. She has never hurt anyone. She is honest, kind, beautiful, talented and compassionate. Help her, protect her and guide her. Bring her abundance and love. Grant her peace, happiness and serenity.

23rd April 2006, the day before Good Friday

Correlations

Entries from 14th to 28th April 2006

14th April (Friday): Fanding called me this morning to say he'd decided to leave Pingxiang at the last minute. He couldn't stay at the hospital any longer, the psychological pressure was unbearable. To protect him from the seeds of depression taking root in him, I told him to return to Guangzhou. He dreaded the moment when he'd have to say goodbye to Grandmother and was worried that she'd be even more determined to be euthanised after his departure. I told him he'd regret it later if he didn't go to see her one last time. In the evening, he called me from the train. It had been raining heavily for several days, but the sun was out when he went to the hospital. Grandmother was talking about her funeral with her sister-in-law, who was almost 90 years old. They are like sisters. Seizing on the opportunity while her attention was distracted, he said to her: "Grandmother, I'm leaving." Not realising that he meant he was leaving for Guangzhou, she calmly nodded her head. He told me he was grateful to God for allowing him to say goodbye to Grandmother in such a warm, intimate and natural way.

God heard my prayers last night. For this, I am deeply grateful.

15*th* April (Saturday): Fanding arrived back in Guangzhou safe and sound. I asked him for a favour. Tomorrow is Easter Sunday and I asked him to attend Mass at Dongshan Church for me. He agreed.

16*th* April (Sunday): I must find a subject for the symposium. Fanding sent me text messages with encouraging excerpts from the Mass: "May the spirit of the Risen Christ reside in our hearts. May the spirit who resurrected Christ also live in our mortal bodies."

17*th* April (Monday): I'm staying in the Shenzhen Building in Beijing, waiting apprehensively for Fanding's calls and text messages. God knows how long Grandmother can hold on. My inner restlessness makes me thirsty all the time.

18*th* April (Tuesday): Fanding sent me a message from Pingxiang: Grandmother sat up on the bed today and had a bite to eat. A miracle.

19*th* April (Wednesday): Fanding called me to say that Grandmother is physically and psychologically unstable. Our family in Pingxiang told him that Grandmother was sharing a room with a 70-year-old woman. She and her husband have high blood pressure but no serious health problems. The social workers of their unit are very thoughtful, and the husband and wife are well taken care of in two separate hospitals. The day after we heard that Grandmother's condition had worsened, the husband suddenly passed away. The wife left the hospital to make funeral arrangements. At the hospital, they were saying the heavens were taking people back. Grandmother, who was supposed to leave, had been retained on Earth, whereas the husband, who only had hypertension, was taken away. To me, it was just pure coincidence. The popular belief is that the heavens take people by making them come back in a car or on a boat. When a car or boat is full, they must wait for the next one.

20*th* April (Thursday): My aunt called Mother to tell her that Grandmother was in hospital. It's the "high season" for depression. She takes alprazolam at night, but only sleeps for two hours. Everyone is in a bad way, and there is nothing I can do about it. Three women from three different generations are all depressed at the same time.

21*st* April (Friday): I called Mother at home in Maoming. The cleaning lady said my parents had sent money to Grandmother in hospital. I was relieved that I didn't have to talk to Mother. When I'm going through a depressive episode, I can't bear listening to Mother complain. This thought has crossed my mind more than once: Go on, let's kill ourselves and put an end to it all.

22nd April (Saturday): Back in Guangzhou. The thought of having to call Mother makes me depressed. I try to change my negative way of thinking through cognitive therapy. I keep telling myself: "Don't call her before you're psychologically ready. Be positive. If she's capable of going to the post office to send money to Grandmother, then she's fine. Stay positive. *The Power of Positive Thinking*."

23rd April (Sunday): Since I came back from Beijing, I have been tired, restless and uneasy. Fanding called me to remind me not to mention Grandmother's cardiac problems or depressed mood when I talk to Mother on the phone. I didn't talk to Mother on the phone. This afternoon, I went to Dongshan Church to find some peace. Some verses from the Bible: "Blessed are the poor in spirit, for theirs is the kingdom of heaven. Blessed are those who mourn, for they will be comforted…"[1] Remember this: "Blessed are those who mourn, for they will be comforted."

24th April (Monday): Talked to Mother on the phone. I was treading carefully, like a soldier moving through landmines. Her voice was tired and hoarse, but normal for someone who is weary and restless. She didn't have her piercing voice that grates on my nerves. She said: "Grandmother is over ninety years old. It's not her death that frightens me, but it upsets me that she's suffering." As I hung up, I thought: "Grandmother, for you, it's harder to live than to die."

25th April (Tuesday): So agitated. Feel burning in my stomach and intestines. Don't feel like doing anything and my lethargy annoys me. Trying hard to stay alert and be normal and not let negative thoughts have the upper hand. But a slip in my attention and the dark soul of depression rears its head and screams: "I'm going mad! Let me out!" After a moment's hesitation, I conjure up all my strength to tame the dark soul in me. Exhausted, I pause to catch my breath. Why can't we just let ourselves go over the edge? We all need to, from time to time. Isn't it inhumane to stop people from doing this? No, no, no. I don't want to go over the brink. There is too much at risk. I am recovering from depression. It's just a fleeting moment of weakness. I am capable of self-control. Pull yourself together. No more negative thoughts. Be constructive. I read an article on Cong Fei's memorial service in the press.[2] It made me think of the "Volunteer Workers' Union." Am I right to think that volunteer workers and philanthropists like Cong Fei can only exist in a city like Shenzhen? Because the people of this city need love and know what it's like to live without it. They know that to step onto the path of love, you need to give.

26th April (Wednesday): Grandmother sleeps all day and refuses to eat.

27th April (Thursday): My aunt read the letter my mother had written Grandmother out loud to her. Grandmother listened quietly. When my aunt finished, she asked: "Was that alright?" Grandmother nodded. My aunt read it to her again and asked: "Are you happy?" Grandmother nodded. It reassures me that Grandmother is only half-conscious. I hope she stays in this state of peace and quietude. Longevity doesn't necessarily lead to happiness. True happiness brings joy and health.

28th April (Friday): I sent Grandmother some delicacies to eat: bird's nest, *chongcao*,[3] chocolate, sweets. I so wanted to go to Pingxiang to see her and talk to her. But Mother and Fanding were against it, saying my presence there would complicate the situation, but they were in fact worried I would relapse into depression. It made me feel even guiltier. I thought of secretly going to Pingxiang, but it would send Mother into hysterics. I am praying. May my prayers bring hope. "This is […] how we set our hearts at rest in His presence."[4] Amen.

28th April 2006
Hidden behind my screen of vegetation
(But in reality, I am curled up inside the ear of a cat)

Complementary Notes

An episode of depression is coming. I can feel it. I am a bundle of nerves, my thoughts are confused, and I can't concentrate. I am negative, and my thoughts are scattered, going haywire inside my head. I keep praying to keep insanity at bay. Make it go far away from me.

TWENTY-TWO

Diary
Tuesday, 29th July 2003 10:50 am

I can't think straight; the analytic abilities of my brain are malfunctioning. It's the medication. I stood in front of the public toilets, trying hard to decipher the signs for men and women: Which are the toilets for women? My brain was unable to coordinate with my senses: sight, sound, touch and smell. Even now as I'm writing this, my hand and brain aren't synchronised. I can only express 40 percent of my thoughts. Is it the depression or the antidepressants that are destroying my brain?

No use worrying about it. Continue with your therapy and watch out for any changes.

Other than that, I feel quite good. Couldn't make an appointment with Dr Xiao for Mother yesterday. According to Wang Tao, a CT-scan would rule out the possibility of a tumour, and if Mother doesn't cough blood anymore, then there'd be nothing to worry about. Sometimes the capillaries in older people's lungs are fragile. They burst easily, but it's not a serious problem. His advice is to have a lung X-ray once every six months and to monitor closely for any changes.

Fanding, my parents and I all agree not to rush things and to let Mother rest while waiting for an appointment with Dr Xiao. To reassure my parents, I made a point of going over to their place in Junya Residence this afternoon and brought some work along. Fanding joined us after work, and we discussed this in a calm and constructive manner.

I felt the Holy Spirit was with my family this afternoon. My anxiety subsided, and I felt less nervous in front of my parents.

Zhou Xiaobin is going to a meeting in Yunnan Province. He suggested we spend a few days together afterwards. I've never been to Yunnan, and as I want to go to Lijiang, it'll be an excellent opportunity for me. But I tire easily these days, so I wonder if I'll have the strength to go. I'll speak to Dr Gong about it. Will I have the energy to get myself into tip-top shape to travel?

Lord, guide me. With Your encouragement, I'll be well enough to travel. But if You do not wish me to travel, let me know. Show me Your intentions. I may not be very bright; my soul is immature and my faculties of understanding are poor. Help me open up my heart and understand.

A few days ago, this thought struck a chord in me: When you are confronted with many problems, look to God to guide you towards the first step of solving your problems.

O Lord, my Father, help me towards the first step. Let me follow You and move forward.

Notes

I can't write. I'm worried about Grandmother who is in hospital and it's affecting my writing. In today's "Notes," I'm going to talk about why Grandmother has never fallen prey to depression, unlike me, who's fragile, depressed, and nervous most of the time. But I don't have any clear-cut ideas about how to go about it.

Another depressive episode is on its way. I can feel it.

Or maybe, just maybe, I should think of it this way: I am simply not in a good mood. I won't slip back into depression. I must have a positive outlook. Quick, use cognitive therapy to cut off any negative thoughts.

It hasn't been good these last few days. I am like two different people. From the outside, I seem normal. People say I look healthy again. I say: "Yes, I'm well again. The worst is behind me." But I feel anxious, restless, overwhelmed and weary. Sometimes when I'm talking or laughing, it suddenly strikes me that I am not normal but mad and that I should pull myself together by talking and behaving in an exaggerated way or run around like a headless chicken to stimulate my nerves. I hate myself! Hate, hate, hate Li Lanni! I hate everything she says. This is going nowhere. I might as well smash my skull against the wall. I think of Li Lanni and her three budgies. She is guilty of having committed unpardonable things. Stop thinking about it or you'll go insane.

I must drive out these negative thoughts. I'm going through a distressing period and we're bang in the middle of the "high season" for depression. Don't be afraid, Li Lanni, calm down. Let me explain.

Your grandmother is a model and a psychological crutch for you. The crutch is broken, leaving you lurching. Do you remember how, as a child, Mrs Gao of the small courtyard was a maternal figure for you? She was plump, had a strong personality and was warm, kind, candid and loyal. During a very difficult period in history, she embodied all the best qualities that a Chinese woman should have. When you were 12 years old and living in the small courtyard, you realised that your mother lacked maternal instincts and that the other women were peculiar. To you, Mrs Gao was the embodiment of an ideal mother figure. You knew if a disaster were to happen, she would save all the children of the small courtyard. It pained and upset you when Mrs Gao had her first nervous breakdown.

It's like when Grandmother fell into a state of depression; Mrs Gao's depression left you feeling lost and bewildered.

Do you remember the last chapter of your novella *Courtyard of My Childhood Years*? You wrote: "If ever I had a step-mother who beat me, I would run into the middle of the courtyard screaming for help. I know Mrs Commander in Chief would come and save me. But I never thought that one day she would return to her native village to till the lands. I never thought the families of the small courtyard would leave..."

Today, you must face up to the pain of leaving your childhood once again. It's an inescapable reality on your path to adulthood.

29th April 2006

Correlations

Excerpts from *Courtyard of My Childhood Years*

6

Mrs Commander in Chief liked to make spring onion pancakes. Basted with oil inside, the pancakes, made up of fine, transparent layers, were crispy and golden on the outside and broke up easily in your hands.

Mrs Commander in Chief was the head of the canteen in her native village. She always found a way to buy lard. And as she was never embarrassed to borrow money, she always had the means to buy it.

Mrs Commander in Chief was in her early thirties. She was buxom, had rounded hips, a large face and head, and thick braids. She liked to wear her thick, straight, silky hair in a braided chignon or braided behind her head. She walked around the courtyard in her floral trousers and short-sleeved men's undershirt with black sesame-dot patterns on the back. Her breasts were round and full, and she had four sons: Lujun, Haijun, Kongjun and Junjun. Lujun's father was 10 years her senior but was shorter than her.

There was a guava tree in front of her house. It was thin with small sparse leaves and had not borne any fruit. Mrs Commander in Chief often nursed her youngest son beneath this tree. He was puny, had a jaundiced complexion and looked like his father. He looked pathetic, curled up in his mother's arms. His mother needed her hands to work, so she kept him squeezed under her armpit, like a cob of corn. He didn't cry or utter a sound of protest, his eyes darting left and right, as if lost in thought.

The baby's face was half buried in Mrs Commander in Chief's breast. She gave me a comb and said: "Nizi, can you comb my hair for me? It stimulates the circulation." She would put cooked peanut oil on her comb and it made her hair smooth, shiny and slightly scented.

"My husband went back to his native village to look for a wife," she told me. "My long thick braids caught his eye. I had ebony black hair then. When I undid them, they would fall loose over my shoulders like a nymph. Ah... all the young girls were in love with him. At the time, he was the head of a battalion and earned a good living..."

At times, I would get angry with her.

When she made spring onion pancakes, my brother would stand next to her in front the stove. She would give him a big piece, which he would eat with his head down. Stroking his hair, she would say with a smile: "Do you want to be my son? You'll have pancakes to eat every day."

His mouth stuffed full of pancakes, my brother would nod approvingly. Tickled, Mrs Commander in Chief would keep on stroking his head, saying: "Slowly, my son, eat slowly."

It would make me blind with anger. She already had four sons and wanted to buy my brother with her pancakes. And my brother was going to betray his family for some spring onion pancakes. So I refused to eat her pancakes. When he had finished eating, my brother would say: "Mrs Commander in Chief, I'm going home."

"Already? Don't you want to be my son?" she asked, laughing.

"No, I don't want to anymore," he answered candidly.

Whenever my brother wanted to eat pancakes, he would say to Mother: "Mother...I want to be Mrs Commander in Chief's son. But don't worry, I won't betray you. I'll come back when I've eaten enough."

"If someone give you lots and lots of things to eat, or lots and lots of money, would you betray me?" asked Mother. "Would you denounce me? What would you do?"

"I'll beat him to death."

"If your father and sister were to denounce me, what would you do?"

"I'll beat them to death!"

"My angel..."

Mother would then kiss him on the head and he would kiss her cheeks, both of them smacking nosily.

7

Xiao Yuzi's mother had gone out with her grandmother and sister, Xiao Shanzi, leaving the dirty laundry to soak in a large basin by the lake.

Taking a wash board and a huge bar of Tramway brand soap, Xiao Yuzi and Xiao Lingzi jumped into the basin and played there for two hours. When their mother came back and saw that the basin was frothing with foam, she put her hand into the soapy water and pulled the girls out.

Xiao Yuzi's mother had a certain charm to her when she disciplined her children. Her mouth was no longer hanging to one side, she had rosy cheeks and her face glistened lightly with sweat, as if she were wearing make-up for an opera performance. She knew how to give a slap in the face. Once, Xiao Yuzi was left deaf for a few days after a thrashing.

Xiao Lingzi was crafty, always hiding behind her elder sister and wailing at the top of her lungs like a trumpet.

Xiao Yuzi was as skinny as a dried roasted duckling. Her arms were thin, like the bad-quality sugar cane that Cantonese street vendors couldn't sell. She never cried, never tried to run away from her mother's beatings. But her spindly, hemp stalk-like legs would tremble.

Sitting on the edge of the bed and holding Xiao Shanzi in her arms, their grandmother said: "Go on, hit her. Harder. Three days without a thrashing and she goes scrambling up on the roof. Three days without a hiding and she goes climbing up walls and trees."

Their grandmother had bound feet and wore child-sized Jiefang shoes. Her hair was tied up in a bun; she had thin red lips and there wasn't a shred of kindness in her eyes. She never talked willingly to the children of the courtyard and smoked Fengshou brand cigarettes.

Mrs Commander in Chief was holding her son in her arms. Red-faced, the child was pointing to Xiao Yuzi's house and thrashing his legs. He wanted to go into the house and was babbling: "Hit! Hit!"

Xiao Yuzi was bleeding from the nose. Red-black blood trickled from her nose like thick snot and dripped from her chin onto her blue floral top. She wiped the blood away with the back of her hand. Still sitting on the bed, her grandmother gave her a piece of cloth and Xiao Yuzi wiped her face with it. Her blood-smeared face made my flesh crawl. I hid behind Mrs Commander in Chief, who was clucking disapprovingly.

"You're going...to buy me...new clothes..." bawled Xiao Yuzi. She was wearing Xiao Lingzi's clothes, which were torn and had never been mended.

"You're...going to...buy me..." she sobbed, wiping her bloody hands on her mother.

Seething with anger, her mother grabbed an axe from under the bed and screamed: "I'm going to chop you up, you dirty little brat!"

Mrs Commander in Chief dashed into the house and thrusted herself between Xiao Yuzi and her mother.

"Easy, easy..." she said, taking the axe away. "It's only soap. What's more precious, money or life? I'll buy you some more. We lived very well before, without these foreign soaps..."

Xiao Lingzi scarpered out the door like a mouse. Pushing Mrs

Commander in Chief aside, Xiao Yuzi's mother kicked her daughter in the back of the knee. Xiao Yuzi fell to the floor.

"You! If you ever try again…" said Mrs Commander in Chief, her face hardening and leaning towards Xiao Yuzi's mother. "If you ever try again…A tigress never eats her cubs…If you dare…"

Xiao Yuzi's mother mumbled to herself. She was incapable of speaking, either from fear or from anger.

"Stop, stop. You're frightening the baby," said the grandmother, glaring at them.

"Who knows what I have to suffer…" Xiao Yuzi's mother sobbed and collapsed onto the floor, hitting her head against the bed frame. "The old, the young…All of them…Let's finish it once and for all…"

Mrs Commander in Chief tried to pick her up, but she refused to move. Xiao Shanzi was shrieking, as if to encourage her mother to stay on the floor.

Mrs Commander in Chief threw me a glance and I took Xiao Yuzi outside, pulling her by the sleeve. I was afraid to touch her hand. She was thin as a rake. Her hands were so frail, and her palms were cold and damp. She was like a tiny gecko.

15

As Lujun was running into the small courtyard, Mrs Commander in Chief caught him, pulling him by the ear.

"You dirty brat, what've you been up to at school? You've been annoying your teacher and bullying your classmates…"

"No! Never!" cried Lujun, his head hanging to one side and his face twisted in pain.

Mrs Commander in Chief tugged even harder. "No? No? Well, your teacher's just been here."

"That motherfu… I'll deal with the old bastard tomorrow. How dare he…ouch…ouch…"

"I'll teach you, little idiot," said his mother, grabbing a broom and starting to hit him with the bamboo handle. "Well? Your teacher can give you a hiding if he wants. You respect your teacher, you dirty little brat. Do you hear me? Do you?"

She rained blows on his thighs and legs. Snuggled up against his mother's armpit, the baby was watching this closely. Lujun ran up the steps and hid behind the Chinese chestnut tree in front of Xiao Chun's house, hurling insults at his teacher:

"Tomorrow he'll see, that old bastard, son of a…"

Mrs Commander in Chief chased after him, almost hitting Xiao Lingzi and Xiao Yuzi, and shouted furiously: "You want to make trouble for your teacher, you'll see, I'll make trouble for you! I'll teach you, you dirty little brat! Where're you hiding? I'll find you. You don't want to study. Well…you're not going to enjoy yourself either…"

In the small courtyard, nobody dared to talk like Mrs Commander in Chief. Born into a poor family of middle-class peasants, she wasn't afraid to speak her mind. But I never thought she would so openly defend the school teacher. Wasn't she afraid that someone would accuse her of being a counter-revolutionary?

Lujun was darting around the courtyard and Mrs Commander in Chief followed behind him, a broomstick in her hand. It was highly comical.

22

"Those motherfu… Damn those bastards," Mrs Commander in Chief ranted, standing at the kitchen door. "Of all the public servants, why should he be sent to the countryside to till the land? Is it fair? Is that how you treat honest folks?"

Xiao Yuzi's mother took a step forward, as if she was about to say something, but Mrs Gong, who was knitting, gave her a small jab with her needle. Xiao Yuzi's mother touched her cheeks nervously and pressed Xiao Lingzi against her. I looked up at Mother. She was watching Mrs Commander in Chief with sympathy but dared not say anything.

"You're not going to work in the fields," said the man with a pockmarked face, forcing a smile. "Once you get back to the commune, you'll be assigned work…"

"There's a saying," Mrs Commander in Chief interrupted. "To be transferred into the city, there's room for talk; to send a demobilised soldier to the country, out of the question!"

Mrs Commander in Chief's baby was shrieking, as if he were being strangled.

"According to the regulations and his public servant status, he can go back to anywhere he wants. You understand? These rules have been set down by the organisation," the man with the pockmarked face explained to everyone who was present. "It's no good getting angry with me. Have you talked to the organisation about it? You were educated by the Party, how can you talk like that…"

"Talk like what?" Mrs Commander in Chief asked, her lips growing pale, the muscles above her cheekbones twitching. "He was a soldier for all these years and now they have no use for him, so they're kicking him back to the country? Damn you, it's not fair. You just watch out, you reap what you sow!"

The man's face darkened, while the others grew pale.

"Don't talk nonsense," said Mother Hu, pinching Mrs Commander in

Chief to shut her up. Then, taking the man aside, she said: "She doesn't mean what she says. She's uneducated, you know. She's just a homemaker and doesn't understand anything."

At that moment, Lujun's father burst into the courtyard and, grabbing his wife by the arm, shouted: "Get back home, stupid bitch!"

Mrs Commander in Chief struggled to free herself, but in vain. So she put her baby, who had stopped crying, down on the ground.

"Are you a man or not? You're just a coward. They cut your balls and you say nothing…"

Her husband slapped her on the mouth to stop her from talking and grabbed her by the hand to take her home. She put up a resistance, but he was stronger. Her braids had come undone and strands of dry brittle hair covered her eyes.

All the people in the courtyard tried to separate them and, in the confusion, Mother and Xiao Yuzi's mother were both punched in the face and doubled up in pain. Mrs Commander in Chief's children, Lujun, Haijun and Kongjun, were crying for their mother.

Mrs Commander in Chief ripped a button from her husband's jacket. He dragged her home, pulling her by the hair. She was crying and squinted her eyes in pain.

I was upset. A woman like Mrs Commander in Chief would never cry.

The door slammed.

I heard her crying inside. Her weeping rose higher and higher up in the sky, as if to drown the sun with her tears.

23

Lujun's father entered the courtyard.

He was dressed in black civilian clothes, like an old peasant. Head down, his hands behind his back, he walked with a slight limp, as if the ground were uneven.

Lujun and Haijun took their younger brother to greet their father. The youngest child was wearing a red knitted top; his buttocks were bare, for his trousers were wrapped around Kongjun's head. Mrs Commander in Chief followed behind. The *guasha*[1] had left unsightly red-purplish marks on her neck and forehead. Her head was slightly sunk between her shoulders. She was wearing a light blue Chinese jacket made of soft supple cloth. Her long, shiny braids were hanging down behind her buttocks. They were so smooth and lustrous that day. She had combed her hair with peanut oil.

27

I heard faint footsteps and looked around me, but saw no one. The gnarled longan tree was like an old woman bent over in pain, her arms outstretched reaching in the darkness for her lost children.

Our house was the only one that was lit up in the small courtyard. And if I opened the door? Was Mother still crying? I stood in the silence of the courtyard wondering.

A long time ago, I had thought that if one day I were to have a stepmother and if she were to beat me, I would run out into the middle of the courtyard screaming for help. I was certain that Mrs Commander in Chief would save me. But I never dreamt that she would leave and return home to work in the fields. It never occurred to me that the families in the small courtyard would ever leave.

Mrs Commander in Chief's family was the first to leave. They left in the dead of night without saying goodbye.

Complementary Notes

Many years have passed, and I still laugh whenever I think of the episode of Mrs Commander in Chief and the school teacher, who was probably surprised to have been welcomed so warmly in a courtyard inhabited by military families. The Revolutionary movement had destroyed the pride and dignity of every teacher. They had become used to being despised and trodden on. He must have been startled to be greeted by a smiling face and a pair of eyes filled with kindness.

The teacher didn't stay long with Mrs Commander in Chief. The men's undershirt she was wearing had milk stains in front and sweat stains in the back. She had an ample bosom and rounded hips. The teacher straightened himself while talking to her in the courtyard and then left hurriedly. Soon after, her son barged into the courtyard, head first into the lion's den.

As Mrs Commander in Chief was giving her son a good hiding, I cheered her on, shouting: "Go on! Yes, go on!" For her son was a bully, who harassed the weak and grovelled to the powerful and was extremely unpopular with the younger children. I was outraged by the injustice of it. Also, it had been a while since I had seen someone come to the defence of a teacher and to openly side with him. I was troubled, excited and confused all at the same time. From that moment on, Mrs Commander in Chief was, to my eyes, someone fiercely loyal and fair. She was truly a mother figure, an angel and a saviour to the children of the small courtyard.

When her husband hit her and she was crying, I felt as if it was me who'd been dealt a blow on my head.

The star of happiness became a shooting star and then faded away. Only a few fireflies were left glowing in the dark night air of the small courtyard.

TWENTY-THREE

Diary
Wednesday, 30th July 2003 11 am

After my third surgical procedure for cancer, I had to be psychologically prepared for any eventuality. I've been intending to draw up a will for quite some time. In a depressed mood these last few days and this idea came niggling back.

Feeling up to the task today, so will get down to it.

LI LANNI'S WILL:

1. If ever I am in critical condition, please don't save me. Let me go peacefully. I hereby ask my family and doctors to respect my wishes.
2. If, as a result of an accident, I am in a coma, please let me die. This will be proof of your love and that you want to save me.
3. Following my death, the money in my bank account will go to my parents. It is to secure them in their old age. Zhou Xiaobing and my parents will jointly inherit my apartment in Shenzhen. The proceeds from the sale will be divided in equal parts between them.
4. Zhou Xiaobing and Li Fanding will each own 50 percent of the copyright on my literary works. My manuscripts will go to Li Fanding.
5. Regarding my personal belongings, Zhou Xiaobing and Li Fanding can keep the valuable objects, if they wish. The rest can be thrown away.
6. It is my wish to be cremated two days following my death and my ashes scattered into the sea. It will not be necessary to inform my friends or my colleagues of my passing, so as not to bother them. I do not wish to have a memorial service, flowers or ceremonies of any kind. I sincerely believe that my true friends will always remember the joyful moments we shared together.
7. I want my parents, husband, brother and friends to know this: I did not die in pain nor fear. I was happy. I will be in heaven and my

prayers will forever be with you. May God bless my family and my true friends.

Li Lanni
My identity card number: 440301XXXXX

30th July 2003 at midday at
Room number XXX of the second XXX of
Sun Yat-Sen University at Guangzhou

Notes

The will is still valid.

Up until now, I haven't felt the need to change anything.

As I was drawing up the will, I was lucid and at peace. No sadness, no worries, no regrets.

There is nothing much to say in the face of death.

I am now prepared for all eventualities. I've tidied my things and settled everything there is to settle. I've given up on controlling what is out of my control. My conscience is clear. I don't owe anyone anything. I am free of worries.

I want to take nothing with me.

When I'm transferred from the hospital room to the mortuary, don't change my clothes or dress me up in my favourite outfit. The hospital gown in which I breathe my last breath will do just fine. Don't cry for me. Don't burn any ghost money for my afterlife. Don't commemorate me.

At the beginning of the 1980s, I had a close brush with death during one of my stays in hospital. I had a glimpse of death. Death is gentle. It was a strange experience and opened a path to my real self.

Sometime after I had drawn up my will, one day, I received a call from Cheng Wenchao. He told me he had talked to his wife, Xiao Fu, about his last wishes. For his funeral, he had chosen a photograph of him smiling and the theme song from the film *Titanic*. He didn't want his friends to be sad and he didn't want to be remembered as being unhappy. I said to him: "I understand. Me too, I've drawn up a will and picked a portrait photo." He carried on talking, crying softly: "I want...my family and friends...to always remember me...smiling." I said: "I understand. I've also got a photo of me smiling."

That day, we talked only about his last wishes. He was so considerate of others and had planned everything down to the last detail. He described what his funeral would be like, how he didn't want to trouble his friends and how he tried to take the pressure off his daughters. To stop him from losing himself in his own thoughts, I kept interrupting him to bring him back. I told him that I didn't want a funeral service and that my portrait photo wasn't for my funeral. In the end, I just couldn't get through to him; he was talking about himself, and I about me.

When he passed away, many of his friends came to his funeral and delivered moving eulogies. People knew the Cheng Wenchao who was strong, but he never opened up about his problems and his inner pain. As a neighbour and family friend who, like him, had cancer, I could see his pain. You grow stronger through pain and suffering; and your pain is greater because you're strong.

When I was drawing up my will, I didn't know how much longer I had to live. I am convinced that you should write a will to prepare for any eventuality. It's liberating and allows you to live without illusions.

5th May 2006

Correlations

Excerpts from *"The Green House by the Lake"*

Nausea. Heaviness in my chest. Numb lips.

I loosened the valve of the drip chamber to speed up the flow of the solution. I hate perfusions. They bring me down, as if the liquid is seeping into my heart. It drips into my body, drop by drop, slowly, excruciatingly.

The perfusion bottle was almost empty. I ripped the cannula from my arm, got out of bed and put on my shoes.

Suddenly, everything faded in front of me.

White mist rising…rising…

I'm lying on a beach. Pink seawater is rising, covering my knees, waist, chest and neck.

Get up. Run!

But I can't move.

Pink waves are sweeping across the blood-red sea, and red seawater is lapping at my chin, mouth, upper lip…I am numb with cold…the blood-red sea keeps on rising…rising…

I feel heavy.

Get up and run! Now!

I am exhausted and drained. I can't move. I don't want to move.

I want to live. Live.

I need air. I'm going to die. Someone help me.

I want to live. I don't want to move. I can't move.

I can't breathe. I'm struggling. Nothing.

The world is blurred. A void.

A spirit shoots up into the air.

I'm floating.

A cool wind is blowing. A stretch of endless blue. Such a soft, pure, soothing blue. I am happy. I feel light. I no longer have a body, just a handful of thoughts in my head. No memories, no attachments, no fear, no...

I float in purity towards an infinite, immense, mysterious blue...

I'm floating at the frontier between two worlds.

The medical staff gave me emergency first aid. I was brought back down to earth.

[...] Slumped against the wall, I felt drained. But my heart was filled with blue light. A secret had been revealed to me. Now I know where I come from and where I'm going.

I don't know what mysterious force it was that kept me alive, but I am eternally grateful to it. It showed me a sign.

When I look back, I realise that all is insignificant and transient. I will always be me. Nothing in the world can change that. Nothing can change me, not even death.

Life is but a prologue to death and death is but a prelude to life.

[...]

February to March 1987

Complementary Notes

I was hospitalised in the middle of the summer of 1982. My transaminase levels were low for no apparent reason and I was put under perfusion every day. Everything was going well until I wanted to speed up the flow of the solution and loosened the valve of the drip chamber, resulting in an accident...

Suddenly I was endowed with supernatural powers.

As I described, I was floating in an endless blue when suddenly I felt the prick of a needle and had the sensation that I was falling, like a shooting star.

Afterwards, the nurse said I was "whiter than the bed sheets" and that I was "inert as a corpse." They were unable to measure my blood pressure and my heart rate was 16 beats per minute. They gave me an injection to stimulate my heart, but my body was stone cold. The lady doctor who did my electrocardiogram came from the same native village as my father. Her daughter and I were in high school together. But even she didn't recognise me, and it wasn't until she signed the papers that she recognised my name. Slightly embarrassed, she said I was unrecognisable.

According to the doctors and nurses, I had lost consciousness, but I could hear and see the medical staff giving me emergency first aid. A lady doctor said: "Her body is cold. Quick, bring a blanket...one more." I saw...no, I can't say I "saw," because I wasn't "seeing" with my physical eyes, but with the eyes of my mind. Years after this incident, I watched the film *Ghost* and saw how after the main actor died, he left his body and carried on living in another dimension from where he could see and save those living in ours. For me, it was déjà vu. Except for the fact that the actor in the film was still in his body, whereas I was made up of only a handful of thoughts. I was what you'd call a spirit. I read something about this a few years ago. Scientists weighed people who had just died and discovered that there were a few grams of difference in their weight just before and after death. They put forward the theory that these few grams correspond to the weight of the soul. It's also said that just after death, the brain is still conscious and that our consciousness fades out gradually. Apparently, our hearing is the last of our five senses to disappear. I am not qualified to comment on the veracity of this information, but based on my experience, I think there's a grain of truth to it. Much is still unknown in our universe. Too many things are beyond our understanding. We can neither prove nor disprove hypotheses such as these. Just because we can't see an electric current doesn't mean it doesn't exist.

TWENTY-FOUR

Diary
Thursday, 31st July 2003 12 pm

Had a dream about undergoing surgery again.

I was hurrying to the airport with my suitcase. When I arrived, the flight was delayed. A lot of passengers were waiting, and no one knew when the flight was scheduled to leave. Since the waiting lounge was full, I waited outside on the tarmac with a few other passengers. I was worried I would miss the announcement and so preferred to stick around.

When we finally boarded the flight, I was exhausted.

We arrived in Beijing at night. Instead of going to a hotel, I went to see someone I knew quite well. Zhu Xiaolin, I think it was. I arrived at her place and thought to myself: "Didn't she go to England? How come she's back in Beijing? Her apartment is small, untidy and a bit Spartan. It looks like she's expecting me, but she's not a very good host."

I explained to her that the oncologists at the Beijing University Hospital told me to come to Beijing for surgery and that I'd like to stay at her place while I had my X-ray exams. She replied: "You can stay for one night, but you must leave tomorrow. I hate people disrupting my routine."

I thought: "She's normally quite sociable. She's invited me a few times, but why has she become so unpleasant?" Annoyed, I wanted to go to a hotel, but after some thought, I told myself not to be impulsive and that perhaps she was having problems and couldn't host any guests.

Cheered by this thought, I told her that I would in all likelihood go home after my X-ray exams the next day, because an operation wouldn't be necessary in the immediate future. The doctors had probably made a mistake and I'd fly back to Guangzhou the following evening. All the while, I kept reassuring myself: "Don't panic. Wait and see what happens after your appointment tomorrow. If you have to wait a few days for the results, then you can go to a clean and comfortable hotel."

I was tired, but calm and collected.

When I woke up, I took my dream to mean that I had made positive progress in my therapy.

So far, I've dreamt twice about undergoing surgery.

In the first one, I was in a remote city where I didn't know a single person. I felt terrified, miserable and lost. Suddenly I saw Hu Ququ, broke down in tears and said: "Ququ, I've got cancer."

In the second dream, a doctor informed me that I was to be operated on immediately. I searched for all sorts of excuses to delay it for as long as possible, but the doctor wouldn't have any of it. Holding on to his white coat, I cried and begged him: "Please, I'm scared. I don't want to be operated on!"

Oddly enough, since my cancer was diagnosed, every time I've underwent surgery or chemotherapy, I've never shed a tear. But I've cried a few times in my dreams.

The psychiatrist at the North Shenzhen Hospital has an explanation: My ability to keep my emotions under control is too strong, leaving me unable to express my fears and hurts. These emotions are embedded inside me and find their way into my dreams. I should be aware of this and try to deal with my emotions to keep depression at bay.

I am not ready to go back in time and relive my feelings after my operation in February 2000.

I sincerely believe this: "God intended it for good to accomplish what is now being done."[1]

Notes

I dislike reading back through the "Diary" section because it forces me to face up to the Li Lanni who is sick. I keep reminding myself that I should reread it just to have a better understanding of Li Lanni during the difficult times in her life. In my head, I know I should, but can't bring myself to do it. Can't. Don't want to.

As a reader, I reject Li Lanni's writings. As a writer, I refute what she writes. A few days ago, I was going to tear up two-thirds of the "Diary" section, but I chickened out. Like I said, it's my wish to leave a testimony to psychiatrists and psychologists.

When I was in Beijing a few days ago, I was talking to my friends Tian Huiping, Du Li and Li Mei. I was complaining that the "Diary" section of my book was worthless, just rambling stories about my nightmares. I asked them if I should delete half of them from the published version. They all said I shouldn't.

They're right. Keeping a diary is therapeutic. As an observer, I would also advise the author to keep the writing as spontaneous as possible. However, I have to reread the "Diary" section once or twice before starting to write the next chapter. But I am unable to take in every word and sentence and always end up skimming through the texts. Also, the muscles of my face tense up; unconsciously I frown and purse my lips. My face takes on various expressions: boredom, helplessness, resentment, disdain and bitterness. I wouldn't want to look at myself in the mirror. I must look atrocious. Watch out or you'll end up with a grumpy, dour face. Take a deep breath. Tap your head and face to relax the muscles. Don't screw up your face when you write. Everyone. Sit up straight. At ease. Smile. Rest.

Mother just called to say Grandmother has been discharged from hospital. She's now in a nursing home.

I said to Mother: "That's great. Going to a nursing home is a good idea." She said: "I thought she'd refuse to go, but she finally accepted the idea. She said: 'I'm home at last.'"

Grandmother, there are far too many things I can't say to you. In the silence of my heart, I honour you, pray for you, learn from you. The taste of life is slowly dissolving in my mouth.

8th May 2006

Correlations

Excerpts from the text messages between our family in Pingxiang and my brother

30th April 2006:

Grandmother's condition has been steadily improving these last couple of days. The doctor has just left. He said if she continued to improve, we can start preparing for her to be discharged from hospital.

Anecdote: after Grandmother ate the peaches, she said: "That was good." After her walk, she said: "That was nice." At bed time, she said: "It's nice here."

3rd May:

When Grandmother finished the bird's nest and *chongcao*, she said: "It's so thoughtful of Fanding and Lanni to give them to me. I'll eat it all and I won't die. But these delicacies are expensive. When they were little, they loved eating pumpkins and lotus roots. They don't want to eat such expensive food, but they gave them to me instead. Thank you."

5th May:

Grandmother will probably be discharged from hospital tomorrow. Today I told her she'd be going to a nursing home. She seemed quite happy about it.

Complementary Notes

A cousin wrote these text messages to Fanding. To put my mind at ease, he forwarded them to me. I was planning to visit Grandmother during the May 1st holidays, but the family is against it. They say Grandmother would be too wound-up and the family at the other end would be too tired to cope. I'll wait and see.

Another bout of depression is looming on the horizon. I can feel it in my bones. I feel guilty and blame myself for not having Grandmother here in Shenzhen with me, so I could look after her. I had thought of renting an ambulance to bring her here so she could live with me, and I could hire help to take care of her. But it wouldn't have worked. I don't know what to do.

The current dosage of antidepressants isn't having much effect. I'm fighting against the Li Lanni who is sick. I should pretend to behave normally. I can't do this anymore.

TWENTY-FIVE

Diary
Tuesday, 2nd September 2003 4:15 pm

Had another dream about school exams.

I was sitting in a classroom when someone announced that there was going to be a maths exam. A wave of fear and panic came over me, for I knew I'd fail. A classmate sitting at the same table said: "Don't worry. You're right next to me, I'll give you the answers." I was worried the teacher would punish us, but after some thought I said to myself that the teacher would take pity on us and let us off the hook. That put my mind at ease.

Then, just as they were about to give out the exam papers, a school supervisor (a fat snooty middle-aged woman) decided to move us to another classroom and change the seating. She was playing around with us.

I felt a rush of anxiety. Changing the seating was chaos and someone (the dunce of the class, most of the time) was always pushing me into a corner, so I ended up not having a table. I didn't know where to put myself, nor how I was going to sit for my exam.

Suddenly, I thought: If I fail the exam, it won't be the end of the world. Take one step at a time. Seeing there was an empty seat, I sat down at the corner of a table, ready to start. Just then, I heard people cheering outside the classroom. A student came running in, shouting: "The exam is cancelled! We can go!"

Breathing a sigh of relief, I ran outside. In fact, the exam session was fake. It was staged by Fatso, who took malicious pleasure in playing around with the students. She was glaring disapprovingly at the students, who were jumping up and down for joy, as if they had been absolved from their sins.

I sighed to myself, thinking: "She abuses what little power she has. If she ever becomes a public official, she'd make people's lives so miserable."

Been having dreams about exams for the last few months. I am much less anxious than before, but still feel vulnerable inside. When will I sit for an exam with confidence in my dreams? When can I face up to my anxieties serenely in real life? You mustn't give up.

I felt so discouraged yesterday. In the morning and afternoon, I prayed. I prayed to God to let me go to heaven. There's too much suffering in life and I want to die. The sooner the better. I am disappointed with my family and I am tired, weak and caught in a dilemma. I wish to rest in the arms of God. I said to Him: "I can't go on like this any longer. If You are willing, let me finish my journey in this life. There is nothing to keep me here. Lord, do according to Your will."

God gave me His answer through a person on the phone. He wants me to serve Him and be a guardian angel that brings comfort. I know that the purpose of my suffering is to one day be useful to Him, to become a noble instrument, an angel that comforts. But I am weak. Faced with my illness and hardships, I run away.

Shame on me.

At dusk, I took a walk to the northern gate of the city. It was hot and muggy. There wasn't a breath of wind and the sky was laden with grey clouds. Suddenly, a cool wind blew from the river, dispersing the clouds, uncovering a patch of blue sky above my head and blowing my sadness and worries away. I felt so strongly the presence of God. He was protecting, comforting, guiding and helping me.

Notes

When I started on my medication, I was hoping it'd only be for three months. But now, three months on, I'm still on them. Six months, one year, two years... three years later, I'll still be taking them, and I'll still be going to the doctor. It is a never-ending fight.

Specialists say that symptoms of depression often reappear in the six to nine months following a remission. If the symptoms continue, then there is 90 percent chance of a relapse. You must continue to take the full dose of medication during the six months following the relapse [...] In some cases, patients must take medication for the rest of their lives.

Well, that's encouraging. Taking medication for the rest of my life, I'd rather not think about that. I feel like the weak side of my personality is about to take over. Shut the door, otherwise I'll go into free fall. I am like Sisyphus, condemned forever to keep pushing a rock up a hill, and just before reaching the top, the rock comes rolling back down again. He pushes the rock up to the top and it rolls back down, he pushes the rock to the top and it rolls back down...

I'd be better off thinking about my maternal great-grandmother and her first name: Xigu.

I love her name. It makes me smile every time I think about it. I see a picture of a chubby young girl of about five or six, smiling innocently.

My thoughts turn to my ancestor, the provincial examination scholar who gave his daughter the name Xigu. He was poor, but proud, honest and principled. Unable to raise enough money to go to the capital for the metropolitan exams, he overcame his disappointment and earned his living as a private tutor. He lived by the principles held by provincial intellectuals over a century ago.

Which brings me to this: I've never tried to find out about the dreams and ideals of my mother, grandmother and great-grandmother. Is it because I unconsciously think they didn't have a right to have dreams and ideals of their own?

My theory: Xigu's dream was to be a devoted wife and mother; Xiaotao's was to study at university and become a teacher; Lanlan's was to be a good soldier.

When Nizi was in her second year of primary school, her dream was to die on a battlefield and be decorated posthumously to bring honour to her family.

13th May 2006

Correlations

Excerpts from "Names"

It is written on my birth certificate that my first name is Xiaolan.

When I was two years old, my grandparents, who lived in the northeast, said that I could have any other name except for Xiaolan.

Many, many years ago, my grandfather had a younger sister called Xiaolan. She died at the age of 16 without having found a husband. According to local customs, the bodies of unmarried young women could not be buried in ancestral graves and must be cremated in the countryside.

Xiaolan died in the depths of winter. After her cremation, her ashes were put into an urn, which was then buried in the countryside.

One day, at 5 o'clock in the morning, Xiaolan came back home crying: "Big brother...I'm cold. Why aren't you taking care of me?" At dawn, my grandfather returned to the place where Xiaolan was cremated and found a piece of bone that had been forgotten. A gust of wind had blown away the ashes covering the bone. That was why Xiaolan came home crying. Grandfather picked up the bone and put it inside the urn. He never dreamt of Xiaolan again.

Many years later, his only granddaughter was born in the heart of winter. As the Chinese character *lan* was part of my mother's name, she called her daughter Xiaolan. But my grandfather dreamt of Xiaolan and my name was changed. Grandfather said: "We'll call her Ni instead." At school, some of the unruly boys would sing every time I walked past: "We have come to Nanni Bay...la la la...beautiful Nanni Bay...la la..." The other boys, roaring with laughter, would sing along: "...So beautiful Nanni Bay..." I would cringe with embarrassment. Putting my hands over my ears, I would shout: "I hate my name!"

In recent years, people have started consulting books on anthroponymy before naming a child to find out the celestial, terrestrial and human attributes of a name to get an idea of the destiny awaiting a person with that name, as well as his/her chances of success in life.

Out of curiosity, I bought a book on anthroponymy and discovered that the meaning of my name is related to the proverb: "If you work at it hard enough, you can grind an iron bar into a fine needle."[1]

Intrigued and apprehensive at the same time, I wondered: "How much longer am I going to be 'ground?' And what if I break into pieces before becoming that 'fine needle?' Maybe it's my fate to never become a 'needle' at all."

First month of the lunar calendar of the year 1994

Complementary Notes

According to the book on anthroponymy, the number of strokes in the characters of the name "Li Nanni" brings more happiness than the one in "Li Lanni."

At the time, people were talking about *qigong*,[2] its supernatural powers and the notion of *qichang*.[3] Some of my friends said the character *lan* in my name wasn't good and that the magnetic field of the character *nan* was better. I have no clue what *qichang* is about, but going by the literal meaning of the character *lan*,[4] I tell myself: "An orchid has a hard time surviving in the ecological environment of a city. Even if it does, it can't flourish, because orchids must live in remote places where the air is pure. Its scent belongs to nature and isn't for the enjoyment of man. Its capacity to adapt is poor, and it can be easily destroyed in an urban environment. The character *nan*[5] is very different. Words with this character have connotations of happiness and prosperity, like 'wind from the south' and 'southern nation.' Even *nangua*,[6] compared to other vegetables, are richer in nutrition and have a stronger flavour."

All that said, my subconscious rejects the name Li Nanni. It flatly refuses to have anything to do with it. For example: my blood group is B, but if I receive blood from group A, it'll cause a break down in my body. My psyche only recognises Li Lanni and rejects any other name, like when someone enters the wrong user code; the machine doesn't react and freezes up.

In that case, Li Lanni it is.

TWENTY-SIX

Diary
Wednesday, 3rd September 2003 11:10 am

Tropical storm Rhododendron is sweeping through the Pearl River Delta region. According to the weather forecast, maximum temperature would be around 29 degrees. We can finally breathe.

[...] (*Author's note: deleted passage*).

I never talk about my disappointments. Maybe it's impossible to talk about them. There's no point.

In the past, I've felt hurt, vulnerable, insecure, sad and humiliated. Maybe it's all related to my cancer.

I feel sorry for him and pray to God to guide, help and bless him. But he insists on wallowing in his own depravity. He's beyond help.

God helps and comforts me and has shown me the way. I must strive to be better. He teaches me and says: "For this is my doing;"[1] "God intended it for good to accomplish what is now being done."[2] I believe in the word of God.

Each hour and every day, I thank the Lord for His love and compassion and for the comfort He brings me. "Blessed are those who mourn."[3] These are the words of God.

"I love you, Lord, my strength."[4] Lord, I know that You love me, with a love that is true and eternal, that You would never hurt me, never leave me, that Your love will be with me always. I am a woman blessed, a child of the Holy Ghost. You protect me. With You by my side, what am I to be afraid of? "When he giveth quietness, who then can make trouble?",[5] "If God is for us, who can be against us?"[6] Yes, that's right. "Do not be anxious about anything."[7]

"He gives strength to the weary and increases the power of the weak."[8]

"Those who hope in the Lord will renew their strength. They will soar on wings like eagles."[9]

O Lord, my heart is now at peace and filled with joy.

O Lord, my Spirit and my Guide, I love You!

Notes

Mother called me to say she was going to Pingxiang to see Grandmother. But Father is worried she'll be upset and fall ill. They're fighting again.

They fight but can't stand being apart. A lot of my friends' parents are like this.

I imagine Xigu's parents wouldn't have had these kinds of marital problems. A woman must obey her father; married, she must obey her husband; old, she must obey her son. These are the "Three Obediences and Four Virtues," a set of moral principles that governed a woman's behaviour and which came under heavy criticism at the turn of the last century. They were the golden rules many generations of women had to abide by.

My great-grandmother's father chose for his daughter a husband who came from an inferior branch of an important clan family. A scholar without ambitions, he was honest and trustworthy, and earned a good living as an accountant. Xigu was plain, honest and simple-minded. Her husband was a handsome man, but temptations of the flesh were few, giving Xigu a relative sense of security. She was widowed young, but her inner world was that of peace and acceptance. People said she was naïve, inward-looking, absent-minded and obtuse.

This reminds me of a story from antiquity: A man by the name of Hundun was born without the seven orifices of the head. His two friends, whom he had previously helped in the past, wanted to pay him back in kind. They opened up seven holes in his head, so he could use his five senses. But he died as a result of having seven holes bored into his head.

Sometimes I think that Xigu being simple-minded and obtuse wasn't such a bad thing. Her father tried to plan out her life, so she could be happy, but he had no control of his son-in-law's destiny.

Ten years ago, in Shenzhen, I often heard women say: "If a marriage is too harmonious, it'll make the gods jealous." It made me laugh. At the time, relationships between men and women were unstable and it was fashionable to say: "Have you... divorced yet?" Several of my acquaintances asked me this. Even an old family friend, who had lived abroad, asked: "Are... you divorced?... Oh...it's a hassle, isn't it?" She had divorced in Shenzhen. At the time, women who were divorced, those who were going to divorce, and even those who weren't going to get divorced all told me that loving couples who are committed to each other didn't exist.

They hinted that I should prepare myself psychologically for a separation, a break down in my marriage or other emotional damage, and that I should be careful. Grandmother taught me an old saying in Pingxiang: "Even when you live to be ninety-eight years old, never mock the lame nor the blind."

Xigu's husband died a sudden death. The villagers wondered what this mother of three, weak and with no skills, could do. But Xigu rose to the occasion and found a way out for her family.

First, her daughter, who was already betrothed, was married off. Then, with the small sum of money she has saved, together with money she had borrowed, she paid for her son to finish his education.

Her daughter's father-in-law, also a provincial examination scholar, was a magistrate of the district of Zhangzhou in Fujian Province. Xigu was confident that her daughter's in-laws wouldn't treat her badly. Anyhow, it was better than staying with her and living in poverty.

Her daughter became a part of the Zhang family. For the first few years of marriage, every day she cried in a corner until her eyes were red and puffy. Her mother couldn't help her. Her husband, who was studying in Beijing, had found himself an admirer and had stopped writing to her. When Xiaotao began the proceedings to file for a divorce, Xigu was powerless to help. Fortunately, her lack of perception protected her from seeing how deeply hurt her daughter was. Her belief in marriage and family was blind, a pillar that propped up her inner world. Her husband had died young, leaving her with loving memories of their marriage, and she stayed faithful to him even after his death. The tragedy that struck them came from the outside and didn't undermine her belief in family and conjugal happiness.

In all the books written by psychiatrists that I have read, they say that more women suffer from depression than men, but, on the other hand, the rate of suicide is higher among men.

I think the number of men and women suffering from depression is about the same. But from a biological, psychological and ideological point of view, women are more vulnerable, and their resistance is weaker. Take this example, for instance: Women catch the flu easily, whereas men only fall ill from time to time. But when men come down with the flu, they become very sick. Women go to see a doctor, but men hold out until they develop something more serious, bumping up the rate of death among men.

I haven't seen the statistics comparing the number of men and women who suffer from depression. There are probably at least 10 percent of women suffering from various degrees of depression in the more developed countries.

Women in developed countries are under tremendous pressure. It's also the case for women in the more developed regions of China. Support is virtually non-existent, making them more vulnerable.

In major hospitals, you see more women than men, both in the wards and in external consultation. But half of these women suffer from psycho-affective disorders. They complain of aches and pains everywhere: blood vessels, joints, liver, gall bladder, kidneys, digestive system, meridians, uterus, breasts, ears, nose, throat, eyes, brain, nervous system. Their somatic illness is tied to their mental sufferings and problems stemming from their family and interpersonal relationship. Most women are unaware of this. They cry, sigh and hide behind their illness. Some of them are vaguely aware of this, but influenced by traditional thinking, they close their eyes, cover their ears, shut their mouths and continue to shuttle between the different hospital services, going from medical examination to another: biological analysis, Doppler, CT-scan, electrocardiograms, physiotherapy.

These women are more fortunate than Xiaotao. They can run away from themselves and hide behind their illness. Xiaotao had nowhere to go or hide. She had to take care of the house. Alone, she suffered in silence and in despair. Her marriage was an empty shell. Even many years later, Grandmother is reluctant to talk about this period of her life. She only said: "For a whole month after the birth of my children, I wasn't allowed to have even one egg! Not one!" Her family in-law wasn't poor, which made her even unhappier. She cried until she had no more tears left. That is why her first born died before the age of one. Xiaotao wanted to die, but she thought of her mother and brother. Women like Xiaotao had sad and wretched lives.

Regardless of their nationality, race or the era in which they live, some women live their lives in mental pain. Whether they are stupid or intelligent, rich or poor, strong or weak, they endure undue sufferings. Pain is part of their destiny.

23rd *May* 2006

Correlations

Excerpts from *Depression: An Undiagnosed Illness*

Mothers suffering from neurosis pass their genes to their daughters. They all have one thing in common: When their daughters need them, they are incapable of satisfying the emotional needs of their children [...]. Those who have written on this subject are reluctant to point the finger at the mother [...]. Mothers who have not developed a solid and stable notion of the self inhibit the personal development of their daughters, instead of encouraging them to be independent. This affects not only how the daughters will later develop intimate, stable and loving relationships with a man, but it also makes them vulnerable to depression.

Ursula Nuber (Germany)

Complementary Notes

Some of my friends also had tense relationships with their mothers during their childhoods.

I know a woman who is an executive in a foreign-owned company. Highly competent, honest and beautiful, she doesn't, however, have the skills to deal with family relationships. After her divorce, she drifted further and further away from her son and was unable to stay in a stable relationship with a man. She tells herself that she is attractive and pleasing to men, which is true. But after showering herself with compliments, she loses confidence in herself again. She asked me, insisting that I should be honest with her: Was she attractive? Was she pretty? Did her personality scare people away? I didn't know whether to laugh or cry. Then she talked to me about her sad childhood. Her mother was a brilliant woman who felt no affection for her daughter. She didn't spend much time with her daughter and when she did, she criticised her appearance and behaviour. The more my friend needed her mother's love, the more she felt her mother scorned and mocked her. She would have tantrums, fight with her mother or do things to make her mother proud, but to no avail. I think it's because of her conflicted relationship with her mother that, as an adult, she is unable to assume her role as a wife and mother. She paid a high price for her mother's shortcomings.

There are common threads in the stories that my friends tell me. As children, they had difficult relationships with their mothers. These mothers were the first generation of career women in China. They're usually attractive, hold a professional title, are ambitious about their political career, are extremely professional, keep their home in good order, wear the trousers in their marriage and are slightly obsessive about cleanliness. The boundaries between their private and public lives are clear cut, and they're more caring and considerate to people outside the family than to their own children.

Which brings me to these questions: Do these relationship problems stem from the mother or the child? How many families in China suffer from such dysfunctional relationships? Does our DNA change from one generation to the next?

TWENTY-SEVEN

Diary
Thursday, 4th September 2003 11 am

Can finally talk about the feelings that have been bottling up in me.
[...] (*Author's note: deleted passage*)
    Yesterday around 12:40 pm, I had a sudden urge to go outside. So I switched off my computer and walked for half an hour in Xiju Gardens. The typhoon had moved on and the rain had stopped. Several people were reading on the benches. I strolled along the wet green cobblestone paths, holding the silver-grey umbrella I bought at a Laiersidan shop. A sudden light rain shower brought a sensation of freshness that penetrated to my core.
    At that moment, I felt God was with me. The Holy Spirit had led me to that place where I received comfort and strength from our merciful God. Suddenly, I was overwhelmed with an odd sensation of being in communication with a divine force. It dispelled all the despair and despondency locked up inside. My mind became lucid and I felt energy running into my limbs like an electric current. My sadness melted away and the world around me was bright and in focus. The Lord said to me: "My grace is sufficient for you."[1] I live in the grace of God and no longer under the burden of my sufferings. Life is beautiful.
    I thank God and the Holy Spirit for the divine revelation They bestowed on me. I have received the strength and courage to live. God gifted me with life and soul. He created me, forged me so I could serve Him. The process of creation is filled with pain. He made me endure hardships. Among his children, He chose the ones He loves the most to praise His name. The more gifted the child, the more arduous is the task. Only thus will he or she be of valuable service to God.
    We are in the first half of September. It's time to put my thoughts in some sort of order.

POSITIVE THINGS:

1. Recently I've enjoyed either meeting up with friends in Guangzhou and Shenzhen or talking to them on the phone. As the Chinese saying goes: "Human relationships are tasteless like water, but beautiful like wine."

2. My parents are well. My relationship with Fanding and his family is good. Li Jiean is a sweet little girl.
3. Sleeping in the study gives me a sense of freedom. The quality of my sleep has improved.
4. The weather isn't so hot.
5. After resting for a few days, I feel physically and mentally stronger.
6. After increasing the dosage of my medication, the side effects are wearing off.

NOT SO POSITIVE THINGS:

1. Still can't read, write or think properly.
2. Still recovering my strength, so exercising and swimming is out of the question.
3. Still irritable and restless.
4. Still have communication problems with others.
5. I feel under pressure whenever I want to start writing again. I have high expectations of myself but lack confidence, so I chastise myself, which makes me even more anxious. I must change this.
6. Since I haven't checked my emails for six months, my account has been cancelled and I don't know how to reactivate it. So annoying.

My computer didn't freeze even once today, which is surprising.

Notes

Two of my friends – a man and a woman in two different lines of work - called me yesterday afternoon to ask after my health. The man told me about a suicidal friend of his, who is part of the social elite in Beijing. He asked me what kind of antidepressants his friend should take and if he could buy them over the counter at the pharmacy. I told him only specialists in hospitals could prescribe such medications. But he said his friend couldn't go, afraid other people would find out.

It's quite common for people to worry about this. Society in general wants its elite members to be strong. While minor ailments like a cold don't ruin their image of being in perfect health, it's unacceptable for them to be tainted with the slightest mental illness.

I didn't know what to say to my friend.

Less than five hours later, I received a call from my woman friend. She wanted some advice for her friend, who is well-off and goes abroad regularly.

But she hasn't seen her friends for the last six months. She's afraid to go out, avoids people and has lost interest in life.

I had mixed feelings when I hung up.

I was glad that society is becoming more aware of the phenomenon of depression. In 2003, when I was first diagnosed with depression, no one could give me any practical support. Today, friends help and support each other. It's the first step on the road to recovery.

I was sad, however, because I was told about two new medical cases in the space of just a few hours, which means the number of people suffering from depression is increasing. Both refuse to see a doctor and to take medication, thinking they can come out of it by themselves.

The Bible says: "There is nothing new under the sun."[2]

A sentence from Zen Buddhism: "Light can dispel a thousand years of darkness; intelligence can enlighten a thousand years of ignorance."

Laozi said: "Do not drift away from virtue, for through it we return to the wisdom of a child."

24th May 2006

Correlations

Excerpts from *Depression Explained*

Those who help their friends suffering from depression should be patient, attentive and understanding. At times, you may feel that all that you do is useless and that whatever you say falls on deaf ears.

When people are in a state of depression, they are afraid of losing their friends. They become difficult and can be a burden for others. As a friend, the best thing to do is to not change your behaviour and show your willingness to help them.

When they talk about their problems, you do not necessarily have to come up with solutions. Just the fact that you are listening brings them comfort and support.

You should keep this in mind: your friends are sick. It takes them twice as long to do things, and everything is blown out of proportion. A sesame seed can take on the proportions of a watermelon. Under the effects of depression, they have a distorted view of the world. It may surprise you to know that what you do for them, no matter how insignificant it may seem, is perceived to be of tremendous importance. Your help and support play an essential role in their recovery.

Act in good faith. If you help them out of obligation, then it could only have negative consequences for both parties.

Gwendoline Smith (New Zealand)

Complementary Notes

Lately I've been surfing the internet again, after having stopped for three years. On the first day, I came across a message asking for help on a forum on psychology in China: "My friend is depressed, how can I help her?" Here's the summary: A 23-year-old girl, a brilliant and sociable university student, recently fell into a depression, perhaps due to problems related to work or a boyfriend. She shut herself up at home, lost interest in life and suffered from insomnia. Her neighbours, classmates and friends tried to talk her out of it but in vain. The person who posted the message, not knowing what to do, asked for advice on the internet. After reading the message, I replied straight away: "You should take your friend to see a doctor specialising in psychiatry or psychology." Then, as I continued to read the thread of the conversation, I realised that several days after the first message, the friend posted a second message to say that her friend had left this world. The girl had died suddenly in circumstances so sad that all her friends were in shock. The friend couldn't accept the girl's death. As I read the message more closely, I realised the incident had taken place two days before I wrote my message. I then wrote another message to apologise and said: "If, in the future, you notice a depressive tendency in a friend, you should take him or her immediately to see a medical specialist." I stressed the importance of consulting a specialist because my own experience was strewn with pitfalls.

Going through the other messages on the website, I saw two other messages that were a cry for help. The first was from a mother who was asking for help for her child suffering from depression. The second was from a 21-year-old university student who was asking for help dealing with her suicidal tendencies. All this weighed heavily on my heart.

The harvest is plentiful, but the workers are few. What to do?

TWENTY-EIGHT

Diary
Saturday, 6th September 2003 11 am

Have to increase the dosage of my medications again.

Dr Gong added buspirone, an anxiolytic. He's going to keep on increasing the dosage of alprazolam until I feel better. Seroxat stays the same: one and a half tablets per day.

The dosage was reduced too drastically and affected the quality of my sleep. My headaches are due to stress and anxiety.

Dr Gong thinks I have a mental block when it comes to medication. I am scared of the side effects and don't trust doctors enough. He advised me to do a psychological test and monitor for any side effects for the next few months.

Current diagnosis: moderate obsessive-compulsive disorder, moderate depression and mild anxiety.

You're improving, Li Lanni. Look at the results. Don't give up.

A LIST OF HAPPY THINGS:

1. Reactivated my email account.
2. Talked to Xiao Han on the phone. We discussed the idea of writing a script for a television series with psychiatry as its central theme. She'll ask around to see if Li Ting and Du Li would be interested.
3. Sent two boxes of moon cake by post to Grandmother. The service is quick, and she'll receive them in three days' time.
4. Increasing the dosage hasn't made the side effects worse. It could speed up recovery.
5. Went to the Baijia shop to have my digital photographs from 1984 printed out. They're old photos I had taken of Zhou Yang and other friends and are the only souvenirs I have of the time when three generations of writers were gathered together on the same day at the same place.

Positive things have been happening every day, so there is no reason to brood over negative ones.

My obsessive-compulsive disorder is on a mental level. Negative thoughts go round and round in my head.

It's a bad habit I've acquired throughout the years. But it's never too late to change.

Notes

Grandmother is dead.

At 10 o'clock this morning, Fanding arrived at the university unannounced. There was nothing unusual about him, except that he was unshaven and looked tired. I told him I would accompany Mother to Pingxiang in the middle of June to visit Grandmother and that I planned to stay for 10 days in a hotel near the nursing home. Looking down and without saying a word, he listened to me chirping away about my plans. Then he shook his head and closed his eyes. I still hadn't caught on. Fanding said: "You won't need to do that." Still not catching on, I asked: "Why not?" His eyes were filled with tears and he said softly: "Grandmother is dead."

I looked up and sighed. I said nothing. And I didn't cry.

On 19th May, at 11:30 pm, the nurse found that Grandmother wasn't breathing. She immediately called the family.

Grandmother, I miss you.

27th May 2006

Correlations

Excerpts from the SMS correspondence between the family in Pingxiang and my brother

Family:

Elder brother, pray for Grandmother and for her journey into the next world. She is free...

Family:

Elder brother, Grandmother will be cremated tomorrow, and the funeral will be the day after tomorrow.

Family:

Grandmother will be cremated shortly. She will soon step on the path to heaven. Let us pray for her.

Fanding:

Have a safe journey, Grandmother.

Family:

Elder brother, we're burning a joss paper house for Grandmother. Let's picture her smiling happily.

Fanding:

Don't forget to burn her a house with air conditioning.

Family:

The funeral has started.

Fanding:

It's cold here in this world. Grandmother, don't come back.

Complementary Notes

There are a lot of things to say, but I don't know how to say them. And it's not for want of trying. Perhaps the wiring in my brain has broken down. Or maybe it's because my thoughts are clogged, causing a dysfunction in my brain, mouth and hands.

I need time.

Please don't make me.

TWENTY-NINE

Diary
Wednesday, 17th September 2003 5:10 pm

Splitting headache.

Was tossing and turning during my afternoon nap. Every time it happens, my head and throat hurt. Strange. Told Dr Gong I'd see the specialists tomorrow morning. After my appointment with the psychologist today, I saw a Chinese physician. I asked Dr Chen to refer me to a gynaecologist. I hate pelvic ultrasounds. Drinking all that water bloats up my stomach. But I can't get out of it. I'll go when I have more time on my hands.

Talked to Chen Zhihong on the phone.

Being independent means I never talk to my friends about my problems, so they never know when I need help. Since they know very little about my professional life and situation in general, naturally I feel misunderstood. It's a vicious circle.

My friends are more intelligent than I am. They have foresight, high-flying careers and finely-honed social skills. In the past, I've often felt inferior compared to them and have had a complex about it. But I've come to accept myself and am learning to build confidence and self-esteem. I've chosen my friends well, because they accept me as I am. I've become more aware of my qualities and understand that God gives us friends to help us.

Notes

Not in the mood to work.

Mother is here in Guangzhou. She can't stop talking about going to see Grandmother in Pingxiang. It keeps her busy. She loves to talk to me about her trip: how she's going to get there; the things she's going to take with her; how long she's staying there; how much money to give to the medical staff; how much money to give to Grandmother; what to say to the staff so they'll be nice to Grandmother. She called the family in Pingxiang to ask them to take good care of Grandmother and tell her she'd be there soon.

I wanted to break the news to her, but my father and brother are against it. They're worried she'd be so upset that she'd get sick. I try to change their mind and force myself to talk to Mother about her trip as if nothing has happened: which hotel we'll be staying in; finding a better nursing home with air conditioning; the least tiring way to go to Pingxiang – by plane and then by coach, or by train.

Mother said: "When Grandmother was in critical condition, she wasn't ready to leave this world, because she wanted to see us before passing away. I'm her eldest daughter. She said to the nurses: 'My eldest daughter is ill. She's ill.' She said that because she wanted to see me. She wants to see you too, because she wants to know why you're sick and why you haven't written anything for years. Since Fanding went to see her, you haven't been and she's worried. The family says that what she fears most is seeing her children die before her. Lanni, I know it hasn't been easy for you these last few years, but come with me to see Grandmother, just to reassure her, so you'll not regret it later. You can go home after two days and I'll stay on, depending on the situation. Also, don't waste your money, you've earned it with your sweat and blood. Be reasonable. Don't forget to do as I said. Otherwise, once we get there, we'll end up being so neurotic that we'll both get sick. Promise me."

In spite of myself, I promised her. I agreed to everything she said, even though it was breaking my heart.

My family has a very odd tradition: We have a habit of keeping secrets from each other. When my grandparents were accused of being counter-revolutionaries, the grandchildren were kept in the dark. I was operated on twice for cancer and I didn't know. My husband, brother, family, friends, superiors and colleagues didn't know. And now that my grandmother was dead, we have to keep it secret until the very last moment. It makes me so angry. What kind of thinking is this? I can't understand this so-called love. It's not love, because it hurts other people. Are we psychologically so vulnerable and fragile?

Not only is this true within a family, you also see it in a given society and nation. In the name of love, we refuse to speak openly and honestly. Things become murky and opaque. We lack self-confidence and we run away. We lie to others and to ourselves. We become far too sensitive and our nervous system starts to malfunction. Our mental resilience erodes away from one generation to the next. Does this have anything to do with our psychological DNA? Has a century of social upheaval modified our mental DNA?

It's the survival of the fittest. A law of nature. Family, country, nation and universe are all governed by natural laws.

17th June 2006

Correlations

Chronology

19th May - Grandmother passed away in the night.

20th May - (Morning) Fanding was told Grandmother had passed away.

27th May - (Morning) Fanding told me.

3rd June - My parents arrived in Guangzhou. They were preparing for their trip to Pingxiang.

9th June - I told father.

11th June - Mother went to the station to enquire about the train schedules and price of tickets.

14th June - The family talked about how to reserve berth couchettes.

15th June - Mother decided that father should stay behind in Guangzhou and that she'd go to see Grandmother with me. We discussed the option of hiring part-time house help to take care of father or whether he should stay with my brother instead.

16th June - Fanding and I agreed to break the news to Mother as soon as possible.

17th June - Fanding asked a doctor about how to give emergency first aid, in case we'd need it for Mother. Father suggested not to say anything until the end of the month and to let Mother slowly find out for herself.

Complementary Notes

Reality makes me nervous and anxious. I am afraid of the moment when I have to face up to Mother. We'll both spiral into depression. Who will save whom then? What should I do if Mother goes to pieces from the emotional shock?

THIRTY

Diary
Friday, 19th September 2003 11:40 am

Feel weak and light-headed. Went for my oestrogen blood test this morning and to my appointment with the Chinese physician. Dr Chen said she couldn't feel my pulse and that I suffered from patterns of Deficient Yin and Deficient Energy. The antidepressants have a toxic effect on the organs, resulting in a dysfunction of the Fluids. She prescribed me three different types of medication and told me to come back on Monday. Time is needed for the body to regulate itself.

Yesterday, I saw the psychologist and gynaecologist. Dr Gong reduced my intake of Seroxat by half a tablet at night. I take the second tablet of buspirone after my evening meal and she increased the dosage of alprazolam at midday. Dr Huang prescribed me five days of progesterone. She'll establish a second diagnosis when the results of the blood test come in. She suggested I should take up knitting or embroidery.

I left the Chinese herbs simmering on the stove for too long. I do silly things when my head is up in the clouds. Stop. Take a break.

Notes

I rarely write down the dialogue in my dreams, for I am afraid of facing up to the freedom and reality of my dreams. That's why the nocturnal Li Lanni thinks the diurnal Li Lanni is incapable of writing.

In the past, I deliberately omitted from my writings the painful memories that haunt my maternal grandmother's family. Reading through them again, they strike me as worthless scribblings. I am no more than a chronicler who records superficial facts, a weak-minded person who only knows how to embellish reality. I don't understand my grandmother. At the start of the Cultural Revolution, it was taboo to talk about her family. Even when the Cultural Revolution was over, it remained taboo in the family's subconscious.

There were rumours about my maternal grandparents: My grandfather and a group of teachers were photographed with Chiang Kai-Shek at Lushan; during the Cultural Revolution, my grandfather was sentenced to death by a popular "dictatorship;" on my grandmother's side, a young member of the family in every generation committed suicide...I never had the courage to ask: "Is all this true? But why? What's the truth?"

I never dared to ask. It was a sensitive topic with my mother and grandparents. They were fearful, like criminals in ancient China who had the word "condemned" branded on their foreheads. Regardless of the government or dynasty that was in place, the word "condemned" remains indelible. And the "crime" eating away at your insides becomes an organic lesion.

When I was a child, I often heard Mother crying in her dreams. I would wake up with a start and lie in the darkness listening to her weeping through the wall. Worried, Father would wake her up and tell her she was having a nightmare. When he was away on duty, it fell upon my brother and me to wake her up. We would shout on the top of our voices: "Mother! Mother! You're having a nightmare!" We would hear her mumbling on the other side of the wall and the crying would stop. Silence would return, and I would lie awake for a long time afterwards wondering what kind of nightmare she'd had.

When I was in my second year of high school, I dreamt that Mother was dead and her corpse was lying on a wooden door. I felt very upset when I woke up, and unable to talk to my family about it, I told my teacher who said: "Don't think any more about this dream."

As an adult, I often have nightmares where I weep and shout. But these cries and tears never go beyond my dreams and never bother anyone. They're prisoners of my mental world. Others have no idea of the terrifying situations I find myself in.

I never talked to Grandmother about it and I don't know if she had nightmares.

It's only now that I understand this: If you don't understand a person's dreams, you will never understand him or her.

Erich Fromm taught me this piece of truth a couple of days ago.

It's a source of relief that I don't have children. For my child would have been psychologically fragile. Even if he or she were happy in his/her daily life, his/her dreams at night would have been filled with disquiet and unease.

In Chapter 25 of *Courtyard of My Childhood Years*, I described the confrontation between my mother and me, and also the beating she gave me. I talked of the wounds we inflicted on each other. After reading the manuscript, my brother "snitched" on me and told Mother, who then threatened me: "Don't you go spreading such nonsense about me. If you don't stop spewing your lies, I'm going jump off a building." Under the watchful eye of my brother, I deleted the incriminating passages, but my true feelings remain buried inside. I tried my best to play down the conflict in our mother-daughter relationship. But every time I reread my story, I am engulfed by hate towards Li Lanni the writer. I hate her for dressing up lies and falsehoods.

In my memory, our fight was violent, the wounds deep and the aftermath painful. You never wash your dirty linen in public. There is a guiding principle that runs through our traditions: "Never tell all to your family or to those whom you respect." This moral code cannot be questioned, and it's impossible to change a code of conduct forged by popular tradition. We've been taught to praise and admire our parents but are unable to understand the pressures and hardships society, history, illness and life's misfortunes impose on them. We turn a blind eye to their mental problems and lack the courage to hold out our hand to them and face the inner conflicts our society creates in us together. Our parents feel lost, alone and despondent. Their children also feel lost, alone and despondent. Are child-parent relationships 100 percent sincere, trustful, happy, healthy, free of regrets and above reproach? Are we certain we can continue in this kind of parent-child relationship? Are we 100 percent sure that our mental DNA doesn't conceal some kind of defect or pathology?

When we love someone, we put our trust in him/her and accept his/her virtues and shortcomings, and we talk to them honestly about their mistakes. When we love a place, we can talk objectively and without reserve about its positive and negative aspects.

I don't know how to write anymore.

Sitting in front of my computer, a wave of nausea hits me, and a feeling of distress wells up inside. I can't concentrate. My pulse fluctuates between 48 and 43 beats per minute. My heart rate is so slow that I can't do much except move around in my apartment. I feel worse lying down. I can't breathe, and my heart feels as if it's going to give up. I can't sit still, either. I feel I lack oxygen and must plunk myself either in front of the fan or the air conditioner. And I slouch. I know it's unsightly, but since I suffer from a Deficiency in Energy, I don't have enough strength to hold myself straight. What the hell, I'll just walk with a stoop. There's nothing I can do. I'm becoming addicted to coffee. A cup of strong coffee speeds up my heart rate a little and stimulates my brain, which has gone numb. But I can't drink a lot of the stuff, because it diminishes the sedative and sleep-inducing effects of the antidepressants. I won't tell the doctor, otherwise he'll increase the dosage.

It's been a month since I've started hiding at home. I avoid talking on the phone, taking any calls and seeing people. And I try not to do anything that would deplete my energy reserves.

The positive and negative thoughts are fighting each other inside my head. Whenever I think of my budgies that I "murdered" 10 years ago, enormous feelings of guilt come over me and I wonder if I can ever redeem myself. Is there divine retribution for what I've done? When I was little, someone threw a broody hen from the second floor of our building. The hen was old. It couldn't fly and fell to its death. I was the culprit. And to this day I still haven't owned up to this heinous act. A few years ago, I bought a Chihuahua. On the day I brought it home, I put it out on the balcony in the evening while I went out to eat. It must have caught cold, for it fell sick the next day. I took it to a veterinary clinic, but it died a week later. I was too cowardly to even say goodbye to it, so I gave some money to the staff at the clinic to have it buried. I was guilty. If I hadn't bought it, it wouldn't have died. I was selfish. Why was I so cruel? Once when I was little, my little brother snitched on me. I asked someone to beat him up. What else? Shut the door. Shut the door. I can't. Negative thoughts are gushing out of me like water roaring out of a broken dam. What if it wipes out all my self-therapeutic work? I refuse to relapse into another depression. I want to be healthy again. I must. But I'm obsessed with one thought. A soundless voice keeps repeating and urging me: "Go on, do away with yourself and your mother. For the sake of everyone. You'll be doing your mother, brother, and father a favour. And you. It's the best way out." Positive thoughts, please, please help me! Help me overcome this! Li Lanni, snap out of it. Shut down these negative thoughts. Stop thinking of the budgies, the broody hen and the Chihuahua. Stop accusing yourself. You've already repented for your sins and you have a clear conscience. The Bible says: "[He] forgives all your sins and heals all your diseases."[1] Li Lanni, wipe out any thoughts of sin from your head! Don't let yourself be devoured by negativity. Watch out. Be on your guard. Repeat this: "Be strong and courageous. Do not be afraid; do not be discouraged, for the Lord your God will be with you wherever you go."[2] Remember this always: Let positive thoughts fill up as much space as possible in your brain. Let in the light. Let the light chase away all the dark shadows in you.

In the night's deep darkness, I close my eyes and try to rein in my thoughts run amok. I repeat over and over again: "Give me light. And more light. Unchain yourself from worries. I am filled with joy. My soul is filled with happiness."

14th July 2006

Correlations

Excerpts from *Courtyard of My Childhood Years*

25

"Nizi, go and wash the rice."

Mother was rummaging in the camphor wood trunk. She was packing, for we were moving to a new place. My brother and I were in the upper bunk reading. I wanted to finish the novels and comic books I had rented for 55 cents before leaving.

[...]

"Nizi, go wash the rice and sort out the vegetables. Do you hear me?"

Then she stood in front of the bed and raised her voice:

"Stop reading your stupid books. Get down from there! These damn books will bring nothing but trouble and we'll end up having everything confiscated from us."

My books made Mother very nervous, as if she were afraid of being accused of sheltering a counter-revolutionary. She was worried sick someone would find out that my grandmother was a landowner.

I ignored her, wanting to finish my paragraph. Irritated, she climbed onto the bed, about to snatch my book away, but I scrambled down, holding tightly onto my book. She was livid and swept up all the books on my bed and threw them outside. My brother jumped down and rushed outside in an attempt to save his comic books.

"If you dare bring them back into the house, I'll tear them all up!" Mother threatened, shaking a book at him from the doorway.

"No, no, please don't," pleaded my brother, running towards Mother, who pushed him away.

"I've already warned you not to read these books. If you carry on, I'll burn them," she said, looking at a box of matches on the window sill.

"No, please don't! I'll have to pay a fine and I don't have money," I begged, snatching the book away and throwing it under the bed. My brother followed suit. The bed was low, and an adult would be too big to crawl under it.

"Oh, I see. You're ganging up on me now," said Mother, seizing my hand and pushing me towards the bed. "Go on, get under the bed. You're going to take every single one of those books out, one by one!"

"No!" I shouted, wrestling my hand out of hers. But her grip was too strong, and I thought of a curse that never failed to work. I screamed at the top of lungs:

"Your grandfather was a landowner! Your family had a house. Your father was banished to the country by the revolutionaries...You...you're a landowner!"

Mother let go of my hand. Aghast, she remained still for a second and then slapped me hard on the face.

"Shut up! You're...a liar. What do you want to do? Where's your heart? So young, but so cruel...you," she said, pointing to my brother. "Get me the cane. Now! Hurry up..."

My brother reluctantly fetched the bamboo cane Mother used to discipline us and gave it to her. She closed the curtains, locked the door and, hitting the cane against her thigh, said:

"The cane is good, it doesn't break any bones. I want you to suffer for a few days and we'll see if you dare to disobey me again. Do you hear me? I'm your mother. I won't hurt you, but you're going to remember this…"

"Mother, no…Not today, next time…" my brother begged.

Before he could finish, I felt a blow on my arm. Trying to see if it had left any red marks, I felt two more blows on my leg. I darted to the door and unlocked it.

"You want to run?" asked Mother, hitting the cane against the door frame. "Go on, leave, but don't come back. Believe me, I'll do what I say."

My brother and I had never once run away during one of our hidings. Mother liked to say that if she couldn't give us a good thrashing, she would be sick.

"You hate me, don't you? You're cursing me, aren't you? You want me to die, don't you? Well, you know what? I'm not going to."

She was looking at me strangely, as if she were staring at something above my head. She raised her hand and immediately blows rained down on my brother and me. It hurt. It hurt so much. Sharp, burning pain was searing through my body.

"Mother, Mother, please," begged my brother, crying, his arms wrapped around his head as he ducked the blows. "Stop…please…We won't do it again…"

Mother stopped and said, glaring at me:

"Look at me! You have so much hate in your heart. What have you got inside your head? What did you say to me just now? You think I'm afraid of you? Let's all die together. I can't take this anymore!"

Then she slapped me. My mind was blank. I was doing all I could to hold back my tears. She wanted me to beg her for forgiveness, but I wasn't going to.

Father was at the door. She let him in and quickly locked the door behind him.

"What's going on?" he asked.

"She accused me of being a landowner. She was going to denounce me and destroy me!" said Mother, the veins on her temples swelling up. "If I didn't teach them a lesson, they would have brought us trouble."

Putting his arm round her waist, he said:

"Don't be angry. Go and get some rest."

"No! She's going to apologise. This girl is bad and cruel. It's getting worse by the day and she's setting a bad example for her brother."

She suddenly raised her voice and shouted:

"Look at me! What did you accuse me of just now? Say it! Say it!"

Her voice was loud and high-pitched, mounting in crescendo. My thoughts became cloudy and confused and my head felt as if it was blowing up.

"You're a landowner! You're scared other people will find out about your family background. Your grandfather was a landowner. He gave your father lots of money to study at Qinghua University. I know everything about your family and I'm going to tell everyone!"

"Very well. You've vented your spleen," she said and then cuffed me.

Blind with rage, I started kicking and pulling her hair.

"I can't take this anymore! Let's put an end to this once and for all!" she screamed through her tears. Then she seized me and threw me against the wall.

My father and brother struggled to separate us.

Everything was spinning around me. I slumped against the wall and slowly collapsed onto the floor.

27

I walked slowly into the meeting hall and sat down on a chair, hugging my knees against me. I didn't feel much pain in my body, head or face, just a burning and stinging sensation.

I wasn't hurt. Mother had given me a thrashing, but I didn't feel hurt.

Never once did she say to me: "My precious, my darling, my flesh and bone, Mother loves you." Not once.

[...]

I heard faint footsteps and looked around me but saw no one. The gnarled old longan tree was like an old woman bent over in pain, her arms outstretched reaching in the darkness for her lost children.

Our house was the only one that was lit up in the small courtyard. And if I opened the door? Was Mother still crying? I stood in the silence of the courtyard wondering.

A long time ago, I had thought that if one day I were to have a stepmother and if she were to beat me, I would run out into the middle of the courtyard screaming for help. I was certain that Mrs Commander in Chief would save me. But I never dreamt that she would leave and return home to work in the fields. It never occurred to me that the families in the small courtyard would ever leave.

Mrs Commander in Chief's family was the first to leave. They left in the dead of night without saying goodbye.

When Xiao Yuzi left, she couldn't stop looking behind her. She was holding a small earthen pot used for marinating vegetables, but inside it contained dried meat. Xiao Yuzi's mother was walking briskly with Xiao San on her back. Both mother and daughter were chubby, and their white skin made them look like wild fat mushrooms from afar. Xiao Yuzi had bendy legs and, tottering behind them, she resembled a tiny ant following a mushroom.

[...]

It was cold. As I was tightening my jacket around me, I noticed the sleeves were short. I had grown, I would be 12 years old soon and in a few days' time it would be my turn to leave the small courtyard [...] (Author's note: The following passages were deleted at the time of publication).

I walked out of the courtyard, leaving my childhood behind.

Leaves of the rose apple tree fell on my shoulders. Autumn was coming to an end. Only a few dark red fruits were left on the tree. I touched the thick bark of the trunk and a ripe rose apple fell on the ground.

The tree was 100 years old. It would have to wait 900 years before returning to the quintessence of the earth.

I picked up the fruit and rinsed it under the tap. Its skin had burst, revealing the flesh inside, its faint scent penetrating deep into my heart.

Holding the rose apple in my hand, I went into the big courtyard.

A blind man was walking past the front entrance.

He had a long head, long arms and legs.

His clothes were mended with patchworks of grey and inside his blue-green canvas bag was a tin canister containing crunchy peanuts. The metallic tip of his walking stick was going tick tick tick as it tapped on the ground. In his old man's voice, he was crying out in measured cadence:

"*Nan...ru*[3]...pea...nuts..."

Tick...tick...tick...tick...

A pause and then:

"*Nan...ru*...pea...nuts..."

Were his cries going to last through the night?

Standing at the entrance of the courtyard, I looked around me. Where was I to go?

The mist was rising.

In the hollow of my hand was a ripened fruit of the rose apple tree.

8th December 1990

Complementary Notes

Over 10 years have gone by and I still think about the passages that were struck from the story. Because they were deleted, they have become even more deeply rooted in me than any of my writings, erupting into my memory, wearing down my resistance until I have no other choice but to incorporate them into this book. It is like a jammed film roll that keeps projecting the same sequence on the screen: a 12-year-old girl standing in front of the entrance to a military base. It is night. A blind man is walking on the streets tapping his cane on the ground. He is carrying an old tin canister, crying out in Cantonese:

"*Nan...ru...pea...nuts... nan...ru...pea...nuts...*"

When I was a child, there were always what you'd call in Cantonese a *manggong*[4] or a *mangpo*[5] selling *nanru* peanuts and *manggong bing*[6] on the streets. They never directly approached the customers, instead walking the streets with the same measured cadence and calling in the same flat voice. They were an emblem of the city.

How is it that this image was so deeply etched into the memory of a 12-year-old girl? More so than those of major national events or historical figures? Even to this day, I have no answers.

The fact that I included the above excerpt from my novella *Courtyard of My Childhood Years* in this chapter reveals a need in me to escape from reality, to go backwards in time and find solace in my memories of the years spent in the small courtyard, because I feel confused and under pressure. I need to hide.

THIRTY-ONE

Diary
Saturday, 20th September 2003 12:30 pm

Received a call from Lü Lei yesterday around 3 pm. He said Gao Hongbo was in Guangzhou and that they were going to play ping-pong with He Jiqing. I went over to watch the match on the ninth floor of the cultural building in the military zone. Gao Hongbo won. He said he'd like to invite the "Chinese Women Association" to dinner next week. In the evening, I had dinner with Gao, Lü, He and Liao Hongqiu at the guest house. We were Vice Governor You's guests. He was with his former secretary Wang and his current secretary Chen. Today Gao, Lü and Liao went to Zhaoqing to look at Duanxi inkstones. I was tired, so I stayed at home.

Notes

My method of self-therapy: Take a deep breath, slowly, gently, and repeat: "I... am...happy, I am...feeling...better...I am...making...progress..."

My brain is exhausted. I need a break.

I thought I could stop my medication after three or six months and live normally again. I'm sick to death of it. It's enough to try the patience of a saint. I'm *soooo* fed up! I mean it. I'm sick of telling myself ad nauseum that I'm happy and feeling better. Enough is enough.

The treatment is going on forever. After being stuffed to the eyeballs with pills, now they tell me I have "mild obsessive-compulsive disorder." Really? I don't feel like it. Who made up all these psychological tests? I haven't been cured of my depression and now they announce that I'm sick with something else. How am I supposed to be positive? If I have obsessive-compulsive disorder, then everybody else must have it too. Who isn't sick? I don't get it. At all.

I don't believe a word of these psychological tests. Guidelines are set by professionals in other countries, but do they apply to the Chinese? Do psychologists and psychiatrists understand the Chinese mentality, or their political, cultural and historical background? But then again, even if these tests were written by Chinese doctors, I still wouldn't trust them. When is the medical community in China going to pay more attention to mental illnesses? I'm not an expert in such matters, but I can say that they haven't even started. Maybe in 10 years' time? It takes five years to become a general practitioner. What kind of results will 10 years of research yield? Who knows, maybe those who have written these tests are themselves suffering from obsessive-compulsive disorder.

Every time I think of the words "obsessive-compulsive disorder," a sense of outrage hits me. They disgust me! People often say I am easy-going. But that's because my personality has been deformed and remoulded over the years. Since nursery school, I've been forced to never speak my mind and to repress my thoughts. I was afraid of being punished and ostracised. From an early age, I've been forced to hide behind the label "easy-going," a kind of golden protective armour. I made myself wear a "good girl's mask," like at a fancy-dress party. I adapted my thoughts, speech and behaviour according to the situation and my environment. Over the years, I've learnt to modify my personality to fit the circumstances of the moment, for fear I might be considered a bad student. But the truth is, I was the dunce of the class.

Inside me lies a Li Lanni who is suffocating. It's only at night in her dreams that she can slip out to breathe through a crack in the consciousness. This Li Lanni despises the other Li Lanni.

I just remembered a strange dream I had in 1986, which I wrote down upon awakening. At the time, I was studying at the Lu Xun Literary Institute in Beijing. It was the first advanced course on literary conferences held at the Institute. I was in the "junior class" and most of my fellow students in the "senior class" were in their last semester and had already received literary awards. I felt my dream had a meaning but didn't know what. I showed my fellow students of both classes the write-up of my dream, but they weren't interested. Maybe it's because my dream touched on a taboo. For I dreamt I was with a fellow student of the Va ethnic minority. We were both standing on a platform, naked, answering questions.

It's only now that I understand the meaning of this dream. The Li Lanni who is locked up inside wants to come out into the daylight.

At midday, while rummaging around at the bottom of my bookshelf at home in Guangzhou, I found a write-up of a dream I had 20 years ago. It was written in black ink on graph paper that had yellowed with time. It was dated January 1987, but I remember having this dream at the end of 1986 when I was staying at the student accommodation of the Lu Xun Literary Institute. Reading it 20 years later is disconcerting, because it plunges me into a twilight world of half-forgotten memories and I feel I'm drifting between a state of wakefulness and sleep. It was like a sign or message from the Holy Spirit. Looking back, I think this dream was a premonition of the next 20 years of my life to come. It predicted my life plagued by cancer and depression, how I was to lose my sense of self, how ashamed I would be of myself before accepting my vocation as a writer.

It reminds me of the dreams of Baoyu, the main character in the novel *Dream of a Red Chamber*, and the music Shenying Shizhe heard in his dreams.

Regardless of one's level of culture, every Chinese person has the ability to glimpse their destiny through their dreams. Our approach isn't analytical like Freud's, nor is our understanding of the unconscious as sharp and penetrating as those in the western world. We have neglected our mental world. Because we've been too busy.

In recent history, we have suffered humiliations at the hands of external enemies and social upheavals that have destabilised our motherland. Chinese people's priorities are of a pragmatic nature: how to survive, how not to go hungry and how to have male descendants. In this context, a country's destiny is also that of an individual. When a country is at war, divided and torn by popular uprisings, how can we even dare to dream? What right do we have to go exploring our unconscious? A collective isn't endowed with a conscience that can shape the lives of individuals. You have no right to talk about your dreams.

We're at the dawn of a new century and should forge a new chapter in history. We can now penetrate into our dreams, dispel the fogginess and search for the colours and music that are ours.

We shouldn't be afraid to strip bare our minds and bodies and unveil the purity of our souls in all their splendour. We should no longer hide, nor be ashamed of ourselves, nor let ourselves be destroyed. Truth must be told, and we must never force ourselves or others to do otherwise. Love thy neighbour as thyself. Be conscious of your own sense of worth. Respect the individuality of mankind and of life.

Sudden thought: If I were back at the beginning of my first year of primary school, I'd write an essay on my aspiration to be able to dream, review my dreams and analyse them.

May the guardians of my destiny teach me, use me and allow me to perceive in my dreams my premonitions and future destinies. May I have the ability to write down the omens and meanings of my dreams with awe and wonder. Lord, let me become a witness to Your power and love.

15th July 2006

Correlations

"Dreams"

I stood up, stark naked, at the back of the classroom. I wanted to walk up to the platform.

Looking down, I glanced at my body: white. It was dazzlingly white. I was pleased with myself. I walked forward, barefoot. The floor was cold.

Someone was walking next to me. It was a classmate of the Va ethnic minority. She was chubby and had beautiful brown skin.

A bright and glaring light shone from the bottom of the platform.

I had forgotten what I was going to say and was trying hard to remember. I think it had something to do with me being naked.

My classmate knelt down, and the platform hid half of her body. I was feeling weak at the knees and wanted to kneel too.

Standing in front of the blackboard, I couldn't hear what I was saying, nor see what I was writing on the blackboard. I think it was something about the splendour and beauty of the naked body.

How come my classmate was now dressed? Me too, I wanted to cover myself up. I really did. Suddenly, I was wearing a light jacket and was tugging it downwards.

Again, I've forgotten what I was going to say.

A rowdy mob burst into the room.

"They say we'll get an eyeful in here!"

"You're starkers! Have you no shame?"

I was cold and wanted to throw up.

(Here the dream broke off. I only remember darkness and chaos and a terrible feeling of shame.)

Far away I heard orchestral music. The ground I was standing on was slightly sunken.

I had a vague feeling there was some kind of meaning: that I was part of the orchestra, and the person standing on the sunken ground wasn't me. The beautiful girl in the orchestra was me.

I heard soft music. It was me playing a musical instrument.

I thought I saw a silhouette in the distance.

Yellow. Graceful. Svelte.

Was that me?

But who is me?

I am ugly, stupid and dirty, aren't I?

I want to see that yellow colour again!

(The dream became blurred. I wandered through different places, but it was foggy and it annoyed me.)

I heard music coming from the hills. The sound of this soft music had something very special about it.

I walked up the hill. It was crowded on top and people were scattered in clusters of three or five around a fire. I put a chicken wing on a fire to roast and waited patiently for it to cook.

Someone was strumming away clumsily on the guitar and humming an old popular song through his pursed lips. Magic was in the air.

Some were playing a game: "White handkerchief, white handkerchief, throw your white handkerchief behind your friend, don't tell him and catch the handkerchief quick." The white handkerchief flew across the fire like an ectoplasm.

The top of the hill was flat. A building, which resembled a town hall, was under construction there. The first floor had just been completed, but progress was slow. I didn't like the look of the building. I was weaving in and out of the scaffolding poles, which had been painted red.

Suddenly, an enormous machine loomed up over the side of the hill. It was a gigantic Caterpillar truck with glaring lights.

I had completely forgotten why I was there.

I looked around me and wandered off.

Night had fallen. I followed the others and started descending the slope.

A man I didn't know called out to me: "Did you find it?"

It jolted my memory and I remembered why I was there. I quickly turned back.

But the others stopped me.

"It's dark. She was here just now."

They pointed at the fire.

A musical instrument made of yellow paper was burning in the flames of the dying fire. Bits of paper were lying on the glowing embers.

I couldn't find her.

No, I couldn't find her.

Complementary Notes

I believe many people have already had this kind of dream where, like me, they find themselves at an impasse. I told a number of people about my dreams and even showed them the write-ups, but they weren't interested. I never mentioned my dreams again. We're all afraid of being laughed at, of being made to look a fool, and then we complain no one listens to us. Tired and disappointed, we shut up.

THIRTY-TWO

Diary
Monday, 22nd September 2003 10:30 am

I listened to a sermon at the Crystal Cathedral that was broadcasted on *Hour of Power*. There were three types of love discussed:

1. I love, because I want you (desire, etc.).
2. I love, because I need you (marriage, etc.).
3. I love, because you need me (transcendence, spiritual love).

Xiao Lübo went to a science conference where more than 4,000 psychiatrists took part. On the last day, three of them talked about three types of beliefs: faith, hope and love. Hope can give rise to miracles. Love can help us become nobler and overcome failures, and prevent us from falling.

I am glad Li Pingping called me.

I bought a copy of *The Wisdom of Menopause* by Christiane Northrup, a well-known American gynaecologist and president of the American Association of General Practitioners. According to her, having a pet helps us relax.

I cleaned out over 300 viruses from my computer. Not bad.

Notes

My initial plan was to spend the first part of this book talking about the four different generations of women in my family: my great-grandmother, my grandmother, my mother and me.

My intention was to explore the psychological history of these ordinary women from an ordinary family, who were fortunate enough to have received a basic education. They weren't born into the lowest strata of society, nor into a powerful and privileged family. Their stories are like those of thousands of other families in China.

I thought Grandmother would live to be 100 years old. Our family's Chinese doctor, himself getting on in years, used to tell her every time he took her pulse: "Grandma, with this heart of yours beating the way it does, you'll live to 100."

My depression is a motivating force that has prompted me go back in time and explore the mental history of my ancestors. Did they suffer from any psychological disorders? Did my brother and I inherit their mental DNA? How does it affect my brother's children and their children? Is there a link between my depression and genetic transmission? Should I continue to dwell on my painful experiences? How should I live my life?

Early this year, I had a sudden urge to call Grandmother to check some facts with her. But since she can't hear very well on the phone, I planned to visit her in autumn to have a quiet chat with her.

When she was in hospital, I asked my brother to give her a message. He said to her: "Grandmother, you have to wait for Lanni. She's writing a book on you, Mother and Grandfather. She's doing this for you. You have to wait for her."

The first few days after Grandmother was admitted into a nursing home, her pulse was normal. Our Chinese physician said: "Grandma, you'll live to be 100."

Grandmother, I truly believed that you'd live to be 100 and would read this book. I'll hurry up and finish it by the end of the year for it to be published next year. Grandmother, I want to talk about your pain. Grandmother, I always believed that of all the people in our family, you were the most gifted in expressing yourself in writing. But you never had the chance. And I, who never wanted to write and don't have your talent, have become a writer.

Too many thoughts are jostling in my head and my brain has stopped functioning. I don't know where I am anymore. Maybe it's a dream? Who's in this dream? You or me?

16th July 2006

Correlations

Excerpts from *Courtyard of My Childhood Years*

13

"The teacher said we have to write an essay about our family history this week. Father, when are you going to tell us about our family?"

"Ask your mother," replied Father.

He didn't like to talk while he was having his dinner.

"The teacher said that our family status wasn't 'revolutionary soldier' but 'agrarian reformer' because of Grandfather."

My parents glanced at each other, as if they shared a secret.

"Why can't we put down 'revolutionary soldier?'" asked Mother, nibbling on her bread bun. "Your father is a soldier. Tell your teacher…"

"It's because your father is a middle-class peasant," Father interrupted.

Father was lying!

"No, Grandfather is a poor peasant," I insisted, looking at Mother, hoping she'd nod in agreement.

"Your grandfather is a middle-class peasant," she said.

"How come? I don't want to be a middle-class peasant," I shouted, overwhelmed by a sense of shame and anger. "Why did he have to buy land? Why isn't he a poor peasant?"

I was livid. Grandfather was stupid and bad. My parents found it amusing, which infuriated me even more.

"He didn't know there was going to be agrarian reform," said Father.

"I don't want to go to school anymore. I want to be a poor peasant," I wailed, stamping my feet. "All my classmates are poor peasants…"

"Come on, we're going to be late," said Father, slinging my school bag over my shoulder.

"No, I'm not going. Grandfather is a *fat ugly sow*!"

Smack!

It was the first time my father had ever slapped me.

I didn't cry. I was boiling with rage inside, but my body was cold. I was speechless, on the verge of tears.

"What's wrong with you? Why did you hit her?" shouted Mother, rubbing my back.

My eyes were blurred, and my thoughts confused. My throat was dry, and the tip of my tongue was tingling. Cold tears ran down my cheeks.

"I hate Grandfather…" I uttered finally.

My insides were throbbing so much with pain that I couldn't move my head.

"I want to be a poor peasant!"

Father looked away. Holding a bowl of congee between his hands, my brother was looking at me in dismay, the corners of his mouth pulled downwards, as if he was about to cry. Mother wiped my face with a wet towel and led me towards the door.

"Go on, go to school. Say sorry to Father later."

Outside, holding back my tears, I looked up at the trees and told myself: "Smile. You must smile." I forced myself to smile, but the skin on my face felt tight and unnatural.

I was stinging inside.

Father had hit me.

A father's duty is to protect his children. Anybody can hit a child, but a father, never. Instead of taking the road to school, I wandered off to the main street. I walked along the fast lane, hoping someone would run me over with their car. I wanted to end up in hospital, my body wrapped up in bandages. Then I wouldn't have to go to school. But cars were few and far between and the drivers were honking and shouting: "Get out the way!"

Father once said that my brother was fished out of the sea and that I was found on a pile of rubbish. I so wanted this to be true, because then I would no longer be the granddaughter of a middle-class peasant. But inside the camphor wood trunk was my birth certificate on which was written the place, date and hour of my birth, as well as the names of my parents. I so wanted… Grandfather to have found Father in a sorghum field.

14

I could smell the pig's heart, jujube fruits and *danggui*[1] of the medicinal decoction simmering in the pot.

I didn't understand why Mother always frowned when she drank the decoction. I had taken a sip from the bowl and didn't find it too bitter. She would shake her head while eating the pig's heart, two deep wrinkles would appear around her mouth and she would say: "It tastes horrible."

My brother and I watched her drink, and he would say:

"Mother…let me drink it for you."

"No, it's not for little children," she'd say. "It makes them restless."

Mother would add eggs and lean meat to strength the medicinal effects of the decoction. Sometimes she would ask us:

"Do you want to have a taste?"

"No, no. It's for you, because you don't feel well," we would answer, backing away. My brother would screw up his face to show that he disliked the bitter smell.

After the decoction had been boiled twice, my brother and I would eat the leftovers. It was a happy moment for us. Mother would pour the leftovers into a big porcelain bowl. With our chopsticks, we would first pick out the jujube fruits, then the lotus seeds which were soft and had a faintly perfumed taste. But there were too few of them, leaving only a light impression on me. On the other hand, there were lots of *danggui*, which were sweet and tasted strongly of ginseng. The goji berries, cooked to a pulp, were bland. The *huaishan*[2] was hard and tasteless. The *danggui* was bitter and just two or three pieces would make the tip of your tongue tingle.

We ate all that we wanted and left the rest. But we thought the Chinese doctor was mean, because he prescribed too few goji berries.

It was fun being sick.

Mrs Gong poured the hot water into the pot and put more coal into the fire.

"Nizi, have you heard from your father?"

I was distrustful of Mrs Gong, because she was always asking me difficult questions.

It had been two weeks since Father had left. Even Mother didn't know where he was.

"Don't forget: Never say anything to anyone about it," Mother said to me. "If someone asks you, don't answer."

I nodded.

"Nizi, I'm worried your father might have gone to Vietnam. We've sent soldiers there to fight for the Vietnamese, but it's a secret."

Xiao Yuzi's mother came into the kitchen, holding a pot in her hands.

"I don't think so," she said. "People get killed in wars. If we're going to fight in another war, they'd tell the families, wouldn't they?"

"What are you cooking here?" asked Mrs Gong, lifting the lid of the pot. Then, seeing what was inside, she turned pale and exclaimed: "Yuk!"

Xiao Yuzi's mother snatched the lid out of her hands, put the pot in a stainless-steel pan in which she added some water.

"It's a delicacy. It tastes even better with ginseng," she said.

"How did you…but there are several placentas in there."

"Getting hold of them wasn't easy. There's an old nurse who works at the gynaecology ward. She used to be thin as a rake, but after eating this, she's now round and plump and has rosy cheeks like a young girl's. They even asked her to give blood to patients who had operations…"

Mrs Gong covered her mouth with a handkerchief, waving her other hand in front of her, as if to say no.

Complementary Notes

The excerpts above serve to illustrate two things: how family background can have a negative effect on a child; and the psychological impact Xiao Yuzi's mother cooking placentas obtained from abortions has on a child.

I broke a taboo by writing about my family history. We were forbidden to talk about my mother's family. As soon as we moved into the small courtyard, we had to hide the fact that Mother could read and write. It made me very nervous.

At 11 years old, I was a wild and unruly child who knew no limits. Up until I was nine years old, I was proud of my mother who was cultured and educated and sang beautiful songs. But her neurosis set in a year later.

My outer environment, as well as my inner world at home changed. My parents never explained to me why they had disappeared from my life for a year without giving me any news. They never said they loved me. I was in great need of their love, but they never once said to me: "Lanni, Father and Mother love you."

I tried to guess what they were feeling inside by observing their behaviour. But I never trusted them. These two adults had let down a child of 11 years old. I didn't love them and didn't want their love, because they didn't love me. All they cared about was that I didn't make trouble for them.

They never made the effort to create a warm family environment for their children. When there were thunderstorms, they never comforted or protected their children, never held their hands, saying: "Don't be afraid. We're here for you." They never told their children that after a storm, a beautiful rainbow would appear in the sky and that thunderstorms were a part of life.

Xiao Yuzi's mother hit her child over a bar of soap. Almost every week, she was at the wash-house rinsing the placentas, thick and heavy with blood vessels. The water gushed out of the tap, tainting the water of the wash-house red. I didn't understand why adults wanted to have children, nor where children came from.

Gathered around the wash-house, the women said: "Children come from this red bundle." Puzzled, I asked: "It's the flesh of a child?" I kept pestering them to answer my question. Some said yes, others said no. "Is it the flesh of a human being?" I asked. After some thought, they replied: "You can put it that way."

There was only one wash-house in the small courtyard where we washed clothes, dishes and vegetables. There I had my first lessons in life. Without having washed the placenta entirely of its blood, Xiao Yuzi's mother would cut it into small pieces before cooking it.

Seeing there was still blood on the placenta, I asked Mrs Commander in Chief: "Why? Do placentas tonify the body?"

She replied: "Who knows? She wants to eat meat."

In the communal kitchen, every family had their own gas stove where they could put their pots and pans. The kitchen was another place of learning for me. The families would talk and gossip while doing the cooking. One day, Xiao Yuzi's mother left something stewing on the stove that smelt of jujube fruits. The women guessed it was placenta and said it smelt good. They envied Xiao Yuzi's mother for being able to get her hands on the placentas and for having the guts to eat them.

Afterwards, Mrs Gong told the others: "These placentas come from the abortion ward. There are several of them in the pot." I didn't know what an abortion was, but from what the women were saying, I tried to guess what was in the pot and imagined Xiao Yuzi's mother eating the little legs and elbows that were inside the placentas. None of the women said she shouldn't eat them. Only Mrs Commander in Chief said: "How could she eat those things?"

This placenta business was beyond my comprehension and troubled me so much that it remains carved into my memory.

Xiao Yuzi's mother was pretty, except when she smiled, and the corner of her mouth would droop. She was kind to me, smiled at me a lot and never scolded me for no reason. Apart from her always hitting Xiao Yuzi and eating placentas, of all the women residing in the small courtyard, she was one of the saner ones. Her mother, originally from Tianjin, smoked like a chimney. A woman of few words, her eyes were cold and hard. No one knew anything about her. In retrospect, I think these four generations of women – the grandmother, mother, Xiao Yuzi (I don't know if she is still alive), Xiao Lingzi and her daughters – all had serious mental issues.

Among the children of the small courtyard, I wonder who, apart from myself, would remember the tainted red water of the wash-house?

THIRTY-THREE

Diary
Friday, 26th September 2003

Had a lovely evening with the "Chinese Women's Association" yesterday. We had dinner, drank tea and enjoyed the view from the patio of the 27th floor of Hotel Yuanyang.

The Chinese medicine makes me restless. My tongue has a thick yellow coating. Impossible to tonify.

Notes

There's a story behind the "Chinese Women's Association".

Over 10 years ago, at dusk, on the 16th day of the 8th month of the lunar calendar, Zhi Hong, Zhang Mei and I met up at Ququ's place. According to the newspapers, the full moon that night would be exceptionally round and luminous and there wouldn't be another full moon as bright and beautiful as this before the end of the century.

We had planned to go to Baiyun Hill to admire the full moon.

There were four of us, all women. We couldn't get there without a car and the place wasn't safe for unaccompanied women. So we looked for a man with the following criteria: He must own a car, have a driver's licence, be elegant and chivalrous but not annoying.

We made a round of phone calls without finding a single suitable candidate. No luck there.

We joked: "Well, it *is* quite boring, going to admire the full moon with four girls. *And* you have to be a driver and bodyguard. Who in his right mind would want to inflict such a punishment on himself? We're no dainty flowers and certainly no cutesy little birds! Just a bunch of old maids!"

Then someone suggested: "From now on, we'll call ourselves the 'Chinese Women's Association.' We'll get together, go wherever we want and do whatever we want. It's as simple as that." The "Chinese Women's Association" was born.

Looking back, I realise this event played a particular role in my personal development. A woman needs women friends who come from the same social stratum but with different personalities, who support each other.

Specialists advise depression sufferers to turn to their friends for help, be with people with a positive mindset and avoid those who are negative.

During my recovery from depression, talking to my friends from the "Chinese Women's Association" brought me a sense of freedom and helped me forget about my worries.

When I was hospitalised for a surgical intervention in 2000, I remember thinking: "There's no need to tell them I'm stuck in a cancer ward. I don't like people taking time off their busy schedule just to come and comfort me. They're already so tired and stressed out." Then in my mind, I would exaggerate the fatigue my friends would feel and blow it out of all proportion until it left me completely exhausted. In hindsight, my behaviour was somewhat pathological. Maybe it's related to my obsessive-compulsive disorder.

My childhood experiences taught me how to face up to my illnesses and inner pain.

They say elephants who are wounded or are about to die isolate themselves from the herd to either heal or to die. I admire this character trait.

At the age of nine, I felt rootless in this chaotic world. I had no sense of belonging, neither in primary school nor within my own family, nor in the army, nor anywhere else. I felt ashamed and worthless, and like I was wasting people's time. Social situations made me nervous and tense.

Whenever I go through a difficult patch in which I feel psychologically vulnerable, unwell, and anxious, all I want to do is hide in a corner where I'll see nothing, hear nothing, say nothing and do nothing. At moments like these, I'm like a magnet drawing energy from the void around me. It's my only way to be normal again.

When I'm in hospital, seeing other patients in my room receive visitors makes me feel lonely. I think of my friends and start to feel sorry for myself. But my reason comes to the rescue, acting like a software antivirus. A firewall immediately pops up, shielding me against my weakness. I say to myself: "Your friends are busy, they don't have time to come to see you. But it's just as well. You should be happy for them. It means they're doing well in their careers and that they're moving up in society. You should be proud that your friends are so accomplished. Be glad to have such human richness in your life."

Am I being dramatic, comparing my reason to a software antivirus? Isn't it pathological to keep on reassuring myself? I admit, I do have mental issues. I'm broken beyond repair.

Writing is part of my therapy. Li Lanni is under observation.

I just remembered something rather curious. Photos taken of me these last few years are blurred, especially my face. According to a popular belief, those who are near death or should have died but have not yet passed away have within them a mysterious force that prevents their souls from leaving their bodies. Their photographic images are fuzzy, because their physical bodies are still on this earth, but their soul is already wandering in the next world. I think Li Lanni dwells in this dimension. The old me is dying while the new me is coming into being. It follows then that images of me are hazy. We still know so little about life and our universe. Just go with the flow.

I was going to talk about the "Chinese Women's Association" but was sidetracked. Maybe there's a reason for it. All the women in our "Association" are accomplished, complex and determined in the face of adversity.

Correlations

Excerpts from *"Where's Home?"* [1]

A few years ago, I went on a trip to the countryside with Li Lanni. We spent a week together in a fishing village at the foot of the mountains [...] In the country, we had dinner early and would spend most of the evening sitting on the terrace outside the house, enjoying the view of the sea and mountains. At sunset, no more boats could be seen out at sea. From time to time, birds would fly above our heads, heading towards the mountains hazy with mist. One evening, I said to Lanni: "Birds, like us, have a home to return to. I often feel very serene at the end of the day." Lanni said softly: "Often at the end of the day, I feel lost and fearful."

Hidden pain, buried so deep inside, invisible and unspeakable, affects you all your life. With no sense of belonging, Lanni roams aimlessly [...] She uses stark and plain language to describe the feelings that surge from the depths of her being, which quickly dissipate into nothingness.

Her delicate sensitivity. Her unfathomable pain. How much strength would it take for her to heal? Her inner life is rich and tumultuous. It serves her writing well but is detrimental to her health. At times, her smile betrays her fragility, giving a glimpse into her being eroded by despair [...].

Chen Zhihong "A few words on Li Lanni"

Complementary Notes

In 1995, I published a collection of autobiographical essays under the title *Life in Shenzhen*. Zhihong's article was the preface. Its title "Where's Home?" reflects my inner world.

The "Chinese Women's Association" is quite flexible. If you don't have time, you don't turn up; if you have to leave early, you just go. At each gathering, there are at least three or four women and seven or eight at the most. We talk about all sorts of things with openness and candour. Sometimes, we might even give the false impression of bickering amongst ourselves.

"You think if you die, the earth will stop turning. Well, think again. You're not that important."

"No, no. Frankly, if you want to sleep with him, go ahead. Stop being coy."

"Go home and sleep. Get an early retirement. Enjoy."

"It'll teach you."

"Okay, talk. Spit it out. Use me as your garbage bin. Vent your spleen."

"Don't be so stupid. You've made a name for yourself but you're clueless."

At the "Chinese Women's Association," we don't beat about the bush. We talk about anything and everything.

THIRTY-FOUR

Diary
Friday, 10th October 2003 10:50 am

Had a wonderful time during the National Day holidays. Spent it with good friends and the ambience was warm and happy. My energy level was low, but I enjoyed the friendship, sun, sea and good food.

I was worried I wouldn't make it through the holidays because of my depression, but it turned out well. Back in Guangzhou, I slept for two or three days and recovered my strength, and I'm back on my feet again.

Had a nightmare on the night of 29th September. Here's the write-up:

I entered a building that had just been constructed. I was walking, and looking around, I saw a residential building behind the first one. There wasn't a soul in sight. Taking a deserted pathway, I arrived at a village. I said to myself: "That's strange. I never knew there was a village here."

Judging from the behaviour of the villagers and from the style of their clothes, I guessed it was the early 1980s. Was it a place modern society had forgotten? Some middle-aged Hong Kong women were practising martial arts with the villagers.

On the side of the pathway was a stone slab with the words "Lixiang Village" engraved on it. As I was wandering through the village, I came across a huge cemetery with numerous headstones. Further along was a white-bricked one-storey house with black roof tiles and a wooden door. I thought to myself: "Why build a house next to a cemetery? It's creepy."

Out of curiosity, I asked the villagers about the local history. They took me to the village head, an old man. He told me the village had no history. I asked: "Does the village have any historical records?" He said there weren't any.

Night was falling. The expression on the villagers' faces changed and there was a strange look in their eyes. I was scared and wanted to leave, but they stopped me. Alarmed, I wanted to make a run for it and began to walk away quickly. A podgy woman with short hair from Hong Kong ran up to me. She said she knew me, but I didn't know her. She said she wanted to leave with me. Suddenly, she threw herself on top of me, her teeth poised to sink into the veins of my neck. Terrified, I screamed: "A vampire!" I was shouting and fighting her off.

When I woke up, I was shaking like a leaf. It was cold in the hotel room. I prayed: "Lord, grant me peace. Stay by my side." Then Satan left.

What's the meaning of this dream?

Notes

The landscape of this dream seemed so real, far more so than my everyday reality. Because in real life, sometimes I am absent-minded, lost in my daydreams; sometimes I feel so ill that I see and hear nothing. But everything was so clear in my dream. The images, in three dimensions, were sharper than high-definition pictures. My memory and concentration were good; my senses (sight, sound and touch) were heightened; and my brain was functioning with remarkable efficiency. I was in better shape than in real life.

There is a popular belief that people with a weak constitution, who are therefore prone to illnesses, are more likely to attract malevolent spirits. Similar beliefs are found in many mythologies.

I grew up on a military base, so I am not superstitious. But there is something strange about this dream.

Is the universe made up of several dimensions?

Are there parallel worlds in this mysterious universe of ours?

Are there other forms of life inhabiting a world which has a higher frequency than ours?

Research is carried out on paranormal phenomena, parapsychology, premonitions, clairvoyance, and other related sciences. Scientists make new discoveries all the time. As for the earth's energy vortexes, I am not qualified to comment on them. Our knowledge and understanding of science and superstition change from one era to another.

What I wanted to say was that I am not superstitious. In fact, I am against superstitions and hate the way they mess with our minds. But my dream has been troubling me. Maybe my attitude towards the world we live in is immature and ambiguous. I am riddled with doubts and questions. And I am like a pupil who wants to put her hand up to ask a question but is afraid of being laughed at. I want to ask the teacher: "What is superstition? What isn't superstition?"

Lixiang, the name of the village, is troubling. I don't even know if it exists in real life.

The grey stone slab was on the roadside at the entrance of the village. It came up to my waist. The words "Lixiang Village" were engraved in simplified characters and painted in red.

Why was the village called Lixiang? I've never been to such a village in my life and the name doesn't ring a bell.

The hotel I stayed in was on a mountain plateau in peaceful surroundings. It's been open for two years and doesn't take outside clients, which were few and outnumbered by the hotel staff. There were no other villages or buildings in the vicinity. The view was lovely and there was nothing suspicious that caught my eye. But I made no effort to find out about the history or the legends of the region.

It didn't interest me.

The fear I felt in the night dissipated at sunrise. Everything was back to normal again, except for a few brief moments when I felt uneasy. Suddenly, a scene from *Green Snake*, a film directed by Tsui Hark, came into my mind. The actresses Zhang Manyu and Wang Zuxian were in an imaginary Chinese mansion. Another time, a still from the film *Rouge* popped into my mind. The actress Mei Yanfang was looking for her lover, played by Zhang Guorong.

There is nothing to be afraid of.

Look at it this way: There is a world of here and now and a world beyond. From time to time, those of our world go over into the next world and experience new things. And vice-versa; those in the next world come here to take a break.

28th July 2006

Correlations

Excerpts from *For the Love of Life*[1]

Dreams as a universal language

It is a very particular language. It is a universal language that has existed in every historical and cultural milestone of the history of man [...] Every night, we speak in this language.

The language of dreams is made up of symbols [...] Our language is determined by society [...]. When we are asleep, we are free from the constraints of the struggles of our daily lives. No longer do we need to control or defend ourselves, nor to obey others [...] Our unconscious no longer holds any secrets for us. It unveils itself to us in our dreams, revealing what is hidden from us in our waking hours.

Erich Fromm (United States)

Complementary Notes

The truth is, Erich Fromm's *For the Love of Life* has been sitting on my bookshelf for two years. And I haven't read it. I bought it because it was written by him, without having the faintest idea of what it was about. Leafing through it, I came across the passage above.

　Regarding words like "intuition," "feel the Holy Spirit," and "guided by presentiment," I'm going to talk about what happened to me today: Feeling frustrated sitting in front of a blank page, I randomly picked a book from the bookshelf (I don't believe in coincidence). As I was thumbing through it, I came across the sub-title "Dreams as a universal language." That was exactly what I was looking for. But I am ashamed to say that all I read of this book was this one passage. I don't have what it takes to be researcher. I always manage to find excuses not to read books: I don't have time, or I'm too tired. I am too pragmatic and pretentious. I only read books that are useful for my writing. What an imposter. Shut the door. Quick, shut the door. My sick self is slipping out.

THIRTY-FIVE

Diary
Saturday, 11th October 2003 11:20 am

A list of positive things I did during the holidays:

1. *29th September*: Had a very pleasant lunch at the airport with some friends. Chen Hong and I talked about the time when we were working together on the television series *Sea Dwellers*. The others were amused at our stories and anecdotes.
2. *30th September*: Had lunch at the golf club at Lake Guanlan with friends. Our discussion on dreams shed some light on my understanding of depression. Played golf with Huang Yanglüe in the afternoon. I was losing but resorted to my "secret weapon" and won the game. From midnight until 1 am, I was with friends at the open-air swimming pool at the Venice Hotel. We talked and drank Finnish vodka. Some were tipsy, and it was great fun.
3. *1st October*: Went to Qizhigu with friends. Had a good laugh, making silly comments about Huang Yanglüe's parallel sentences.
4. *2nd October*: Went swimming at Jiediao Beach next to the yacht club. It's the first time I bathed in the sea this year.
5. *Morning of 3rd October*: Went net fishing out at sea on a fishing boat. We caught 100 kilos of fish and afterwards had lunch on the beach at Xiyong village. The fishermen prepared the fish, and it was delicious. But the others preferred oven-cooked chicken, a specialty of the region.
6. *Early morning of 5th October*: Took my friends to the airport. Then the members of the Association of Writers of the Provinces of China gave me a lift home to Guangzhou.

Something positive has happened every day. I give thanks to God.

Notes

Took out the garbage.

Yesterday Ququ called to see how I was. I hesitated and then told her I was about to take out the garbage. But the waste containers were full, and I couldn't empty all of the rubbish. Talked to Ququ, which helped release some of the mental pressure, because she is understanding and mentally stable.

I talked about my feelings about Grandmother's death and my depression relapse. I said I didn't want to live to 100, because longevity isn't what it's made out to be. My grandmother didn't die of multiple organ failure, but from the humiliations and hardships she had suffered all her life. I feel so sad for her. Ququ told me not to dwell on it, and that I should go out and see the others from the "Chinese Women's Association."

I know she's right, but I don't want to go out. My unit called me today to say the Association of Writers of the Provinces of China is organising a trip to Xinjiang province and that there were a few places left. I declined. I'm tired and just want some peace.

It's been unbearably hot this year. When temperatures soar in the regions of Changsha and Nanchang (Pingxiang is somewhere between the two), I say to myself: "Lucky that Grandmother isn't here anymore."

Before when temperatures reached 35, 38 or 39 degrees, I'd start to worry. Because I knew it'd be sweltering inside the small hut on the rooftop where Grandmother lived. It was no bigger than a bicycle shed, but uglier and without air conditioning. There were no trees outside where she could cool off in the shade. And there was no wind. Grandmother used to say: "The heat is awful."

When the temperatures dropped to below zero, between minus five or minus seven, or when it was snowing, I'd think of Grandmother. I lived in Pingxiang during my last years of secondary school. One winter, I fell ill after washing my clothes in icy-cold water. If a healthy adolescent couldn't withstand the cold, then how could a frail old woman?

Grandmother had a sad life. But she lived to a ripe old age and had the pulse of someone who is 100 years old. She was hospitalised for cardiac problems and for a heart laden with sorrow.

When the doctor said she could go home, she had nowhere to go. If she had stayed in hospital, she would have had daily injections that cost over 200 yuan a day. All the money she had was what Grandfather had left her. And she refused to spend her savings and the money my mother, brother and I had sent her. When my brother saw her in hospital, she had lost a lot of weight and had sores on her arms. When she was still of this world, people around her were already calculating the best time for her to die: Passing away at the third *geng*[1] at night would be more favourable to her descendants, while she should avoid dying at the fifth *geng*.[2]

Grandmother never had a house of her own.

Grandfather had studied mathematics, so he had limited knowledge of history and philosophy. He also had a poor understanding of human nature. He was oblivious to how the times had changed. Less and less emphasis was being placed on traditional Chinese values: loyalty, filial piety, etiquette, justice, humanity and compassion. He lived in a pivotal period of history where old rules had been destroyed before new rules were laid down. Still guided by his old set of values, he gave his house away to his family, renouncing his rights in the process. Ignoring sound advice, he gave it to those who he thought were more vulnerable than he was, sacrificing his own self-interest and Grandmother's. He was under the illusion that he'd be happy in his old age, but that was not to be.

My grandparents had nowhere to live in town. At 80 years old, they had no other choice but to return to my grandmother's native village. The children of Grandmother's brother offered them a room with an attached kitchen. On many occasions, I asked Grandmother to come and live with me in Guangdong: "Come and live with me in Shenzhen, you'll be a lot more comfortable." But she said: "Do you know the proverb: 'At seventy, never live under someone else's roof; at eighty, never eat at someone else's table?' Thank you for being so thoughtful, but I can't leave my native land. I can't live anywhere else."

In the mid-1990s, I travelled to a meeting in Changsha. As I had some free time, I took a long-distance bus to visit my grandparents. The town of Pingxiang was out of the way, and I had to take a minibus that stopped off at the small villages. The minibus was packed, and the passengers were squeezed in like sardines. We couldn't sit, couldn't stand up properly, and were huddled together, unable to see even the front of the bus. The road was bumpy, and I felt nauseous from being jolted up and down.

Except for an old bed, there was no other furniture, nor electrical appliances at my grandparents' place. There was an earthen oven and kitchen utensils: a big water container and a bamboo ladle that had been used in the countryside a few decades ago, when I was in primary school. The bamboo stool, worn-out and wobbly, was a hazard.

The daughter-in-law of my grandmother's brother often asked her children to help my grandparents by fetching the water at the reservoir and doing manual work.

I came down with acute gastritis in Changsha and was under perfusion at a hospital for an entire day. Feeling better the following morning, I visited my grandparents, but could only stay for one night at Pingxiang, for I had to return to Changsha for the meeting. I was going to ask Grandmother to put me up for the night. When we finished dinner, it was already dark. I was expecting Grandmother to ask me to stay, but instead she said: "I've seen my little granddaughter. Go on, it's time to go back into town." Taken aback, I looked at them as if to say: "Don't you want me to stay?" They looked uncomfortable, and I realised they were embarrassed. "Don't you want to come back to town with me?" I asked. Shaking their heads, they didn't seem to want me to stay much longer. I sensed that they wanted me to leave.

On my way back to Changsha, I felt so disappointed. Even though I was sick, I went to see them, thinking we could spend some time together. But I was wrong. I spent half a day at Pingxiang. When I went back to the secondary school where Grandfather taught and where he taught me physics, a tremendous sadness came over me. They didn't come out to Pingxiang to see me and didn't call either. Back in Guangzhou, still feeling vexed, I said to my brother: "Don't even think of going to Pingxiang. Grandfather and Grandmother have loads of children and grandchildren, they don't care about us."

Today, looking back, I think I was extremely childish.

I often blame myself for not having been more supportive of Grandmother, knowing full well she had a difficult life.

Mother thinks I lack social skills, am naïve and reckless. Worried that I'd upset Grandmother, she put down a rule: We each look after our own mother. She'd take care of Grandmother, and I'd take care of her. Whenever I meddled in her affairs, she'd start having sleeping problems and fall sick. Worried that I'd get into trouble with Mother, Grandmother would tell me to mind my own business.

I sent Grandmother some money, so that she could install an air conditioner at home. But the family at Pingxiang refused to do it, saying it'd cost an arm and a leg to install electric cables. I offered to pay for the whole house to be rewired, but they said no.

On the phone, Grandmother said awkwardly: "Lanni, don't install the air conditioner. I'll give you back the money." I said: "No, Grandmother. Keep the money. I'll install an air conditioner so you won't be so dependent on the rest of the family. You said you could pay the electricity bills, so why shouldn't you have one?" But she didn't even want me to visit her. The hut didn't belong to her and she didn't want to get me into trouble.

It upset me to think of Grandmother enduring the heat and cold in her little hut. But there was nothing I could do. There isn't one ounce of filial piety in me. I bowed down in the face of pressure and pretended to see nothing and to know nothing. I despise Li Lanni.

Ququ asked me on the phone: "Was your grandmother a difficult person? Did they make her go into a nursing home?" It upset me that she asked such a question. I answered: "My grandmother was very kind. She always put other people first. That's why it breaks my heart."

Tropical storm Gaemi brought rain these last two days. The temperature in Guangzhou went down from 37 degrees to 30. But I'm still restless and moody. I need to be alone.

I keep following the weather report for Changsha, I can't help myself. When the temperature drops, I feel relieved, but sad. When the temperature soars, I tell myself that it's a good thing Grandmother isn't suffering anymore, but I still blame myself.

Li Lanni, are you glad your grandmother is dead and that her suffering doesn't weigh on your conscience anymore? Li Lanni, just because your grandmother has gone to heaven doesn't mean you've been let off the hook. How many elderly people are there in Pingxiang, Changsha, Guangdong and elsewhere in the country who are suffering, perhaps much more than your grandmother? Think of them. "When looking after the elderly members of the family, do not forget those who have no family ties with you. When bringing up children of your own, do not forget those who are not of your flesh and blood."[3] How can I not think of others?

Shut the gate. Please. Let my heart rest, or it will be eaten up with sorrow. There was nothing I could do. It's not just me. There are lots of people whose hearts are in the right place but aren't in a position to help. Don't make me think about it anymore. Grief is strangling, killing me. Let me breathe.

Li Lanni, don't be afraid. Finish your book. Because then you can talk about all the children and the elderly people who are in pain. Your voice will be heard. God is listening to you, "[...] till the Spirit is poured on us from on high, and the desert becomes a fertile field [...]"[4]

29th July 2006

Correlations

"Seven Unclean Spirits"

When an impure spirit comes out of a person, it goes through arid places seeking rest and does not find it. Then it says, 'I will return to the house I left.' When it arrives, it finds the house unoccupied, swept clean and put in order. Then it goes and takes with it seven other spirits more wicked than itself, and they go in and live there. And the final condition of that person is worse than the first. That is how it will be with this wicked generation.[5]

Gospel of Matthew, New Testament, Bible

Complementary Notes

When Jesus was teaching a crowd using the parable of the "Seven Unclean Spirits," his disciples asked him why he had chosen this story. Jesus replied: "I chose this parable because they hear not, see not and understand not...But you, you are blessed, for you have eyes that see."

Negative thoughts caused by depression are like these unclean spirits. To drive them out, I resort to different methods: medication + cognitive therapy + religious beliefs + word therapy. I sit quietly, empty my mind, "clean out" my inner wounds, sweep away the dust and worries that have been building up in me for years and let my heart rest. But these unclean spirits mutate, become more resilient and attack me again. They say that in 70 percent of cases, depression can become worse at each relapse. Such was my experience. I repeat to myself: "Let the light enter your heart to fill your whole self with positive thoughts. Do not allow the unclean spirits to take root in you."

The Chinese of today should read the parable of the "Seven Unclean Spirits" and reflect upon the moral of the story.

Why is modern man capable of inflicting so much pain on others?

In the past, even when we did others harm, we knew we would be subject to the laws of karma. We were brought up in accordance with certain ethical and moral values: humanity and the Confucian notion of filial piety; reincarnation of Buddhism; virtue of Taoism; and the love of one's neighbour of Christianity. There were also popular beliefs: divine justice; good will always conquer evil; those who lack virtue will never have descendants; ill-gotten gains will disappear like water; those who do harm to others will meet a violent death. The minds of many generations have been steeped in the simplistic and polarised view of the world as being divided into black and white, good and evil. Today people say: "Root out all forms of superstition." But this would entail rejecting all forms of belief: pagan gods, Buddhism, Confucianism, Allah, Marx, Lenin, Mao Zedong. There would be nothing to believe in. Our hearts would be empty. An empty house open to an unclean spirit, who would invite seven other unclean spirits in. How could we not become evil? With more people becoming increasingly vicious, how could our society not be evil?

Those who have eyes have a duty to see; and those who have ears have a duty to listen. For the future of our children, wake up.

THIRTY-SIX

Diary
Thursday, 23rd October 2003 12:50 pm

I brought a puppy back with me to Shenzhen. I called it Lele. It means joy and happiness.

As I was walking through the Yuanling Gardens on the afternoon of the 18th, I noticed five puppies sleeping under the sun on the lawn beside their owner. They were one month and five days old and slept all the time. Lele was adorable, so I went to the breeder's place to check out the parents, as well as the conditions in which the dogs were raised. The breeder seemed reliable.

I arrived in Guangzhou with Lele on the evening of the 20th and found out how complicated it was to travel in a taxi, express train and the underground. Lele is a bright and lively puppy and we get along well together. He's a gift from God. I am so thankful.

Lele is settling into his new home. He doesn't do his business around the apartment, is clean and well-behaved.

I am not made for life in Shenzhen. Not one week goes by without me having sleeping or digestive problems. Went back to the Cultural Union's office and saw Mr Dong, the new director. New forms of work organisation have produced good results.

I've been on antidepressants for six months now and my condition has clearly improved. I trust in God to pull me through the valley of death.

Notes

Father said: "Some people, as soon as their bellies are full, want to have a dog. Incredible!"

Midday. Dusk.
Beside the trees and lampposts next to the accommodations for the teaching staff. On a lawn in Xiju Gardens.

A little mixed-breed dog, bursting with energy, was running around happily on the lawn. It was a handsome crossbreed between a Pekinese and a white and yellow Papillon Dog. His little pink tongue was sticking out of his mouth, opened in a smile. His big, round, shiny eyes were darting around.

School children were shouting: "Oh, he's so cute! He's adorable! Woof, woof! Come play with me!"

The little dog tried to catch the butterflies that were resting on the flowers, chased the sparrows at the foot of the trees, chewed on blades of grass and marked his territory at the foot of the lampposts. He was racing around like a horse on his little legs and had a red collar with a matching red leash. A woman was running after him, distraught and out of breath.

She wasn't walking her dog, her dog was walking her. From time to time, she'd shout: "Stop, you little rascal! Stop! Sit! Or I'll spank you! You hear me? Stop, you little tyke! I'm angry!"

This little dog is called Zhou Lele.

Zhou is his masters' family name. I called him Lele, in the hope that, like a medical physician, he'd bring joy to those who suffer from depression through his kindness, wisdom and understanding.

He's a joyful little soul. He plays all the time and enjoys himself even more when his mistress is cross with him. Passersby are amused to see a grown woman being dragged along by a little dog of five kilos.

Friends who knew I suffered from depression advised me: "Get a dog. It'll help with your recovery." But I asked myself: "I didn't want to raise children, so how can I have a dog?" However, books that teach you how to cope with depression often say that a pet can benefit those who suffer from depression. As soon as I was strong enough, I would take walks outside. I'd often think how pleasant it would be to be strolling along with a dog and was quite excited by the idea. Dogs often had starring roles in western films. They're loyal, intelligent, obedient, sweet and affectionate.

I said to myself: "Better fewer, but better. Be sure to weigh the pros and the cons before buying one. The dog must be affectionate, honest, clean, easy to maintain, healthy, and one hundred percent obedient. The dog must not have a big appetite, not need a lot of exercise and not smell of dog."

On my way back to Shenzhen, it was by chance that I came across a litter of puppies dozing in the sun. I was reasonable. I didn't want to have any old dog breed, so I took a glance and was about to walk away.

The breeder said the puppies were one month and five or six days old. That meant they would have been born on 11th or 12th September. No, that wouldn't do, it reminded me of terrorists. I was about to leave.

The puppies have not yet been weaned. Eyes closed, they were sound asleep. There were five of them: two males and three females, and they were no bigger than the palm of my hand. Since they all looked the same, there was no way of telling if they were ugly or pretty, nor what they'd look like later on. I wanted to leave.

I stroked one of them. Its fur was so soft. Eyes closed, it took a couple of steps forward, fell on its side and carried on sleeping. In books about dogs, they warn against buying dogs less than two months old, because they won't live long. I caressed each one of the puppies' heads. They were adorable. I left, pleased with myself for having been so sensible. I switched on my internal system of positive thinking and said: "Well done, comrade!"

On my way home later, I had to cross the lawn again. The puppies were still sleeping in the sun. Two of them were white, two were white with black patches, and the last one was white and yellow. Its fur was silky and slightly wavy, whereas the others had short, smooth fur with hair that lay flat. In books, they tell you not to have dogs with wavy fur, because it might be an indication of some kind of illness.

I was indeed very sensible. There was nothing weird-looking about this little bunch of crossbreeds. Their breeder probably didn't love them very much. Go, you'd better leave. But this little one was totally unselfconscious. He was fast asleep, eyes closed, lying on his back, showing off his belly, oblivious to the crowd gathered around him. It reminded me of the story about the poet who "exposed his belly in the eastern chamber." I imagined a youthful Wang Xizhi[1] displaying the same devil-may-care attitude.

Then...I forgot the rest. I vaguely remember paying the dog breeder.

Zhou Lele turned out to be somewhat problematic for someone like me who suffers from depression. When I'm out walking with him, nine times out of ten, I come home at the end of my tether. Scolding him has become a habit. I've never scolded anyone in my life and don't know how to, either. I feel it's beneath me. Even now, I can't for the life of me remember what I said to Lele. I am so fed up when he pulls on his leash that I'd swear at him. Sometimes I'd be so furious that my stomach would hurt. But it's so silly, getting all riled up by a dog...The more I try to laugh it off, the more it gets on my nerves. What's worse is that I can't control my temper.

Li Lanni is afraid of being alone with Zhou Lele at home. When she is tired and doesn't want to play with him, he whines and stares at her, making her nervous. She runs away, would rather hang around bookshops and supermarkets than go home to face Zhou Lele, who understands human nature so well. There is a communication problem between the two.

A word of warning to my fellow depression sufferers: be careful when you choose therapy involving a domestic pet in the hope that it will help you heal. Already in poor health, you spend a large amount of energy coping with your negative thoughts and behaviour. Would you have enough energy to look after a dog?

A descendant of Xiaotao and Lanlan, Li Lanni refuses to perpetuate the faulty genes that are the origin of the mental illnesses prevalent in this family. She made up her mind not to have children. But she is raising Zhou Lele, because she took him home when he was only one month and five days old. In him, she sees the child that is in her.

Zhou Lele brings out the aggressive tendencies that have been suppressed in her. Thanks to her little dog, she has come to see this side of her personality. If she had had children, they would have followed her footsteps into depression. She can't put the blame on her parents, nor her ancestors. Zhou Lele is the mirror in which she sees the hidden and ugly side of herself.

The books also say that dogs can fall into depression and suffer from emotional wounds.

4th August 2006

Correlations

Excerpts from *Seeing Red and Feeling Blue:*
The New Understanding of Mood and Emotion

[...] People who kill and then commit suicide. It is more common than we think [...] and shows that pressure, depression and violence are closely related.

Aggressiveness and depression – red for anger and blue for depression. Whether it is from a logical or intuitive point of view, anger and depression are two sides of the same coin. Violence is an emotion that is turned outwards towards society, which can lead to criminal behaviour. Anger is an emotion turned inwards, towards oneself.

[...] Experiments show that depressed and aggressive children tend to look at the world with hostility. The difference between these two types of children is that depressed children tend to turn the hostility inward towards themselves, whereas aggressive children seek to put the blame on others.

Susan Aldridge (England)

Complementary Notes

The key words in the above passage are: "kill" and "suicide."

Every day we hear stories of murder, assault and suicide in the media: newspapers, magazines, news programmes. Policemen, journalists, teachers and doctors are up to their necks in work. Professionals whose work is in some way related to homicide and suicide are swamped with work: lawyers, judges, firemen, security guards, television presenters, families of murderers and criminals, families of victims and those who committed suicide etc. But the professionals, viewers and readers can see the word "kill" and not understand the mental illness and the moral crisis that underlie this one single word.

When I was a child, I read a story told in the form of a comic strip: A family had built a house and its chimney was next to a heap of straw. All the villagers said the house was beautiful. However, a neighbour complained: "You have to move the chimney to avoid a fire." But the owner of the house ignored the warning. One day, a spark carried by the wind fell onto the heap of straw. It started to burn, and the house caught fire. To thank the villagers who had put out the fire, the owner invited them to dinner. Those who were injured were the guests of honour, but the neighbour was not invited.

The author's sympathy lies with the neighbour. My thoughts on this: If we don't recognise the fact that "pressure, depression and violence are closely related," and if we don't attribute more importance to mental health, then the "peaceful house" our society has built will burn. There is a risk that whichever way the anger and depression turns, inward or outward, it will destroy our society and ourselves. Today in China, we should take precautions to avoid a crisis stemming from mental health issues.

THIRTY-SEVEN

Diary
Monday, 27th October 2003 5:30 pm

Talked to Peng Mingyan on the phone. Was saddened to hear her father is very sick. After I hung up, I prayed for them both. I believe God will help and protect them.

At midday, I went to the Family Policy Centre for an interview with a housekeeper who'd be working for me part-time. Her name is Li. In the morning, she works for a history professor by the name of Jiang and is looking for a second job. She started this afternoon. She'll help me around the house and take care of Lele: feed him, wash his towels, groom him, etc.

God's blessings are everywhere, bringing me comfort.

The Cultural Union called me this afternoon to say that they were organising a dinner tomorrow evening. It would be a get-together for writers to discuss literary creation and other topics.

The weather has cooled. My health has clearly improved, and I'll start to reach out to people again via text messages. Playing with my dog helps alleviate my depression. So impatient to get back to health.

Notes

In the magazine *Cancer Rehabilitation*, they talk about Jung, who thinks that the collective unconscious is composed of different models: mother figure, hero, sage and saviour, etc. By "model" he means the archetype or universal symbol of a person that serves as an ideal figure.

What did the Chinese maternal archetype look like these last thousands of years? Did it change when our feudal society became a modern one? What kind of changes were there?

Xigu's life spanned two centuries. I wonder if her notion of an ideal mother wasn't in conflict with her emotional needs. She never had to experience the psychological wounds of the revolution.

For the women of Xiaotao's, Lanlan's, and Nizi's generations, as well as for those of the following generations, the maternal archetype conflicts with the maternal figure of our society and our consciousness. History created this phenomenon. These women must go through the pain of "mental re-education." The pain lingers on even to this day.

We live in an era when our mental DNA is changing and going through a process of renewal.

Every one of us is responsible for our lives and destiny. We're just links in a chain that constitutes the human race that has existed for millions of years. We must never underestimate the mental illnesses that plague us at this point in history. Because millions and millions of years later, we will be part of the collective unconscious of mankind.

A woman botanist was born in 1908. Even when she was almost 100 years old, she still went to her office at 8 o'clock every morning. According to the newspapers, Hu Xiuying was born into a peasant family in a village in Jiangsu. Her father died when she was four years old. Her ancestors, as well as her mother, a peasant woman, were all illiterate.

Hu Xiuying said: "I lost my father when I was four years old. I lived with my mother, an intelligent and capable woman. She was the most talented woman in the village." Her mother was her saviour and her "lucky charm."

At the age of six, she entered a Protestant primary school. In secondary school, she obtained a scholarship from a Protestant organisation to study at the Jinling Institute of Science and Social Science for Women. When she graduated, she taught and studied at the University of the United Church of Christ at Sichuan and Lingnan University in Guangzhou, accompanied by her mother. After the war of resistance against Japanese occupation, she won a scholarship to Harvard University where she was able to conduct extensive research. She said: "It's a blessing from God. Thanks to the scholarships, I didn't have to spend a single penny."

Xiuying was a contemporary of Xiaotao.

Xiaotao was born in January 1911, also during the Qing dynasty. Their mothers belonged to a generation of women whose lives spanned two centuries. The emperor abdicated, and the imperial Chinese examination system was abolished. Our cultural DNA changed. The "Chinese spirit" changed. The criteria for "real Chinese women" also changed. Poverty changed Xiuying's mother, but not Xigu, Xiaotao's mother.

Xigu had the good fortune to have been unaffected by the social upheavals. The terror, anxiety and despair brought about by the events that took place at the turn of the century could have ripped apart her mental world. But her insensitivity, a defining trait of hers, protected her.

She was lucky enough to have passed away before she reached 80 years old. On a winter's day in the 1950s, when the family was preparing to celebrate the Chinese New Year, she caught cold at her daughter's home and died of cerebral meningitis.

She was fortunate enough to have passed away before the Great Famine and the 10 years of Cultural Revolution. She had a good life.

7th August 2006

Correlations

Excerpts from *The Spirit of the Chinese People*[1]

The real Chinaman, we see now, is a man who lives the life of a man of adult reason with the heart of a child. [...] . Now if the spirit of the Chinese people is a spirit of perpetual youth, the spirit of national immortality, the secret of this immortality is this happy union of soul with intellect. [...] All great men, all men with great intellect, have all always believed in God. Confucius also believed in God, although he seldom spoke of it. [...] This organisation in the State religion of Confucianism in China is—the *school*. The school is the Church of the State religion of Confucius in China. As you know, the same word "*chiao*" in Chinese for religion is also the word for education. In fact, as the Church in China is the school, religion to the Chinese means education, culture. [...]

The serene and blessed mood which enables us *to see into the life of things*: that is imaginative reason, that is the Spirit of the Chinese People.

Gu Hongming

Complementary Notes

It is written in the translation that Gu Hongming was born in 1857 and died in 1928.

Xigu's father was a few years older than him. Gu Hongming was a great master and an overseas Chinese born into a prominent family. He studied abroad in his youth and became a public official in the imperial court of the Qing dynasty. He was a university professor in the early days of the Republic of China. Xigu's father came from a modest background. He had never been to the capital, had never seen a foreigner and never held an official post. He taught the children in his village.

Why am I talking about this? Because Gu Hongming was part of an intellectual elite. He was highly cultured and wrote a book that influenced many generations. Xigu's father was an intellectual of humble origins. He taught in private schools and wrote poetry and essays, but none of his writings survived. Even his own children don't possess any of his writings. They say he wrote beautiful calligraphy, a skill that couldn't be acquired easily.

In the history of China, which goes back 2,500 years, cultural and moral education fell upon schools and families. It is the foundation on which the Chinese spirit was built. Intellectual elites, intellectuals of modest background and cultivated people all agree that the defining characteristics of the Chinese people are profundity, openness, purity and subtlety. They consider the serenity in which they live their lives as a blessing from heaven. They have the intelligence of an adult, while living the life of a child, meaning a highly spiritual life.

This explains the choice Xigu's father made. He was an intellectual of humble origins and lived his life true to the spirit of the Chinese people. If he had lived 100 years later in our materialistic society, he too would have suffered from depression.

THIRTY-EIGHT

Diary
Wednesday, 29th October 2003 11:15 am

Yesterday, around a quarter past midnight, I felt a heaviness in my chest, which kept me awake. So I lay on the couch, wrapped up in a blanket. The tightness and pressure intensified between 4 or 5 and 8 o'clock in the morning. I took some Xinbao[1] pills, which brought some relief. It's like my heartbeat is erratic.

Recently, reading through the Psalms, it struck me how beautiful the verses are. They're so comforting and uplifting. Two days ago, I came across a verse written by King David: "Yes, my soul, find rest in God; my hope comes from him."[2]

Came back to Shenzhen this afternoon. Yesterday evening, Secretary Li and Minister Wang organised a dinner for the writers in the Paris Room of the Yinhu Hotel. Almost all the Bureau members of the Writer's Association were there. The ambience was warm and convivial, creating a positive environment for creative work.

I am tired and lacking in concentration. Still can't get down to do some serious reading and writing. It's God's way of telling me that I should take a break and enjoy life a bit more.

Every day I feel God's love and blessing. There's only one thought on my mind: I am blessed.

Notes

More on the topic of "mother figures."

It's possible that Mrs Commander in Chief, whom I talked about in *Courtyard of My Childhood Years*, awakened in my "collective unconscious" two archetypes that are closely related in me: the mother and the saviour.

In the unconscious mind of a child, the role of an ideal mother is to protect and save her children from danger. Like a mountain you can lean on, she is healthy, plump and buxom, with thick shoulders, solid arms and legs and a straight back. Her hands are soft and warm, as if she held the sun in her palms. She has wide voluptuous hips, a round belly, large curvaceous buttocks, a large face covered with a sheen of sweat. She has a hard look in her eye, a clear voice, black hair and is always bursting with energy. She can easily carry a child in her arms or on her back while doing the cooking. She likes to make bread buns, chicken thighs, candies, padded jackets and bow ties.

Every day, she compliments and encourages her children; she gives them cuddles and kisses. When she is angry, she shouts, hits the table or the door frame with the cane of a feather duster just to frighten the children, so they scamper off. When she disciplines her children, she explains to them why they are being punished. When their sobbing and bawling have reached a fever pitch, she takes them in her arms and says softly: "Don't cry. Mother is punishing you because she loves you and wants you to be good."

When she has time on her hands, she plays hide and seek with her children. Other times, she strokes their heads, sings songs and lullabies and says: "Mother loves you. You're my precious little ones. I love you with all my heart." When her children are sick, she stays by their sides to comfort them: "Mother is here. Mother knows how much you're suffering." When her children are scared and call for their mother, she is immediately by their sides. She hugs them close to her when they are afraid; when it is dark, when there is a storm, when they are bullied; and when they are afraid of monsters and the big bad wolf. She is a mother hen who protects her chicks from the eagle, hiding them under her wings. Ready to fight tooth and nail to save her chicks, she drives the eagle away and her children are saved.

For a child, the father is the sky and the mother is the earth. And the child is the quintessence of the sky and the earth.

I never made the effort to find out what Xiaotao's ideal mother figure would have been.

During the transition from the 19th to the 20th century, the mother-daughter relationship between Xigu and Xiaotao was unclear and ambiguous. This kind of situation is not uncommon. In modern times, school girls looked up to their heroine Qiu Jin[3] – a mother of two children. Their favourite topic of conversation was a western play whose main character is a woman called Nora who left the family home.[4] The spirit of the May Fourth Movement, which changed the entire country, erupted into Xiaotao's world.

Xiaotao felt lost and disorientated. How should she be a woman and mother in this new era? Xigu wasn't the mother figure that she so needed. And she couldn't follow the footsteps of Qiu Jin. The author of the play didn't say what happened to Nora after she left home.

Within her family-in-law's hierarchy, there were her parents-in-law and all the generations that preceded them. As for the generations below them, there were the older and younger brothers and sisters, the uncles and their wives. During the day, she took care of the house: washed the clothes, cooked, gathered the fire wood, gathered grass for the pigs and prepared their food, fed the pigs, chickens and geese. At night she mended the whole family's shoes and clothes by the dim light of the oil lamp.

Xiaotao became a mother at the age of 18. She gave birth to a fragile little girl. It was bad news for a family who had been waiting eagerly for a male heir. She was still unaccustomed to her role as a young mother when the baby died. Would she be able to conceive again? What was the point of staying with the Zhang family? To wait for what? Wait for a divorce? If she left, her family would have lost face and her ancestors would have turned over in their graves. It wasn't until 1933 that she became a mother again. For four long years, she was deprived of everything: children, husband, moral support, hope and love. How did she live through these years of neglect and despair?

She often had nightmares of dead children. Many years later, her daughter, Lanlan, had recurrent nightmares where she saw her child swimming in a river. Suddenly, her child disappeared under the water, and she shouted: "Help! Help!" People jumped into the river, but instead of finding a child, they caught only fish. Beside herself with grief, she screamed: "My child! My child is dead!" She woke up crying.

Many years later, Lanlan's daughter made the choice not to have children. But she too had recurrent nightmares. In her dreams, a car full of children toppled into a drainage canal. All the children died, and their dismembered bodies were strewn all over the ground. Heads, legs and arms were blocking the canal opening. Blood was everywhere, and corpses were piled up one on top of another...

Do we call these "organic wounds?" Would this be an "archetype?"
What is it called then?

12th August 2006

Correlations

Excerpts from the script for *A Hundred Years of China*[5]

1911 - On 10th October of the year of Xinhai of the lunar calendar, the feudal system which had lasted for thousands of years came to an end.

25th October 1915 - The marriage ceremony of Sun Yat-Sen and his secretary took place in Tokyo.

14th November 1919 - In the historic city of Changsha, Zhao Wuzhen, a young woman of 23 years old, committed suicide in a palanquin in protest of her forced marriage.

Twelve days later, Mao Zedong wrote 10 articles in which he severely criticised the feudal system [...]. Five years earlier, this son of a peasant [...] ran away from home in protest of his arranged marriage.

1929 - Wen Xiu, concubine of Emperor Puyi, who had abdicated, announced in a press release that she had asked for a divorce.

Complementary Notes

Given the situation, Xiaotao had no other choice but to give up. During times of crisis, it's your genes that shape your life. She wanted her husband to come back. The Japanese invaded the country, and the family lost all its fortune. Four of her children died. She brought up her grandchildren. She had worked hard all her life, but she was entitled to nothing: neither salary, employment insurance, social aid, social status, compensation, nor respect. She had never experienced the joy and pride of being a woman in a New China. She had lived according to her conscience and her own work ethics and paid good for evil. She taught me this: Love is patience; love never gives up.

THIRTY-NINE

Diary
Thursday, 30th October 2003 11 am

I thank the Lord. "But if he remains silent, who can condemn him?"[1]

Switched on my mobile today and found nine text messages from Shenzhen asking me to return as soon as possible for a literary meeting.

Sunday morning, I watched *Hour of Power*. Reverend Robert A. Schuller gave a sermon on "faith that moves mountains." We must believe that God can move any mountain and unblock any mental obstacle.

1. Patience.

We must learn how wait in today's culture of instant gratification. Be it in the practical or spiritual aspect of our lives, we should go patiently with the flow. Reverend Schuller used the process of photographic development as an example: Before, we had to wait a few days for pictures to be developed... Now, however, with digital cameras, we've lost the habit of waiting. We demand immediate results and gratification. And now we don't even have the time to make ourselves a cup of coffee before going to work in the morning.

2. Perseverance.

With perseverance, we can successfully execute our projects. It is like a farmer who tills the earth, sows the seeds, irrigates the land and put in fertilisers. It takes several days for grass to grow, become abundant and then to dry. We must wait decades before a tree can be cut down to make wooden beams.

3. Prayers.

When human efforts cannot change a situation, prayers can be of assistance to us. Reverend Schuller gave this example: A premature baby girl weighed just over one pound at birth. The doctors said she wouldn't live. She was in an incubator for two months; her parents couldn't touch her, afraid they'd hurt her. They were by her side every day, watching her through the incubator and praying. The baby survived and grew up to be a healthy little girl. When she was five years old, she went to a baseball match with her parents. It rained after the match and the air was cool. Her mother asked her: "Can you smell the cool air?" She replied: "Yes, I can smell God. This is what

I smelt when my head was resting on God's bosom." Her mother then understood that during the two months when she and her husband were watching helplessly over their daughter, she was safe in the protective arms of God.

What a beautiful testimony.

Notes

They say that before children reach the age of one, they are extremely sensitive to their mothers' emotions, and they know the secrets hidden in their mothers' subconscious. If the mother is harbouring suicidal thoughts in her unconscious, then the child's will to live will be diminished, triggering self-destructive tendencies. That was the case for Xiaotao's daughter who died prematurely. Her death liberated Zhang Gongzi.

I borrowed part of the script for the cultural documentary *A Hundred Years of China* and tried to imagine Zhang Gongzi's life in Beijing: "17th August 1928, Qinghua University became Qinghua National University. Luo Jialun was head of the university [...] The 'North Sea' and 'South Central Sea' lakes were opened to the public. The inhabitants of Beiping liked to skate on the frozen lakes. Some were doing figure skating, and the ambience was like that of a western fancy dress party. Students and intellectuals enjoyed this pastime."

Many years later, three characters talk about their lives at the time:

Ni: They say you enjoyed yourself immensely then, spending every weekend at Beihai Gardens…Tell me, what kept you so busy?

Zhang: Er…I was studying.

Tao: He was courting a girl.

Ni: Was she pretty? I heard her father was a public official in Beijing.

Zhang: He was a high ranking official. Ah…

He gave a quick glance at Tao and was silent. Tao said nothing, a hint of scorn in her eyes. They smiled wryly.

Ni: How could she have fancied you? You're not handsome and your face is too long. I don't believe it. Not one bit.

Zhang: Women found me quite attractive then...She would come to the university on the weekends and wait for me. She wanted me to take her out... How could I refuse...

Tao: He wrote to me the first year but stopped after that.

Zhang smiled uncomfortably.

Ni: You could love someone of your own choice. What was it like?

Zhang was about to say something. Tao looked at him, waiting for an answer.

Ni: Forget it. All this was decades ago.

Zhang: Beijing girls are...bold...and...direct...I had my principles, you know...otherwise...I...would have...Well, you didn't write to me either, after a year (*glancing at Tao*).

Tao: I was waiting for you to tell me. I was waiting for that moment when you'd tell me. I wanted to know how you'd tell me (*looking at Zhang*).

Ni: You would have been waiting until you're 100 years old. And you would have lost out.

Tao: If he had said he was leaving me, I would have left. I wasn't afraid. Who knows...I may have been happier...and I wouldn't have been a homemaker all my life.

Zhang: I came back, didn't I?

If I were Zhang Gongzi, I wouldn't have come back.

Pingxiang is a small mining town. At night, the houses are lit up by oil lamps. The latrine is in the pigsty. To do your business, you have to squat down on two wooden planks laid across the pit. The pigs come and nudge their muzzles against you, sniffing at your head, face, arms and thighs. If you aren't careful, you'll fall into the pit. The streets are full of potholes. When you cross the town, the smell of coal sticks to you, and even your snot turns black.

This small town was lightyears away from Beijing.

In 1911, the rules of the university stipulated that a graduate was equivalent to a successful candidate at the imperial examinations. Zhang Gongzi had a promising future: a graduate of Qinghua University, popular with women and living in a society opened to the influence of the West.

If I were Zhang Gongzi, I wouldn't have come hodme.

I could have stayed married. The new generation of women weren't looking for social status. I had a lover in Beijing and a devoted wife at home. Sun Yat-Sen, Chiang Kai-Shek, Xu Zhimo, Guo Moruo et Lu Xun...These famous people were free to pursue their love interests.

It wouldn't have been such a bad thing if Zhang and Tao had divorced. Remarried and living in Beijing, Zhang Gongzi could have worked at a research institute. He would take his morning walks with his birds in a cage, and he would accompany his wife to the opera on the weekend. He lacked the qualities to excel in his career or work in a post sufficiently important to be controlled by the people during the Cultural Revolution. In the 1930s, Xiaotao was a remarkable woman by the standards of a small town like Pingxiang. She would have had many marriage proposals. No matter what line of work she chose, she would have carried it out with competence, humility and dedication. In the 1950s, she could have entered into public service, earned a salary and medical insurance, housing subsidies, a retirement pension, and the right to express her opinions and participate at the International Women's Day symposium. She wouldn't be in hospital at 95 years old, worrying about her life and asking to die by euthanasia.

The last year of university was a turning point for Zhang Gongzi.

Fate came knocking at his door. He was spitting blood and was rushed to the hospital. He was forced to end his studies and return home to recover. This coincided with major family and social upheavals that were happening at the same time: His elder brother was deployed with his troop; his elder sister eloped with her lover to Guizhou; his younger sister was married off; his younger brother left for Yanan with his classmates and died in a car accident on their way to South West National University; and his father died during the Japanese Occupation. His family was broken and ruined; Zhang Gongzi could no longer return to Beijing.

In the autumn of 1933, Xiaotao gave birth to Lanlan. Lanlan's elder and two younger sisters died; a younger brother also died while the family was escaping from the Japanese. Xiaotao mourned the death of her children and buried them. She kept her sanity, thanks to the genes she inherited from Xigu.

This is the story of an ordinary Chinese family. War and social upheavals have erased all traces of any death related to depression.

The "incubation" period for depression in the collective subconscious is longer than for other pathologies. Depression remains dormant for four or five generations before breaking out like lava erupting from a volcano, flowing, spreading and destroying everyone and everything in its path.

It's the universal law of cause and effect.

16th August 2006

Correlations

Excerpts from *Depression: An Undiagnosed Illness*

According to the World Health Organisation, depression gives rise to stress, which is the cause of many illnesses in women. This implies that depression is responsible for a number of illnesses, and even death, in women [...] Illness can be caused by: conflicts in love or marital relationships, infidelity or alcoholism in a partner, loneliness, isolation, disappointment, divorce [...] We have mental "black-outs" [...] Many women use these "black-outs" (they are part of our psychological makeup and are not related to depression) to "forget" about their husbands' infidelities and mistresses. We can also use them to retain the happy memories and escape from our painful experiences [...] In fact, these "black spots" help us to lead happier lives.

Ursula Nuber (Germany)

Complementary Notes

In their old age, Xiaotao and Zhang Gongzi would bicker about who would die first.

Xiaotao's worries: If she were to die before her husband, who would take care of the "old man?" Without her, he wouldn't live for very long. The "old man" was pig-headed but had a soft heart and wouldn't have stood up to being bullied, humiliated or cheated.

Zhang Gongzi's worries: If he died before Xiaotao, people would look down on her and treat her like dirt, because she would have nothing: no retirement pension, medical insurance, social benefit, or home.

After they were reunited, together they lived through major social changes: incessant fighting between warlords, Japanese invasion, Liberation, agrarian reform, the Three-anti Campaign and Five-anti Campaign,[2] the Great Famine, the Anti-Rightist Campaign and the Four Clean-ups Movement.[3] When he was denounced during the Cultural Revolution, he endured so much suffering that he no longer had the will to live. His wife comforted him: "You can't die;" "After the storm comes the calm;" "Don't be scared, I'm here for you." When they were sent to the country to work in the fields, his wife, who was a few months older than him, did his share of the work. When they had no money to buy a new towel, she made one from scraps of cloth. Later, he would say with gratitude: "Without my wife, I would have died years ago."

When Zhang Gongzi died, he left his wife 3,000 yuan in savings. During his final days in hospital, lying in his bed, he would say to Xiaotao: "I don't want to die. If I could live a few years longer, you'd have a better life." He regretted not letting her join the workforce in the 1950s, thinking his monthly salary of 78 yuan would suffice to support Xiaotao all her life.

Many years later, when Xiaotao talked about her "old man" with tears in her eyes, she said: "My old man is gone. My old man is gone." To this day, I can still hear her sigh.

FORTY

Diary
Friday, 31st October 2003 9:56 am

Had a very strange dream in the early hours of the morning. Woke up drained.

In the dream, I met some people, Chinese and foreigners, outside a touristic city I had never been to before. We were heading towards the town gates. There was nothing unusual about the city, except that it looked like the ancient city of Xian with its inner and outer sections. A crowd was gathered in front of the gates. I was only a few feet away from the gates when suddenly there was a series of explosions and bullets started whistling past me. The inner city had been bombed, and there were bodies and blood everywhere. I lay face down on the ground, petrified. I thought I heard someone say they were going to kill everyone inside the city and spare those who were outside. I felt sorry for those inside but breathed a sigh of relief for myself.

Then I was a Jewish woman in the Second World War. Dressed in rags, distraught and depressed, I was on the run, looking for food and a place to hide. People around me kept disappearing and I wondered if they had been sent to a concentration camp or a gas chamber. Then I was out of my mind with worry when I realised that I was running out of medicine. I was afraid to go to a pharmacy, in case I'd be recognised and arrested. But I couldn't go on like this, because I knew vaguely that without my medication, I would die.

Suddenly, I thought: "I'm not Jewish. They can't arrest me. But I've got nothing to prove it." I had to find a way to escape from the city that was occupied by the Nazis. My anxiety began to subside. But when my dog, Lele, woke me up in the morning, I still hadn't found a way out of my predicament.

Still exhausted. My nightmare siphoned all the energy out of me. My head is heavy, and my eyes hurt.

Why did I have a nightmare? I feel fine. Nothing happened yesterday that could have vexed or upset me.

Don't give up. The healing process is slow for your kind of mental pathologies. The process isn't linear, but goes round in spirals, like the whorls of a snail shell. You're bound to regress at some point.

Li Lanni, don't lose hope. To keep on persevering is in itself a victory. You must be strong in the face of challenges. Don't be afraid. Be patient. "Do not be anxious about anything."[1]

Notes

When I woke up, with my eyes still closed, I used cognitive therapy to soothe my nerves. When I have dreams like these, I need to analyse them. My diurnal self is eager to know my nocturnal self.

Maybe the city in my dream was an assembly point for the souls of people suffering from mental illnesses; the corpses inside the city were people who had died because of their mental illness; the Jews who were hunted by the Nazis were people who had fallen prey to depression. Li Lanni, who nearly died, shouted at me to run away as far as possible.

I had to find a way to escape from the city because I was afraid of being sent to a concentration camp or a gas chamber. Terrified and worried sick, I knew I could have been arrested at any moment. I was trapped, but was determined to find a solution.

During the day, I take my medications, read the Bible, practice cognitive therapy, aromatherapy, animal-assisted therapy and food therapy. At night, Li Lanni descends into the valley of her subconscious, attempts to mend her "organic fractures," reinforce her cerebral abilities and hasten the regeneration of her nervous system.

I am fully aware of the following facts: Negative thoughts lead to nightmares; positive thoughts trigger self-help mechanisms. Be confident. The Nazis were barbaric during the Second World War. Better days lie ahead.

22nd *August* 2006

Correlations

"Festival of the Dead"

Grandfather arrived in Guangdong in the winter. His light skin was in stark contrast with the dark complexion of the Cantonese. In truth, he was ghastly pale. His stomach cancer was already at an advanced stage and there was blood in his stools.

I was living in the north side of Guangdong at the time. It snowed that winter. When he saw the snow, Grandfather said:

"Hey little one, let's go back to the northeast in the spring, shall we? Grandfather has sold his house and with the money we can make a few trips there and back."

"But nobody is there anymore. And we don't have a house. Why do you want to go back?" I said.

I fell ill soon after that and spent a few months in a military hospital in Guangzhou.

One night, a few days before the Festival of the Dead, Grandfather came to fetch me at the hospital.

"Come on, let's go," he said. "We said we'd go back home in spring, remember?"

"But will the doctor let me leave?"

"Come on, hurry up. The train is leaving soon."

We hurried to the station. The platform was crowded. Just before boarding the train, I realised that Grandfather had disappeared. The train started to move, and I was running along the platform crying: "Grandfather...Grandfather..."

It was a moonless night. I lay in the darkness, eyes open, feeling numb all over. At dawn, I wrote a letter to my brother, telling him about my dream.

He wrote back saying that Grandfather had passed away the night before.

Following Grandfather's last wishes, Father took his ashes back to the northeast to be buried in a plot of land belonging to the family. Grandfather would not be alone and would no longer be homesick. He was attached to his land and loved his life as a peasant. His soul would never again leave the land he had loved so deeply.

3rd April 1993

Complementary Notes

On the subject of dreams, mental DNA and hereditary genes, I should talk about my father, grandfather and great-grandfather.

Grandfather and I never talked very much. When I was four years old, and again when I was six, my parents and I travelled to the northeast to pay a visit to my father's family. Our stay was short. As I was very young and lacked the intellectual ability to understand, the memories of these two trips are vague. Aside from these two trips, we never returned to Grandfather's native country again.

When we lived in the small courtyard in Foshan, Grandfather stayed with us for two months. When we were on the island of Hainan, he stayed with us for another two months. Then he came to the north of Guangdong. Several days after his arrival, I was admitted into hospital. At the time, I didn't know he was sick and didn't understand what cancer was.

Grandfather was a quiet man. He didn't like to play with my brother and me, preferring to be by himself. We were his only grandchildren. He would smile at our whims and tantrums, but never took much notice of them, gently brushing us aside.

People say he was someone important back home and was much respected by bandits and wealthy families alike. They hated him but couldn't be rid of him.

I often asked him about our family's history. He refused to talk about it when we were living in the small courtyard, because he was wary of the young Red Guards. When we were on the island of Hainan, he lowered his guard and told me about his dream. In his dream, his little sister, Xiaolan, who was dead, came crying to him: "Big brother, I'm cold." The next day, he went to the place where she was cremated and found a bone of hers that had been forgotten. He picked it up and put it in the urn.

Grandfather told me about the fox spirit of his native village.

Intrigued, I asked him if it was a fox with a coat white as snow and if it had nine tails and could transform itself into a beautiful woman. Grandfather shook his head and smiled, reluctant to say more, afraid that I might say something I shouldn't and get us into trouble, for people could have accused us of spreading superstitious beliefs of the bygone feudal world. Once I asked Father:

"People say the influence of shamanism is very strong in the northeast. Is it true that our family believes in the fox spirit?"[2]

"I remember seeing adults interrogate the spirits, but I don't know which ones," Father answered. "They say the fox spirit and the Li family have a history that goes back a long way. She followed the family to the northeast and has been with us ever since. Apparently, she has strong magical powers."

Did the generations before my grandfather also believe in the fox spirit? What kind of dreams did they have? Were their dreams also subject to the laws of DNA? Do these genes undergo changes? If popular culture is prevented from taking root in a society, does it leave footprints in us?

FORTY-ONE

Diary
Saturday, 1st November 2003 11:20 am

Dr Gong said most of the patients at the psychiatric department at the Second Guangzhou Hospital suffer from depression (bipolar disorder included). Other pathologies include: anxiety disorder, obsessive-compulsive disorder (OCD), hypochondria, panic disorder, schizophrenia, somatisation disorder, etc.

People who have bipolar depression are often gifted with excellent writing skills.

Those who have OCD can't stop themselves from washing their hands all the time. They can easily go through a bar of soap, and even when their hands are sore and peeling, they still feel their hands are dirty.

A panic attack has all the symptoms of a heart attack, but the heart rate is normal.

Then there is social anxiety and agoraphobia.

Somatisation disorder is characterised by fatigue and strong anxiety, but biological tests and medical examinations are normal. Some patients aren't given the correct diagnosis, and only two out of 100 receive the appropriate treatment.

An example of schizophrenia: A man had sexual intercourse with a prostitute. After reading an article on AIDS, he thought he was infected. He had HIV tests in several hospitals and all the results came back negative. He refused to believe them and was determined to prove that he was infected.

Some people take a few steps to the left and then to the right, make peculiar gestures a few times over before going through a door.

I'd like to talk about problems related to depression in the form of a television series, but it'll be difficult to produce.

Today, as I was reading the Bible, I came across a verse from Psalms that struck a chord in me and jotted it down straight away: "We went through fire and water, but You brought us to a place of abundance."[1]

This verse reflects my state of mind and the phase I'm going through in my life at this very moment. It speaks for me.

Notes

A few days ago, I attended a meeting at the Yangzhou Hotel. I ate an apple before going to bed. Afterwards, I couldn't stop staring at the knife. My gaze and attention were focused on the point. The knife wasn't in its sheath. I hid the knife at the bottom of a fruit basket, but it was floating in my mind's eye. In the middle of the night, I took it out and, like a sleep walker, walked around the room with it in my hand. Desperate to rid myself of my obsession with the knife, I hid it in a drawer, but in my mind I could see its cold shining blade gleaming in the darkness. It was my OCD acting up again. Thanks to cognitive therapy, I managed to keep a positive state of mind and wasn't spooked by my own behaviour. I had to cover the point of the knife. With a towel? Toilet paper? Or an envelope? I put the knife in a hotel envelope, sealed it and hid it at the bottom of the fruit basket. I stopped thinking about the blade.

When Dr Gong first told me about the obsessions that people with OCD have, I thought it was funny. When the results showed that I had a mild form of OCD, I refused to believe it. What, me? But it's my mother who has severe OCD. The doctor explained that a lot of people have OCD in one form or another. He told me not to think too much about it. Just carry on taking my medication.

I read Pingxiang Secondary School's historical documents. There are two kinds of traditions in this part of the country. The first is the tradition of revolution. When the Aozhou Academy became Pingxiang Secondary School, the students participated more in revolutionary activities. The second tradition is the will to learn. The number of students who left to study abroad rose, as well as those who had earned a place at a top university. I wonder if Zhang Gongzi's father was among those who heard Huang Xing's speeches?[2] Was Huang Xing a revolutionary or an imperialist? When Liu Shaoqi,[3] Li Lisan and Zhang Guotao[4] were at Pingxiang High School, how did the head teacher Zhang view these students? Did he turn a blind eye to what they were doing? Did he expel or issue warnings to students like Zhang Guotao? Or did he secretly help them? We will never know. But one thing is for certain: Zhang, the head teacher, didn't live in an ivory tower surrounded by Chinese Classics. I read that before becoming the town mayor, he had received a new method of education at the end of the Qing dynasty and had studied law and politics in Beijing. He united the old and the new, the right and the left. I wonder what he thought of the Empress Dowager Cixi, the young emperor Puvi, the United League,[5] the Northern Expeditionary Army[6] and the underground resistance. Did he get caught up in the revolutionary fervour? But I think he knew how to protect himself and abstained from siding with the revolutionaries or the counter-revolutionaries.

Zhang Gongzi and Xiaotao belonged to the proletariat. They were ordinary people, fearful, obedient, virtuous and kind. When the revolutionaries were in trouble, Zhang Gongzi bribed the officials to have them freed from prison or have their sentence reduced. Xiaotao travelled some tens of kilometres to visit women in prison and brought them clothes and comforting words.

Lanlan takes after her father. She can't take the hardships of life, likes to study and is incapable of starting a revolution. The irony is that at the age of 16, she left home to join the revolution. According to historical documents: "More than 160 students were on the front line of the revolution." Lanlan was one of them. The school in Pingxiang had a tradition of underground resistance since 1925. She overcame her tendency toward inactivity, a trait she had inherited from her parents, and became a soldier in the Chinese People's Liberation Army.

When Xiaotao was pregnant, she had a serious heart condition and her husband had a stomach illness. Her daughter was already in poor health while in her mother's womb. Her digestive, pulmonary and mental functions were diminished. She joined the army when she was still growing and, as a result, her health declined rapidly.

When Lanlan enrolled in the army, like all the other new recruits, she was told to quickly fill in a form. She was no longer at school, taking her time to finish her exam papers. She didn't understand the meaning of the word "status."

"It means what your family does," someone explained to her.

"I come from a family of teachers," said Lanlan.

"Do you own any lands?"

"Yes," she answered truthfully, remembering the lands her grandmother had owned.

"In that case, you write 'land owner.'"

Without a second thought, Lanlan filled in "land owner" on the form, digging a hole for herself. No, not a hole, a deep, dark well. And she spent the rest of her life climbing out of it. She paid the price of having answered a question with honesty and naivety. Later Lanlan said: "My comrades told me I should never have written 'land owner,' because my father was a teacher. The officials said I couldn't change it, otherwise I would have been accused of lying to the Party and I would have been branded 'reactionary.'" The blood of Zhang Gongzi and Xiaotao ran in her veins. She became sad and despondent. All her life she was prone to depression.

When she was 17 years old, Lanlan was on deployment with the Artistic Regiment. The troop leader gave her a letter, which she then gave to the deputy.

"This letter is for you," the deputy said to her, smiling.

"But I don't know the person who wrote me this letter. Why would someone do a thing like that?" said Lanlan.

Annoyed, the deputy said to the organisation of the Party:

"I've dedicated my life to the army. I didn't get married and I have no descendants. The women soldiers know what their duties are. A teacher who was a comrade or a neighbour of Zhang Gongzi is now the father-in-law of a certain leader. During the sixties of the last century, he was commander of an important military zone. A student became the wife of the head of a division in Ganzhou. Even when there were political changes, no one could touch her."

When she was on deployment, Lanlan used a foot basin as a pot to cook her food in. When she was helping the peasants in the fields, she didn't wear a hat on purpose to make her soft white skin turn dark. She was ashamed of her body, because it wasn't that of a peasant. Every time someone said how delicate she looked, she felt ashamed, upset and worried. She wanted her body, her soul and every gesture of hers to resemble those of a poor peasant and a proletarian.

Lanlan forced herself not to behave like a capitalist, to hide her delicate manners and to not baulk at doing manual work that was strenuous and dirty. But certain traits alien to the working class would slip out of her accidently, like a fox betraying his big bushy tail that it so desperately tries to hide. All her life, she has been forcing herself. All her life, she has never been herself. It is the destiny of a whole generation.

23rd August 2006

Correlations

Excerpts from *On Anxiety:*
How It Takes Root and How You Can Change Yourself [7]

The most common symptoms of obsessive-compulsive disorder (OCD) are: compulsive rituals, obsession with control, mania for cleanliness, isolation, need for perfection...intrusive and repetitive thoughts.

The truth is, every one of our gestures can become compulsive with time. The definition of an obsessive behaviour is the inability to follow our will or beliefs to do or say something. [...]

Behaviour becomes uncontrollable. [...] If we are prevented from doing these compulsive gestures, it could trigger anxiety. [...] It could even cause sadistic or sadomasochistic tendencies.

Verena Kast (Switzerland)

Complementary Notes

The compulsive thoughts and behaviour of Lanlan are discernible in *Courtyard of My Childhood Years*.

Certain descriptions from the excerpt from Verena Kast's book struck a chord in me: mania for cleanliness, obsession with control, intrusive and repetitive thoughts and need for perfection.

These are the psychological footprints the last generation has left on mine.

I'd like to mention as an example an incident that happened recently. My collection of essays *Phoenix in the Rain* had just won the Lu Xun Literature Prize in Guangzhou. Mother said: "I'd like to speak my mind on *Phoenix in the Rain*. It would have been a good book, if you hadn't included *Courtyard of My Childhood Years* in the collection."

Me: What's wrong with it?

Mother: You were critical of me.

Me: You should have read it more closely. There were only a few lines of criticism. I said you were a victim.

Mother: Li Lanni, you're a disgrace!

Mother raised her voice, pointing a finger at me. The tension was palpable. My father, brother and I were stunned.

Me: Okay, okay, I'm a disgrace. But why?

(*in a conciliatory tone*)

Mother: You have a gift for writing, but you write nonsense. You take advantage of the fact that I'm vulnerable and can't defend myself.

Me: How's that? Nonsense?

Mother: You said I put *danggui* in my herbal decoction, but I almost never use *danggui*. I use ginseng.

Trying not to laugh, I glanced at my brother, who was stifling a laugh. Father looked fed up.

Mother: You know my body can't tolerate *danggui*. Li Fanding, don't copy your sister.

Me: Li Fanding, tell me, when we used to eat the leftovers in the decoction, did you see any *danggui*?

Before I could finish, I burst out laughing. Fanding was laughing too but tried not to offend Mother.

Li Fanding: I ate the sweet things first: jujube fruits, *dangshen*[8] and left the bitter stuff...

Me: Since *danggui* is bitter, you only put in a few slices. There were lots of *dangshen* in the leftovers.

I am glad that so far, I don't have symptoms such as "intrusive and repetitive thoughts" or "a need for perfection."

FORTY-TWO

Diary
Monday, 3rd November 2003 10:20 am

Fanding came back safe and sound from Japan. The nanny has left, but it hasn't disrupted his family routine. He sounded relaxed on the phone, so there's no need to worry about him.

Had a nightmare last night. Dreamt that Fanding had asked Mother to organise his wedding celebrations, which were to last for three days. I was annoyed at him for insisting that the reception should be held at home and not in a restaurant. I lent him some money to pay for half of the expenses. While Mother and I were talking, Fanding hid his head under a blanket, pretending to be asleep. He was fleeing from reality, and I was furious. I wasn't tired upon awakening but felt glum and heavy.

I feel worse in my dreams than during my waking hours. It's so annoying. People say I am happy, that I am fulfilled in my family and professional life. But anxiety is so deeply rooted in me that I can't extricate myself from it. It has something to do with my insecurity as a child, my illness and the emotional turmoil I went through during my adolescence.

Today on the satellite television channel Phoenix Television, I watched a program called *Morning News* where they talked about a survey conducted in Singapore: A lot of men have extra-marital affairs after three years of marriage. This is common among white-collar workers who have spent time abroad. In these families, 70 percent of the wives suffer from depression and 30 percent of the children show symptoms of depression.

I suffered severe anxiety in my childhood and youth. If God hadn't saved me, I would have ended my own life. That's for sure. But death wouldn't have solved anything. My soul would have been filled with hatred. Incapable of loving myself and others, my time in this world would have been purposeless and in vain.

We sang hymn number 236 "Moment by Moment" during worship yesterday at the Dongshan Church. I love the following verses:

> *Never a trial that He is not there,*
> *Never a burden that He doth not bear;*
> *Never a sorrow that He doth not share,*
> *Never a teardrop, and never a moan;*
> *Never a weakness that He doth not feel,*

Never a sickness that He cannot heal;
Moment by moment, in woe or in weal,
Jesus, my Saviour, abides with me still.

Lord, these verses speak so truly of what is in my heart.

Notes

Lanlan changed careers. Lanlan got married. Lanlan resigned. Lanlan became a homemaker.

Sitting in the inner courtyard, the women loved to tell children stories. What kind of stories?

Once upon a time... A man was abandoned by his wife. For he had squandered his family's wealth through gambling and his extravagant lifestyle. Someone had put out his eyes and he was reduced to begging on the streets. One day, someone gave him a bowl of noodles, which he wolfed down. At the bottom of the bowl was a strand of hair, which he recognised as belonging to his former wife. He had been begging at her door. Filled with shame and remorse, he jumped into a river.

Once upon a time... A man lived with his daughter, son and second wife. When his second wife gave birth to a son, she no longer wanted her husband's children. One day, the man took his son and daughter to play in a valley far away from their home. Then when they weren't looking, he quietly slipped away. Unable to find their way home, they eventually died of thirst.

Once upon a time... A man, who was a father and husband, was successful at the imperial examinations and became a court official. The emperor gave him his daughter in marriage. The man's wife took their two children to see their father. But the man refused to see them and ordered them to be assassinated. Later, a man of moral virtue by the name of Bao Gong ordered the wicked father to be beheaded. As the saying goes: Better to follow a mother into poverty than to live with a father at the imperial court.

In the courtyard, where the families of the field army lived, every day you would hear stories like these. The army is essentially masculine. A woman's identity is tied to her family. When we use the words "follow" or "belong" in reference to a woman, it shows that her status is inferior to a man's, and this instils a sense of insecurity in her. There is always the shadowy figure of an imaginary enemy lurking in their mental world. Every child who has grown up in that courtyard has heard folk tales of wicked step-mothers.

Once upon a time... There was a step-mother who would get up in the middle of the night. With embroidery needles, she would prick the temples of her husband's child. The child had painful headaches, but the doctors were unable to find the cause. The child died a slow and agonising death.

Once upon a time... There was a wicked step-mother. While the father was away on assignment, she would insert an iron hook into the child's anus and lacerate his intestines. The child died without showing any signs of pain, and the doctors never found the cause of death.

Once upon a time... A father loved the son he had with his second wife more than his daughter from his first marriage. The girl cut off her little brother's penis. Blind with rage, the father hit his daughter and killed her.

This is how suspicion, hate, paranoia and fear, through the medium of folk tales, sow bramble seeds into the children's hearts. These seeds grew, spread and transformed into the nightmares that haunt the lives of many women.

Before changing her career, Lanlan was a performing artist in the army. She was promoted into the army elite. She was thorough, discreet and meticulous. She wrote beautiful Chinese characters and was considered an elite among the elite. She hoped to one day participate in the implementation of a communist society. At the time, people were saying that China would become a communist country in 20 years' time. But this young soldier was so naïve. She led a life of privilege in the army. She was hard-working, and the other soldiers wrote letters to the army's newspaper praising her. When she was sick with her stomach illness, her superiors made special arrangements for her to be treated in a clinic in Tangshan. There she learnt the Forty-Eight Posture *Taichiquan* with a Grand Master. When she was reading in her dormitory, young officers would throw their basketball in her direction to attract her attention. When she did her training in the morning, there would always be an admirer by her side.

One year, 90 percent of the women soldiers were deployed to different parts of China. The sudden and brutal changes that took place during the following years affected her mental balance.

The labourers in the countryside knew at a glance that she wasn't one of them. Her skin was too white, and her voice too soft. She looked frail and delicate; she had a graceful body, long fine arms and legs, and an elegant neck with clear white skin. From her head down to her toes, there was not one part of her that looked like she belonged to the working class. She set about transforming herself. She began to deliberately leave dirt and machine oil stains on her hands and belongings. When she worked outdoors in the summer, she would go bareheaded just to get a tan and have rough and dry skin. When your thoughts become red, the red of communism, then your heart also turns red. Lanlan was lost. If she left the army, overnight her best qualities would become shortcomings. You want to be a Party member? Impossible. To begin with, you don't look like the working class. And you can't even get a tan when you're working outdoors without a hat. And to top it all off, it is written in your file that you come from a family of landowners. Lanlan couldn't stop thinking: I joined the army very young and didn't understand the meaning of the word "status." I made a mistake when I filled out the form. My father was a teacher, so I asked the Party organisation to change my status. But they said: "Your father studied at university, so it means that you come from a well-off, landowning family. Under no circumstances can you change your status now. Your way of thinking is wrong, and you must correct it." Lanlan thought to herself: "I'm such an idiot. At the time, I wrote 'landowner' on the form when, in actual fact, my father is a teacher."

Lanlan has been saying this for the last 50 years and she is still saying it to this day.

The genes of weaklings, specific to intellectuals, run in Lanlan's veins. She wanted to be part of the revolution but lacked the ability to see it through. She had a blind spot: fear of starting a revolution. From a rational point of view, she was all for a revolution. She liked to say: "I joined the army when I was sixteen and was so naïve." She wanted change but spent all her life changing herself. Her life is like a botched gender reassignment surgery. Year after year, month after month, her organs, viscera and Five Organs[1] were being slowly ripped out. Her mind was broken and in need of healing. Change, change, change. She had to keep on changing. She had lost herself and was nowhere to be found. Like someone who has been mutilated and shattered. Reason and emotion had shut each other out. Mind and body were in perpetual conflict. Her pride and her intrinsic self loathed each other. She was condemned forever to live a life of mental pain, without hope of ever healing or finding peace.

12th September 2006

Correlations

Excerpts from *Courtyard of My Childhood Years*

17

"Tomorrow there'll be a school meeting and a struggle session. You've been tasked with bringing the person up to the platform."

My heart was beating away at the thought of this privilege that had been given to me.

"Do you want to know who it is? It's your teacher."

I exchanged a glance with the deputy leader of my team. She had huge eyes, and when she widened them, they would make her face look inhuman.

And when she was surprised, her thick lips would curl back like sheets of rubber.

"In class, she quoted an ancient proverb several times: 'An inch of time is an inch of gold, but an inch of time cannot be purchased for an inch of gold.' She's a capitalist."

Supervisor Zhang's hair had turned white. But no one knew if it was from old age or from illness. There were people at Mother Hu's house, watching from the windows. Mother Hu and Xiao Ling waved at me. Regaining my composure, I said to myself: "Stand up straight and tuck in your tummy. Mother Hu always says that young girls who walk with a slouch are ugly."

Mother didn't come. She disliked struggle sessions, especially when students criticised the teachers. Because when my maternal grandfather was a biology teacher at Pingxiang High School in Jiangsu, he was denounced and beaten by his students. They stamped on his feet, which suffered irreparable damage.

Our teacher, Mrs Liu, looked up now and then, probably out of fatigue. Our deputy leader ran up to her and pressed her hand down on her head. Excited, she turned round and winked at me. I was impatient for my turn to do the same. Suddenly, the crowd began chanting: "Bow your head, confess your crimes! Bow your head, confess your crimes!" Terrified, I could only see a sea of eyes, mouths and faces in front of me. My heart was empty like a school satchel that I wanted to stuff with whatever object I could find.

"Go on, it's your turn," the deputy leader said in a hushed voice and kicked me lightly. "Her hair is oily, and my hands are all sticky."

I touched Mrs Liu's head of grey hair, but I was small and couldn't reach the top of her head. She bent forward slightly for my sake. My hands were greasy and had a sickly smell. It felt as if there was a film of oil on my skin that would be impossible to scrape off, even with a knife. My hands had an allergic reaction, and my palms turned red. They were itching, as if countless ants were crawling all over them. I suddenly remembered the time when I touched some poison ivy in a forest long ago.

I no longer wanted to be the deputy leader of my team. I just wanted to run from the scene and hide in a corner.

Complementary Notes

In the three years that we lived in the small courtyard, Mother was full of worries. She had resigned from her job and become a homemaker. My maternal grandparents, who were denounced in Pingxiang, almost died. Through a stroke of luck, they were sent to the countryside to work in the fields. My father, who was part of the "left wing" and extremely busy, was often absent from our home.

Before the incident in the excerpt above took place, I would often hear stories about couples divorcing. The person who had a low political status was always in the wrong. The ability to obey orders is essential in a soldier. And if his or her work involved dealing with state secrets and the spouse came from a landowning or capitalist background, then the spouse would invariably be driven from their home. Many families were destroyed this way.

For three years, Mother pretended to be illiterate.

She lived with the sword of Damocles hanging over her head, terrified that the neighbours would find out the truth about her family background. She never mentioned her parents and they never wrote to each other. She knew that her father lacked the physical strength to work in the fields, because of his age. He had rectal bleeding and suffered from severe anaemia as a result. Blood would run down his legs and into the soil. Mother was worried sick. She didn't want to get my father in trouble but couldn't abandon her parents. Twice, she secretly sent them parcels from another village and spent the next few days worrying that someone might find out and conduct an enquiry.

It was around this period when her neurosis began to develop.

All day long, she would clean the chairs, floor and windows. She scrubbed the mat until it was in tatters; she scrubbed the window frames until the paint came off. When she disciplined my brother and me, she made sure all the windows were closed, so that no one could see or hear us. At the time, my little brother was only five or six years old, but he was already wise to her ways. She only needed to throw a glance at the windows and he would shut them, put the latch down and draw the curtains, not letting a single shred of light through.

My brother and I were a bundle of nerves. We were petrified at the thought of unintentionally revealing Mother's secret. Children aren't always careful of what they say. Once I blurted out something I shouldn't have, and afterwards I was so scared that the houses and trees around me seemed to swell up. My eyes were like magnifying glasses that amplified everything in my vision. I wanted to disappear from the face of this Earth. For days after that, I was sick with worry, wishing my words could be devoured by the air. I would be on the lookout for any suspicious movements, expecting a disaster to fall on my head.

Every day I thought about how, if someone found out Mother came from a landowning class and Father divorced her as a result, my brother and I would then be forced to choose between our parents. Who would I choose? If I stayed with Father, my future step-mother might try to poison me. But if I stayed with Mother, I might be reduced to poverty and live as a beggar. With no work and no roof over our heads, would Mother try to poison me? I had a bad feeling about this, and every day I would watch out for the slightest change in Mother's moods. Our parents were unable to provide us with a sense of security. Our inquisitive neighbours could easily discover Mother's secret.

Sometimes I felt as if I were a spy, and at other times, an underground agent. I was 11 years old and unruly and rebellious. Mother thought I was a landmine that could explode at any moment.

In primary school, I was the only pupil among my classmates to become the deputy leader of our team. And I was tasked by the propaganda team to escort a teacher, who had been denounced, into "prison." Even Mother was wary of me, saying I was a wolf in the making. But what she didn't know was that I was even more troubled and uneasy than she was. I puzzled over why I had been nominated deputy leader. Even though it was nothing more than a title, my classmates considered my "public official" status superior to that of a teacher. I had never tried to win over my classmates, nor denounced them, nor took any credit for myself. I was neither a class delegate, nor a Little Red Guard, and yet this heavy responsibility fell on my shoulders. I was both happy and wary of my new role. My mother's family were landowners. How could I have become deputy team leader during the Cultural Revolution? Shouldn't I tell the truth? My teacher was denounced publicly. But the ancient proverb that she quoted, Mother said it often too. It was part of our education. "An inch of time is an inch of gold, but an inch of time cannot be purchased for an inch of gold." Grandfather said it too. And yet, the proverb was poison. But I liked it and it was easy to remember. I lived in constant fear that my classmates would denounce me one day. I was like a fox that was trying hard to hide its tail and failing miserably. From time to time, I would feel my coccyx to see if my tail was sticking out. Was I a fox in human disguise?

At the age of 11, I already felt old. I was full of worries but couldn't talk to my parents about them. I didn't know if my mother was good or wicked, because she had moods like my maternal landowning grandmother. She poisoned me with ideas from the feudal age. She said young girls should sit up straight; she forbade me from wearing pretty dresses, visiting my friends and eating my bowl of rice at the front door. I didn't trust my father either. I was convinced that if he were to divorce Mother, he would remarry soon afterwards. Even at eight years old, I could see from the look in the other women's eyes that they liked him. As I was just a child, these women ignored me most of the time. I could tell from the way they talked that they fancied him. Every time there was a woman who talked to my father with a twinkle in her eye, I would hang around on purpose, playing by myself. The more they didn't want me to hear their conversation, the more of a nuisance I became. The fact is, from an early age, girls have an intuition about these kinds of things. At two or three years old, their "collective subconscious" is capable of sounding the alarm: the Big Bad Wolf is here! They would throw a tantrum. Even if they aren't fully conscious of what they are doing, their initial instinct is to chase away the Big Bad Wolf.

All the stories of wicked step-mothers have instilled in me a natural distrust of fathers. Without exception, they all stand by and let the step-mothers torture their children. The weaker ones close their eyes and cover their ears, so as not to see or hear their children being tortured. The crueller ones even give the step-mothers a helping hand to tie up the children, duct-tape their mouths, blindfold them before torturing them to death with needles and steel wires.

When we lived in the small courtyard, I would often wonder if Father was capable of killing my brother and me. The neighbours used to say that when the mother dies, even the best of fathers change and only love the step-mother's children. I believed every word they said. When Mother gave us a hiding, I never dared to run away. For if she dropped dead from anger, a step-mother would come and take her place. And I knew that she would hit me harder than my own mother. But a child who doesn't run away when she gets a good hiding is unnatural. Without a doubt, she will fall sick when she reaches adulthood.

FORTY-THREE

Diary
Tuesday, 4th November 2003 10:50 am

I've been dreaming excessively for the last few nights.

Last night, I heard a shrill voice in my dream calling me: "Lanni!" I shouted back: "Hey!" My brain felt as if it had received an electric shock. In my sleep, I was aware that I was dreaming. I felt disoriented and my body couldn't move, but my mind was awake and I was looking around me, wondering who it could have been. It sounded like Luo Jianlin's voice, but I wasn't sure. Could it have been a stranger? Then I suddenly realised that it could have been me. I've been feeling so lost all these years that I no longer recognise myself, my body, nor my intrinsic self.

It's like I've been sleeping for a long, long time and my soul is sick, plunged into a state of unconsciousness. My body is on autopilot, weak and quivering like a thin sheet of paper, bereft of any creative energy. Did the light of the Holy Spirit shine on my soul last night? Did my soul reveal itself to me? Am I going to wake up? Is my soul going to rouse from its slumber?

I'm seeing the doctor this week. I keep telling myself not to lower the dose of my medication too drastically to avoid any secondary effects. Twenty percent of those who suffer from depression end up committing suicide. For some of them, it's because the dosage of their medication is wrong. Antidepressants have severe side effects. If I hadn't survived chemotherapy, I would have given up long ago.

At a senior control committee meeting a few days ago, I was talking to Cheng Wenchao about the side effects of chemotherapy drugs. He said they made him feel dizzy and that he had trouble reading and writing. It just goes to show that I didn't simply lack willpower at the time. Cheng also said that he had mouth ulcers, and I said I had them too.

Listening to other patients talk about their experience of surgery, chemotherapy, medication and symptoms, I realise that my experience was more traumatic.

It's a shame that I couldn't talk more about my ordeal or complain more about my physical and mental pain. I am afraid of becoming like all these doctors and nurses who are so used to death and suffering that they have become immune, and are incapable of feeling compassion. Medical staff members lack a direct and first-hand experience of illness and pain. When I talk to other patients, they find comfort and moral support in knowing that I've also been through the pain and that they aren't alone in their misfortune.

Today, we enjoy higher life expectancies. Take Song Meiling for example: she lived to 106 years old and her life spanned three centuries. There is a popular saying: "At forty we become lucid; at fifty, we know our destiny."[1] But I don't agree with that, because the explosion of knowledge taking place in the 20th century has changed people's lives. There are now too many things to learn, too many challenges to face and too many things to change...

Do we really become more lucid at 40? Do we know our destiny at 50? But it's exactly at this stage in our lives that, for better or for worse, we're struggling to shape our destiny. We should stay calm and level-headed, make life simple for ourselves, learn how to let go and accept that in life you must lose something to gain something. In short, I will quote a verse from the Bible which sums up my personal experience: "[...] Knowledge of the Holy One is understanding."[2]

Notes

I heard someone calling me several times in my dream. I felt restless and ill at ease. When I woke up, I had chest pains and goose bumps, and my scalp was tingling. I felt disoriented, as if my mind had been driven out of my body and wouldn't be coming back for a long while.

An incident in my childhood comes to mind. We were at our maternal grandparents' home. The heat was stifling that day. My little brother, who was two at the time, was lying in the shade on a rock by the Wanggong Lake, bare-bellied and fast asleep. A troublemaker a few years his senior who lived in the neighbourhood decided to play a trick on him. Pretending to be a Taoist priest, he mumbled a prayer, stamped his feet, pointed a finger at my brother's forehead and spat out a mouthful of "holy water." My brother was frightened out of his wits and fell ill a few days later. The elders of the village call this "driving the soul out of the body by fright." And if the soul cannot be called back into the body, then the person will die soon after. Following the custom, my grandmother walked around the lake several nights in a row, calling out for my brother's soul. My memory of this incident remains vivid to this day.

It was dark. I remember the reflections in the water, the smell of fish and the serpentine pathway winding around the lake. Holding my brother in her arms, Grandmother was walking and shouting at the top of her voice: "Fanding, come back!" From time to time, she would make me call out. The pathway was barely visible. Tripping along behind her, my eyes on her back, I found it difficult to stay on the pathway and shout at the same time. Grandmother, gently patting my brother on his back, said to him: "*Laigu* (the name for young boys in the regional dialect), you must shout 'I'm coming back.'" My brother's head was slumped at the base of her neck. He had a fever and was only half-conscious, but he made an effort to call for my grandmother's sake. Strangely, my brother recovered two days later. To soothe his soul, we walked around the lake shouting for two or three more nights.

The superstitious element of this story aside, from a psychiatric point of view, we have all had similar experiences in which, after a shock or a fright, our minds are confused due to a decrease in the activity of neurotransmitters in our brains. What the popular belief calls "calling back the soul" is in fact a therapeutic method to restore inner peace.

I don't know when I lost my soul. I have no proof to show how it could have been lost. Who can recover it for me? What can I do to make it return?

13th September 2006

Correlations

Excerpts from *Courtyard of My Childhood Years*

24

Father was sick and spent two weeks in bed. The doctor said he had high blood pressure. One day, when he was back on his feet again, he said: "Come on, let's have breakfast outside." That was the first time our family ate in a restaurant.

The fish congee was delicious. The slices of fish, white, boneless and slightly curled at the edges, melted in our mouths. The texture of the congee was fine and smooth. Sprinkled with spring onions that were as green as jade, it gave off a delicate aroma of perfumed rice and fish. My brother ordered a bowl of plain congee to share between us. It had been simmering for such a long time that it was white and creamy like milk. A pinch of salt enhanced its flavour. There was a bottle of salt on the table and we could help ourselves with no extra charge. My brother put in a pinch of salt and then another until the taste was salty and spoilt.

That day, Mother bought my brother and I each an umbrella. Father gave me a *Xinhua Dictionary* and my brother a copy of the comic strip book *The Battle of Weihu Mountain*.

The regional grocery store was filled with porcelain ornaments. I took a liking to a white porcelain bird. Its body was hollow, and you could make it sing by filling it with water and blowing into a hole beneath its tail. Afraid to say that I wanted it, I pointed it out to my parents. To my surprise, Father told me to buy it and Mother even said to buy two.

I remember a story I read in a book: A family lived in great poverty. Unable to feed his family, the father bought some arsenic. He then took his family to a restaurant, and after a copious meal, the whole family swallowed the poison and died.

Had Father been discharged from the army? Were my parents going to divorce?

"Let's get some ice cream for the children," Mother said, stopping in front of an ice-cream parlour.

Father bought four portions of milk ice cream and two scoops of red bean sorbet. Afraid that he might put poison in the ice-cream, my eyes watched his every move. I didn't want to be poisoned.

Autumn was coming to an end, and the ice cream parlour was empty. I was playing around with my ice cream, softening it with a red plastic stick. I had never tasted ice cream before but was unimpressed. My heart felt as if it was slowly climbing upwards towards my ears, where it wanted to hide. It was shrinking, becoming tighter and tighter, like a ball of red hot iron.

"We're going to move. We're going to live on the island of Hainan," Father announced. "There's a Military Youth Division for construction and production over there. A lot of people are working on the rubber plantations."

I closed my eyes. The cold from the ice cream was hurting my eyes, its coolness penetrating deep into my heart.

"We'll be surrounded by the sea," Father continued. "Life over there will be harsher than working in the fields. Brace yourselves for a tough life ahead. Lanni will learn how to fetch water from the well, and as for your little brother, he'll learn to collect firewood in the mountains. There're no electric lights at night, only oil lamps. And there probably won't be any green vegetables to eat, just plain rice with soya sauce."

"I love soya sauce rice with a bit of pork fat," exclaimed my brother gaily. "Can we buy pork fat down there?"

"Father, did you do something wrong?" I asked softly.

"Nonsense," Mother said, glaring at me. "A lot of Father's colleagues have gone down there. It's a position of trust."

"But I like it here," I said. "You can go, give me a bit of money and leave me here. I can take care of myself."

"How can I leave you here?" Mother retorted. "You have to follow your social account. Who will give you authorisation to stay here? Even your school won't take you in."

Father lowered his eyes and started playing with his ice cream with the plastic stick.

"Father, why are we always moving? How many times has it been?" my brother asked. He had finished his ice cream and was now worrying about our imminent departure.

"That's enough, no more questions," Mother said impatiently. "Lanni will leave school next week to help me pack."

Then she gave my brother and me 50 cents each.

"Here's some money. Lanni, take your brother shopping. Buy whatever you want, and we'll count the money tonight to see how much you have left."

Father made an impatient gesture with his hand.

"Off you go, don't bother with counting the money," he said. "Just don't spend all your money on food, get some souvenirs. Who knows, maybe we'll never come back to the city."

Complementary Notes

At a meeting some time ago in Meizhou, I was talking to Jia Zhaojun and Meng Fanhua about depression. Jia Zhaojun said that the "virus" of mental illness and depression was spreading like influenza. Books on this subject talk about "hereditary genes," "biological flaws" and "mental black spots," etc. But it was the first time I had heard of the notion of a "mental illness virus." Come to think of it, depression does seem to be transmitted in the same way as influenza. For depression can be passed on, and it spreads and undergoes mutations like the influenza virus, SARS or the bird flu. It happens within the same family, be it big or small.

An Irish writer suffering depression once referenced Jung, saying that our brains are all connected to the collective unconscious that has developed over many centuries. Each individuals' thoughts are influenced by those of the human race's "central brain." Speaking of the therapy Jung underwent for his depression, he put forward the hypothesis that Jung would have found a way to cure depression if only he'd tried to gain a deeper understanding of his own.[3] But I don't think Jung could have gained an in-depth knowledge of himself. I am convinced that my brain is connected to the collective thoughts of the human race and that I am, directly or indirectly, influenced by the "mental genes" of my ancestors.

In hindsight, I realise that during the period when we lived in the small courtyard, I gave the impression of being a wild and unruly child. I was always climbing up walls and trees and was constantly caught up in fights. I was a little terror and didn't behave like a girl. The truth is, the "mental illness virus" that my mother and her mother's mother had passed onto me was beginning its process of contamination inside me. It was destroying my physical and mental health. My natural instinct for survival triggered my mental immune system, which attempted to prevent the "virus" from spreading. In the struggle between the attacker and the defender that ensued, the neurotic person that I became was born.

On one hand, this child had only been in primary school for a year and lacked culture, knowledge, education and discipline. Her brain hadn't had sufficient stimulation. But on the other, her psyche had already been contaminated by a "virus" and her defence mechanism had become abnormally over-active as a result. She felt that she was in danger within her own family. An unusual look between her parents; casual words spoken by the neighbours; rumours and gossip, half-finished sentences carried by the wind; paper rustling on the ground; she analysed all this with an excessive attention to detail. Unable to withstand the inner tension that this generated, and with nowhere to release the pressure building up inside, she became unruly, disruptive and rebellious in order to attract attention.

During the time when she lived in the small courtyard, she took to seeing death and destruction in everything. She only heard the bad and threatening things. And her memory recorded only what was grey and black.

This is the destiny of not just one child, but of a whole generation.

It is the spiritual desert that an entire race of people must cross.

FORTY-FOUR

Diary
Wednesday, 5th November 2003 11:20 am

Tired to my bones and bogged down with worries. Had an absurd dream. Down in the dumps when I woke up. Maybe I am just being ridiculous.

I was inside a bank, standing at a window, counting a wad of 50 yuan notes that I had just withdrawn from my account. When I came to the last one, I noticed that it was torn into two halves with zigzag edges at three-fifths of the length of the note. I showed it to the clerk, a plump middle-aged woman, and asked to change it for another one. But she refused.

"It wasn't torn when I gave it to you just now," she said.

"I didn't realise until I was counting it," I said. "It wasn't me. Anyway, you're supposed to take back damaged bills."

"We don't take them back under such circumstances. You can file a complaint with the director when he comes back."

Not wanting to cause trouble, I asked her for some Sellotape to stick the note back together.

"I don't have any," she said. "And anyway, it won't do much good."

"Yes, it will. I'll show you. It's easy."

I was lining the two halves up when a gust of wind blew them away. In trying to catch them, I tore them into small pieces. An old man at the next counter stepped over beside me and started to arrange them into a Chinese paper cutting. I panicked and shouted at him, saying it was rude not to queue up. But he was coarse and vulgar and shouted over my voice. At a loss as to what to do, I left the bank and sat down on the lawn, where I carried on piecing the bank note back together. Suddenly the bank note blew up into a red paper cutting the size of a towel, making it almost impossible to stick the pieces together. As if under a spell, the more difficult the task was, the more obsessed I became. I was worn out by my struggle against goodness knows what. Fatso from the bank came over to see me when she finished work. She watched curiously as I tried to stick the pieces together. She admired and pitied me at the same time and offered to give me a hand. As if driven by insanity, I couldn't stop.

What a waste of energy.

When I woke up in the morning and realised it was just a dream and that there were no torn bank notes to piece together, I breathed a sigh of relief. In my slumber, I was telling myself how reassuring it was to wake up, but, lying in my bed, I couldn't come out of my somnolence. Worn out by my dream and unable to move or get up, I scolded myself: "I'm so stupid. I'm not a greedy person, so why did I behave like that in my dream? What was I thinking?"

I'm sitting at the computer. My mind is clear, and I wonder: Is there some kind of symbolism in my dream?

In real life, I sometimes can't help behaving stupidly and doing mindless things that make no sense. At first, I'm not aware that I am being idiotic or that I'm wasting my own time. But then, everyone does senseless things from time to time. When we're stuck in a quandary, we mustn't panic, but stay calm and lucid to have a clearer perspective of the situation and work out whether or not it's worth wasting our energy on it.

Thinking about my dream and my past, I realise that I often waste my own time and energy. I am so stupid. Let me remember this dream, so that I will never again do pointless things like sticking a bank note back together.

Notes

As I was analysing my dream in my diary, I realised that I barely know the real Li Lanni. Maybe the torn bank note is you, mutilated and in shreds. It's your mental world and your life. You are broken and want to heal. It pains you that you've been reduced to a human wreck. And this business about the bank note... You think you're blameless and that it's the bank's fault, the system and its refusal to change the note. You resent the bank because you couldn't assert your rights and regain your dignity, ending up having to put the bank note back together yourself.

In your illness, you began to take antidepressants and keep a diary. It's your way of piecing together a broken Li Lanni. But no matter how hard you try, you'll always be broken.

Your impatience wears you out. There's no hurry.

Li Lanni, I've already told you not to force yourself. It's your OCD acting up again. You are trapped in your own mental blockage.

Even though the bank note was torn, it had lost none of its value. Although the clerk refused to help you, it didn't mean the system itself didn't accept or recognise you.

Find peace within yourself and learn to bide your time. Have confidence in yourself and in the system. "Don't be afraid; just believe."[1]

I know you have faith, but it's not strong enough. That's why the truth, which you dare not face, appeared in your dreams. Your soul is suffering.

Remember this old saying: "A wounded reed does not break; a fading light does not die."

14th September 2006

Correlations

Excerpts from *Courtyard of My Childhood Years*

Three boys came out running. They had something hard and bulky hidden beneath their military uniforms.

"I couldn't find the copper wire. I don't know if there's an electric current or not, but I couldn't find the switch. What a bummer. A purple wire like that, long and thick, could sell for a good price on the market," Little Fatso said, a bead of sweat hanging from the tip of his nose.

"I'll go and see!" said Zhang Xiaoxia.

"Me too!" I exclaimed, standing in front of the wall.

The copper wire was inside a sheath alongside four or five plastic wires. The sheath entered the wall and ran into the military barracks. The copper wire was dangling from the wall; its end had been cut off and the inside was purple, which meant it was worth some money.

"Come on, let's all hold hands, the five of us," Zhang Xiaoxia suggested. "I'll reach for the wire, and if I get electrocuted, we'll all die together, alright?"

"No, no, no!" the three boys cried out in chorus.

"Or we can play stone-paper-scissors and whoever loses will reach for the wire."

"No, no. No way," Little Fatso said. "Next time. And I'll borrow a torch."

"Go on. Get out of here, all of you. I'll go."

Zhang Xiaoxia gave me an empty aluminium toothpaste tube.

"I'll sacrifice my life, if I have to," she said.

"I'll go," I exclaimed, surprised by the words that had slipped out of my mouth. "If I get electrocuted, don't ever tell my mother that I was here stealing electricity with you lot."

18

There was a meal at the big courtyard canteen to commemorate the years of scarcity and rationing. A banana tree had been cut down for this occasion. Its roots have a bitter taste and are an essential ingredient for making wild vegetable dumplings. It serves to remind us of the bitterness of life.

Tiny roots came out of the earth in the hole where the banana tree had been uprooted. Suddenly a handful of fruit candies fell into the hole. I looked up and saw Zhang Xiaoxia. She whistled to catch my attention. She was in her first year of secondary school, had a sporty haircut, loved playing the *yueqin*[2] and spent all her free time practising at home. All the women in the courtyard said the *yueqin* had the power to tame the soul, and that when it came to Zhang Xiaoxia, it was like the saying: "A prodigal son returning home is worth more than gold."

Inspired by Zhang Xiaoxia, Mother spent six yuan on a *yueqin* for me, but I had to teach myself. At the end of two months, I was incapable of playing even the melody of "The East is Red."[3] Mother couldn't believe that Zhang Xiaoxia and I both played the same musical instrument, nor that a girl as wayward as she was could get back on the right track. Mother said: "A dragon gives birth to a dragon, a phoenix to a phoenix, but the offspring of rats only knows how to dig holes."

Zhang Xiaoxia was a phoenix then.

However, according to Mother Hu, it wasn't because of the *yueqin* that Zhang Xiaoxia had calmed down. It was because she had begun her menstruation. Girls who menstruate know what modesty is and dare not make mischief.

21

Zhang Xiaoxia was going to do her military service on the island of Zhenbao.

"It's freezing there," she said. "On the battle field, you have to get down and crawl in the snow. But the snow, it's nothing. I'll be a highly-decorated soldier and become a hero," she continued, standing on the tip of her toes and pushing out her chest.

With her fine, regular features and long legs, she was even prettier than before. Not yet 15 years old, she was already one and a half metres and taller than an 18-year-old girl.

"Will you miss your family? Will you think of us here in the big courtyard?"

"Of course not."

"Will you write to us?"

"No. What's the point? Once I arrive in my division, I won't be thinking of anyone. And you shouldn't think of me either."

We were all extremely disappointed. But then, I would do the same. Once I move to a new place, I will put my past behind me. I don't like the past.

Complementary Notes

What I wrote about in *Courtyard of My Childhood Years* is 97 percent true. As for the remaining three percent, I can't guarantee that my memory is perfect or that the choice of my words is always the best. I changed the names of the people by replacing one character in their names with another.

When I was in my fourth year of primary school, Zhang Xiaoxia was in her sixth. She was pretty and was an unusual character among the inhabitants of the big courtyard. A special unit, the Artistic Regiment, lived in the big courtyard. My father had been transferred from the Maritime Defence Unit to the "left wing" faction of the city. We lived in a small courtyard that was inside a bigger one. The families of the lower middle-ranking officers of the Artistic Regiment also lived in the small courtyard. A few metres further down was the main courtyard. Children of the small courtyard had little contact with the residents of the main courtyard.

Zhang Xiaoxia's father was the head of the Artistic Regiment, and her mother was a military doctor who looked like the cinema actress Wang Xiaotang, especially her eyes, which were slightly bulging. She had a curvaceous body and walked gracefully, always looking in front of her, like a well-educated woman. Zhang Xiaoxia didn't have her mother's beauty, perhaps because of her youth and lack of maturity. If you listened to the women of the small courtyard, you would have thought that out of all the children living in the big courtyard, Zhang Xiaoxia was the unruliest one of them all. But I had never seen her hit someone unprovoked. A tad arrogant, she rarely condescended to mix with the common lot. Extremely agile, she could kick and swing a sharp punch. And from time to time, she would teach the bullies a lesson.

Some years ago, while watching the film *Charlie's Angels*, the agility of the actresses stirred up my memories and I remembered Zhang Xiaoxia at the age of 12 or 13. You couldn't use the word "sexy" to describe her. But her temperament, personality and even the way she moved bore resemblance to the spy character played by Cameron Diaz.

When I met her, I had just moved into the city from the island of Haidao. I was a stranger in a new place and felt lost. The bullies tried to make trouble for my brother and me. To protect my brother, I often had to face them down. Today I realise that Zhang Xiaoxia had acted out of a sense of justice. She took the initiative to play with us, and the bullies, seeing that she was on our side, stopped harassing us. She came from a strict family. Her mother rarely allowed her to play outside, for she had to stay at home to study.

Together we got up to some mischief: stealing white turnips and potatoes from the canteen's vegetable garden and stealing electricity from the dormitory of the middle division. Then there were also the children from the main courtyard; Zhang Xiaoxia was the leader of the pack. Their families were never short of money. These children didn't need to sell aluminium toothpaste tubes and copper wires for money to rent comic books. They did it out of boredom, seeking excitement and challenges. I derived a certain pleasure in imagining that if, one day, I got run over by a car or got killed by a grenade, it would be my way of getting back at my parents. I wanted them to feel grief and remorse for me. That was why I was always up to some kind of mischief: grabbing electric wires, crossing in the middle of the street, climbing rooftops and trees, and generally being wild and reckless.

There was a kind of complicity between Zhang Xiaoxia and me. We didn't play together often, but I remember two conversations we had. The first one was when she told me her grandfather was a capitalist. It was a family secret. Seeing that I was worried about my mother's family, she told me her secret out of empathy. My situation at the time was like that of the Jewish people during the Second World War. Hunted by the Gestapo, they were terrified, hiding in whatever shelter they could find. Then one day, a woman pianist who looks like she belongs to the Aryan race in every way tells you that she is Jewish, making you feel that you are not alone in this world.

In our second conversation, she told me that at night when she was sleeping, her mother would come into her bedroom, take off her trousers, spread her legs… to see. I was young and didn't understand. Why would she be so perverted? No wonder Zhang Xiaoxia hated her mother and joined the army at 14.

I was only 11 years old then and felt angry for her, but my anger was blind.

It wasn't until I was writing *Courtyard of My Childhood Years* that I finally understood. In a world as warped as ours, Zhang Xiaoxia's mother was afraid that her daughter would be at risk of sexual abuse. As a doctor, she tended to see only the dark side of life. She was worried for her daughter and wanted to protect her but went about it the wrong way. I think she might have been slightly paranoid.

During my years in the small courtyard, I often played with three other girls who also lived there. They were a year older than me, and more mature. Once, we were playing in the woods behind the meeting room, sitting up in the tree and talking. Her voice trembling, the skinny girl said: "You know… you have to be careful. There's a pervert living in the big courtyard." I felt alarmed. We were living in the military barracks, so how could it have been possible?

"The last time we went on a trip, he picked me up to help me get down from the car," she continued. "Then he pretended to accidentally touch me… there."

I couldn't bring myself to believe that there were perverts like him. It had never happened to me.

"It happened to me too," said the girl with curly hair. "A few times even. Once he touched my bum. Another time he groped my breasts so hard that it hurt. I was crying, and he stopped."

I had grown up on the island of Haidao, where interactions with people of the outside world were few and far between. These stories made me nervous and ill at ease. I asked the girls how I could tell if someone was a pervert or not. They said you couldn't. You just had to be careful.

The fat girl said there was a doctor at the clinic. Once, he took her inside a hut, pulled down his trousers and told her to touch him there. She refused and started crying. Alarmed, he gave her some fruit candies wrapped in glass paper and told her not to tell anyone. After this, he took her to the hut a second time. He asked her to touch him there and she did.

"It was weird," the fat girl said. "White stuff spurted out from there. It was funny. It was all over my face and I started crying. He wiped it off and let me go."

After that, she always avoided the doctor. When she saw him from a distance, she would run in the opposite direction. She didn't want to be near him.

I was horrified by these stories, which haunted me for several days. Then I understood. Even in places that seemed the safest and the most imbued with the revolutionary spirit, there was always danger and wicked people lurking about.

You could trust no one.

FORTY-FIVE

Diary
Monday, 10th November 2003 10:50 am

I drank some coffee. It's been a while since I last had any because of the side effects it has, like headaches, stomach aches and sleep disturbances. A few years ago, in the mornings and afternoons, I used to always have a cup of Colombian coffee before getting down to my writing. Otherwise my mind would be foggy, and I wouldn't be in any mental shape to work. I love the smell of coffee. Of all the different kinds that I have tried, those of Milan and Paris are the best. In one of my articles, I compared them to Elder Sister Bao and Younger Sister Lin, two characters from *Dream of the Red Chamber*.

Searching through the different therapeutic methods for depression, I found this one: Learn to let yourself go and do as you please. I'm all for it! Do as I please, why not? At least now, at this precise moment, I feel good, happy and not at all depressed. Modern man has a tendency to push things to the extreme. We either let ourselves go so much that we lose control over ourselves, or we impose so many restrictions on ourselves that we are afraid to go forward. This isn't life. Why can't we find the right balance between control and letting go? Maybe we have to experience extreme states before finding the happy medium.

Last Friday, during the consultation with the head physician, Dr Gong told me not to worry and that efficaciousness of alprazolam depended on the dosage. So I went back to taking three quarters of a tablet at bedtime and, sure enough, the nightmares have stopped. It's amazing how increasing or reducing a quarter of a tablet can be so effective.

According to Dr Gong, 20 percent of women worldwide have suffered from depression at least once in their lives. Fifteen percent of men have psychiatric disorders related to depression, panic disorder and OCD. The statistics are horrendous. He also said that, according to the medical profession, a good relationship between a doctor and his/her patient has a positive effect on the illness, as if the illness is halfway to being cured. I think this is especially true in the field of mental health and psychotherapy. No matter how prominent a doctor is, if a patient doesn't trust him/her, the effectiveness of the treatment is reduced to almost zero. In some cases, a doctor's behaviour and attitude are more important than his medical expertise. Therefore, a good relationship between a doctor and his/her patient is essential.

Owing to the population density in China, a doctor is faced with work overload and has many patients to see every day. The shortage of ethical and competent doctors is an indirect consequence of this. Often in my prayers, I ask the Lord to send us more gifted and principled physicians.

Dr Gong told me what his wife and child thought of my book *Life in Shenzhen*. They like reading biographical essays that talk about everyday life. Several doctors have told me that my book reminded them of their childhood.

I remember in 1995, when I was at Bing Xin's teacher's home, she said to me: "Lanni, you must write with your heart." At the time, this truth seemed to me so simple and obvious. But it was only when I wanted to take my writing skills to the next level that I finally grasped the essence of her words.

Yesterday on *Hour of Power*, the Reverend Robert A. Schuller explained Dr Peale's theory of the "law of attraction." It is the ability of positive thoughts to attract positive energy, which then makes positive things happen in your life. Being with people who think positively does the same thing. A positive mindset guides us towards a positive direction in life. It's the same principle as in the proverb: Birds of a feather flock together. A crow attracts a murder of crows; a seagull draws a squabble of seagulls. Negative thoughts push us into a bottomless pit. We must learn to transform positive thoughts into positive actions.

Letter to the Hebrews, Chapter 6, Verse 18: "[...] It is impossible for God to lie." The promises of God are true and trustworthy.

Positive thoughts have the power to bring about change. And faith can move mountains. We must believe in the impossible, take things into our own hands and find a way to succeed. When tragedy strikes, we turn to God and ask Him how He could have let it happen. Answer: It is the will of God. Through tragedy, God transforms the negative into positive, makes possible that which is impossible. But we must have faith.

As an example, the Reverend Schuller told us a true story: An organist had worked at the Crystal Cathedral for 30 years when he fractured an elbow in a car accident and could no longer play the organ with his two hands. However, several composers wrote musical scores intended to be played with only one hand. The organist is currently planning to go on an international tour.

The program's guest of honour was a well-known writer. The organisation in his parish was dysfunctional, and he suffered as a result. He wrote about his experience in his book, which had a positive influence on non-believers, as well as those "in between worlds," namely non-practising Christians.

Notes

Reading the essays of Bing Xin, I realise that it is the background of her stories that interests me most. I am envious of her teacher, who had loving parents. Even though her father was a military officer, he knew how to give love to his child. Her mother was a homemaker and enjoyed physical and mental health. Brought up by such loving parents, a child would certainly grow up to be part of the elite. An elite that speaks the universal language of love.

I don't know if Xigu told stories to Xiaotao in which, following the tradition of folktales, the good are always rewarded for their acts of kindness. Long before Xiaotao was born, in every generation and in every dynasty, mothers told their children similar stories. Tales and fables. Generation after generation, mothers nursed their children while telling them stories of love.

Western civilisation began to make its way into China after the Xinhai Revolution in 1911. Western culture enriched the mothers' milk and, subsequently, the children were better nourished. But Xiaotao's milk wasn't as rich as Xigu's, because Xiaotao had grown up in the terror and chaos of war. The mother's blood essence was unable to produce milk nutritious enough to feed her children. There were no fables nor fairy tales of love. Only sadness and sorrow.

In the era when Lanlan became a mother for the first time, the word "mother" was devoid of meaning. Her comrades of the Revolution all followed revolutionary educational methods. Children no longer drank breast milk snuggled against their mothers. Instead, they drank cow or goat's milk lying on a bed. The mothers, too busy starting revolutions, had no time to nurse their babies, let alone tell stories to their children. But then, what stories had they to tell? The tale of Meng Jiangnü[1] who wept at the foot of the Great Wall? Stories of superstitious beliefs of the feudal era? Or the tale of Snow White, a capitalist? No, it was up to the women at the childcare facility or kindergarten to tell stories of spies or the assassination of landowners.

I was born in the heart of winter. According to my maternal grandmother, as soon as Mother came home from the hospital, she put me in another room, where I slept all by myself in a small bed. Apparently, that was the new scientific method for raising children. My grandmother said it was so cold in the room at night that I was crying like a kitten. But Mother forbade her to pick me up, saying she shouldn't give in to my whims. According to the new method, you should let the baby cry until it is used to being alone and stops bawling. Grandmother asked herself: "Is this the new educational method? If a mother can't cradle her child in her arms or nurse her, then is she truly a mother? When the child grows up, will she feel love for her mother? How can you bring up a child like that? You might as well not have children."

Mother tried to convince Grandmother of the benefits of this new educational method, but to no avail. Mother said: "Communism will take over this country in twenty years' time. We should make a clean slate and do away with feudal traditions and old ways of thinking. Children belong to the people.

And the people will feed and raise them to be warriors as tough as iron. They're the heirs of communism."

Children like these have grown up in a collectivity. Maybe I exaggerate somewhat in likening them to pigeons raised in confined battery cages. Conceived and fed with the same method, they have the same serial number. They all eat, learn, see, hear, think and function in the same way.

Father and Mother were sincere in believing that communism would be implemented in 20 years' time. That their children would grow up in a utopia, where you could do as you wish and obtain what you want. Oppression and social classes would be abolished, and no one would go hungry. Peace would reign on earth.

I have an aunt who lived in the northeast of China. She wanted to marry an officer who lived in a city. Her brother and sister tried to make her change her mind: "China will soon be communist. The city and the countryside will be one. You can live and work peacefully in the village. The countryside will soon be as prosperous as the city."

16th September 2006

Correlations

Excerpts from "Blue Sea, Grey Sea"

When I was a child, I disliked looking at the sea. But the adults in Shoudao always looked at the vast expanse of water with intensity. The canons were positioned facing the sea. It was under surveillance 24 hours a day. For me, the sea was the enemy. Together with the other children, we would imitate the adults doing their military exercises.

We were like weeds growing wild on the island. We were used to the sounds of canons and rifles and the murderous din of military exercises, but we had never heard a tale by Hans Christian Anderson, nor read the essays of Bing Xin, which are filled with so much beauty and compassion. I read Bing Xin's essays for the first time when I was 20 years old. I read the book in one go, starting at dusk and finishing in the early hours of the morning. I put the book down, overwhelmed with emotion. When I shook Bing Xin's teacher's hand, I felt the warmth of her hand passing through her fingers into mine. It seeped into my blood, rising up into my heart and head. Startled and confused, I stammered: "Bing Xin's teacher... the sea... the sea..." At a loss for what to say, my eyes suddenly filled up with tears. I was embarrassed, unable to understand why I was crying. I let go of her hand, wanting to run away. But she held firmly onto my hand and said: "Gently. Come. Come closer." She was looking at me, concerned. There was a profound love in those beautiful eyes that had seen so many changes in the world.

"The sea... What about the sea?" she asked, a kind and caring look in her eyes.

"I... I...," I stuttered, trying to concentrate on my words. "Me too, when I was a child, I grew up in on a military base by the sea."

"Which sea is that?" she asked.

"The sea of Nanhai. It's grey. I feel... so ashamed. I don't like... child... wild..."

Then I broke down in sobs. As she couldn't make out what I was saying, she continued to look at me with the same kind and caring look in her eyes. Suddenly it all became clear. For far too long, I had been harbouring resentments and feeling sorry for myself. I was filled with shame. In the memories of my childhood, I saw grey waves rolling across the sea. At that moment, I tried to focus my mind on the image of the sea, in the hope that a miracle would turn the grey sea into blue.

Spring of 1993

Complementary Notes

The sea that I talked about in this chapter is the sea of our unconscious mind. I'd like to point out that the sea of my childhood is different from that of Bing Xin's teacher. Our notion of love and hate, beauty and ugliness is shaped by our childhood environment and education.

FORTY-SIX

Diary
Tuesday, 17th November 2003 10:20 am

I have a Toshiba notebook now. The old laptop I bought just before the New Year in 1997 no longer works very well. If, in the next few days, I can get used to the Toshiba, then I'll take the old laptop with me to Shenzhen and keep it as an extra.

Slept badly these last few nights. Although I didn't have any nightmares, I felt anxious and edgy in my dreams.

In one dream, I was at a meeting where the participants were discussing extremely boring topics. From time to time, I would have a snack at the hotel canteen, where it was crowded, or just hang around in another room. I wanted to go home but had no transport. I felt stupid and angry with myself. How could I waste an entire day at meetings like these?

Then I dreamt that Fanding was still in high school. But he wasn't working hard enough for his high school graduation exams, because he was being too kind. Every time a girl asked him to help her with her homework or to chat with her, he couldn't refuse. He was wasting his time with them. I was worried that he would lose out and ruin his future. Afraid that he wouldn't make it in life, I berated him for his stupidity.

In another dream, I was constantly looking for something: a place to eat, a road, a station in a strange town, even toilets. I felt insecure and was looking for a place where I could hide and do my business. But I always ended up being spotted. Or, after taking all my clothes off, I would notice there were people around me. I would then hurriedly gather up my clothes to cover myself and search for another place to hide and put my clothes back on.

What do these dreams say about my mental state? Am I going to slip back into depression?

My doctors in Guangzhou and Shenzhen have warned me about the side effects of antidepressants and that I should be careful when taking them for the first time. Generally, an improvement can be seen after nine months. But you must continue to take them for a relatively long time to reinforce the effects and prevent a relapse. If the first treatment takes a year to be effective, then the second treatment will last for three years. A third depressive episode has serious implications, because it means the medication has little effect. This is the reason why the suicide rate for people suffering from depression is 20 percent and not 70 percent. I must accept that I will probably be on medication for a long time. No matter how difficult and annoying it might be, I mustn't give up.

On the Sunday broadcast of *Hour of Power*, the Reverend Robert H. Schuller played a video in which he had a discussion with Mother Teresa just before she died. They were talking about how faith wasn't an empty notion, but a reality. Faith is powerful. We need a kind and merciful God in whom we can trust. Mother Teresa said that it was our duty to give love to those who are hungry, in body and soul, and that it was more difficult to help those who were emotionally empty than those who were physically hungry.

She told this story as an example: She knew a man who was successful. He never went hungry and owned a big house with a large lantern hanging outside. But he wasn't happy. The man shook Mother Teresa's hand warmly.

"It's been many years since I've shaken someone's hand," he said to her.

"You have a big house. Why don't you light this pretty lantern?"

"Nobody comes to see me. What's the point?"

"And if I send a sister to visit you every day, then would you light it?"

"Of course," he replied.

From that time on, he would light his lantern every day, waiting for the sister to come. Several years later, he wrote a letter to Mother Teresa: "I thank you for lighting up the lantern in my heart."

To Mother Teresa, we all need to receive warmth and love.

Notes

When I was a child, I could sing "Love Our Fatherland, Love Our People." But what's the point?

At the time, the notion of love, in the broad sense of the term, was in fashion. My parents liked to say to the Party's organisation: "We must love our fatherland. We must love our people." To the teachers at school, they would say: "Love our Party. Love our fatherland. Love our work." At the gathering of the Red Guards, people would say: "Love our brothers and soldiers." People would say to the head of their village: "Love the collectivity. Love socialism." But my notion of the fatherland is this: mountains, rivers and streams; earth and islands. My notion of the people is this: labourers who sweat in front of furnaces and peasants who plough the land. Even though I've never come in contact with the "people," I've come to know them through movies and magazines.

The island where I spent a part of my childhood belonged to the maritime defence unit, an outpost of our fatherland. Both children and adults were on alert for any attempted invasion by the enemy. It was through the notion of "hate" that I learnt the meaning of being "on alert." It is through a fierce hatred for the enemy that we are able to acquire skills deadly enough to defeat that enemy and protect our fatherland and its people. In the environment where I grew up, the notion of hatred was the cornerstone of our lives. We were never to forget this: If we cannot defeat the enemy, every social class and reactionary faction, and then our fatherland and its people, will be condemned to disappear forever.

On a couple of occasions in the 1980s and 1990s, Lanlan and Xiaotao had conversations like this:

Lanlan: If I hadn't resigned back then, I'd be enjoying an officer's pension today and wouldn't have to worry about my medical expenses. I joined the army too young and didn't understand anything. I regret it now.

Xiaotao: You made that choice. Who could have stopped you from doing what you wanted?

Lanlan: You and Father never taught me anything. I was lost. That's why I was always getting into trouble.

Xiaotao: But no one taught me about life either: marriage, pregnancy. …My mother never taught me any of these things. Look at me, I've been a homemaker all my life.

Lanlan: You never helped me find a husband. I only knew one boy then. We saw each other often, but he had dirty habits like a peasant. I didn't want to go out with him, but no one gave me any advice. Everyone in the army knew we were a couple. I felt guilty breaking up with him, so I let myself drift into marriage.

Xiaotao: Be content with what you have. At least you could choose your husband. I had an arranged marriage. It was my whole life.

Lanlan: I remember one thing you said to me back then. You said there were too many old people in my husband's family and that it'd be hard work burying them all. I didn't understand what you were trying to say. In fact, you were trying to tell me that there'd be heavy responsibilities to bear in his family and many financial problems to deal with. But I didn't have the slightest clue of what married life would be like. My husband would send money to his family every month and we lived on my salary. One year, you had to look after the children to help us make ends meet. It still makes me angry when I think about it.

Xiaotao: You're driving yourself mad. You think too much and it's bad for your health. Be like me. Eat well, sleep well and don't brood. Know how to be content with what you have.

17th September 2006

Correlations

Excerpts from *On the Sense of Anger:*
Incentive for Self-assertion and Self-development

If today you ask people why they are angry, almost all of them would say because their dignity has been violated. We feel the hurt, because our integrity as a person has been infringed upon. The way we react to this violation on our person is telling of the psychological complexes that have developed in us throughout the years. What I mean by complex is the sum of all the unhappy and hurtful experiences of our past and which have accumulated in our subconscious [...] Repressed anger can lead to depression, even cancer.

Verena Kast (Switzerland)

Complementary Notes

I know a good number of women who suffer from chronic repressed anger. They are all, without exception, intelligent, sociable, and have brilliant careers. But they are seriously ill. My maternal grandmother, mother and I belong to this category of women who suffer from a permanent state of repressed anger. It has been passed down from one generation to the next, and when it came to me, it transformed into cancer and depression. I've been hit with a double whammy, so to speak.

In the process of writing this book, things have become clearer to me. It is logical that I should suffer from both cancer and depression. Inevitable even. But what is surprising is that I am still alive.

FORTY-SEVEN

Diary
18th November 2003 10:15 am

I am so stupid. Lele, my little dog, is angry with me.

I was playing with Lele with a colleague of mine, who works part-time. We put him into a cardboard box for rice-cookers and were having fun watching him getting all worked up trying to get out.

Lele is so spoilt. There's no end to his mischief these days. He does his business all over the apartment and bites everything that comes his way. So I wanted to teach him a lesson. He was whining in the cardboard box. Seeing his sorry little face filled me with a sense of satisfaction. He deserved it. We were laughing and clapping away. I continued to tease him even after my colleague had left. Furious, he sprang out of the box. I was crouching; he took me by surprise and bit me on the cheek. I was livid. What if he started attacking people? I had to put him in his place, so I spanked him with a Japanese wooden sandal. But he retaliated and tried to bite me again. I slapped him lightly on the muzzle and he backed away, looking at me sideways with his round black eyes full of anger and resentment. I then went out to buy some books but was upset and shaken. How could I discipline such a recalcitrant dog? When I got home, Zhou Xiaobing said Lele was sulking in a corner and asked me if I had scolded him. Just then, Lele appeared, put his front paws on Zhou Xiaobing's knees and looked at me, wagging his tail. I ignored him, and like a child whose pride had been hurt because he had been wronged, he went sulking back to his corner. Zhou Xiaobing felt sorry for him, went over and found him still moping. My husband then accused me of being unfair to the dog: "Lele didn't like being laughed at, but instead of stopping when you'd had your fun, you and your colleague carried on taking the mickey out of him. His pride was hurt. You smacked him and then ignored him. He's only two months old and didn't understand why the adults were treating him that way."

I came to my senses.

I was wrong. The day before this incident, I'd read how every one of us needs love. And animals, too. Especially dogs, because they are man's best friend. They have their dignity and are living beings in their own right. We should love and respect them. Later, when I was having my dinner, Lele didn't come over, as was his habit. What I love about him is that he has character. I tried to tempt him with a piece of fish. After hesitating for a while, he came over and ate it. It's amazing how much dogs are like us.

Notes

I've been suffering from chronic fatigue for a month now. Even if I don't do much during the day, I feel sluggish and lethargic. Nothing is worrying me, but I feel out of sorts. It's like my mind has left my body to go for a stroll outside and doesn't want to come back. I keep thinking about the ash-grey sofa in my study. I have an urge to crawl under it and go into hiding. When Lele is sick, he often hides under there, curled up against the wall. How does he know...how shall I say it... that it's safe there? I can't find the words to describe my state of mind. I just want to disappear under the sofa. I try to use my reason to control this impulse, but the Li Lanni in my head is yelling: "Why not? What's stopping you? Go on. Then you won't think about it anymore." Today is 13th November. The time is 11:05 am. I am alone at home and Lele is dozing on the window sill. I'm going to switch off my computer, and then I'm going under the sofa. Who knows, maybe it'll be therapeutic.

Okay. It's done. I am out. The time is 11:26 am.

Lying on the window sill, Lele watched me crawl out from under the sofa. His eyes were wide open, but mine were closed, so as not to have to look at him. His eyes were devoid of curiosity, fear, compassion and understanding. I felt there was something there in that look of his, but couldn't put my finger on it.

Under the sofa, I felt as if I were inside the ear of a cat. My forehead was resting on the parquet floor; my hands were on the back of my neck; and my knees were bent in a yoga posture. I could feel my heart beating; my pulse was throbbing in my neck and on the left of my navel. With all my limbs huddled against me, I felt safe. I couldn't see most of the objects in my study: bookshelves, computer, telephone, alarm clock, calendar, etc. All this was hidden from my view, preventing the chaos of the outside world from reaching me. My life suddenly became much simpler. It occurred to me that my behaviour could have stemmed from the collective unconsciousness. Throughout the centuries, in times of war when people's lives were in danger, they would hide under the bed, huddled up, eyes closed, wishing they could disappear through a crack in the ground or shrink to the size of an embroidery needle. It is the same for the people of today. When confronted with danger, like an aeroplane explosion, an earthquake, or bombs, and overwhelmed with helplessness, with nowhere to run, we close our eyes and curl up in a foetal position. It's our instinct for survival.

I read in a newspaper that 23 people out of 100,000 die by suicide. Shenzhen has a population of 9,000,000 and there are 2,000 cases of suicide a year. About 50,000 individuals suffer from mental illness because someone close to them has either committed suicide or attempted to commit suicide.

I think these numbers are too low for Shenzhen. Doubling the figures would bring us closer to the truth. If we include the migrant population, the total population in Shenzhen is estimated to be at 13,000,000. Migrants are particularly affected by psychological problems. Compared to those in the other regions of China, the inhabitants of Shenzhen have a relatively passive lifestyle and are, therefore, more vulnerable from a psychological point of view. In my opinion, those who have lived in Shenzhen for more than 10 years have either experienced depression or some other kind of psychological wound. This is true for everyone, whether they are successful in life or not, be they rich or poor, educated or otherwise. Embedded deep in each of us is a book of confessions.

I've rarely written about Shenzhen in the past, because I had lost my soul. It couldn't find its way back to my body, nor a home in this city. For a long time, my body and soul were out of sync with each other. They were drifting, each on its own, broken and lost. Then they got sucked into a big black hole and were transformed into bubbles.

I was afraid to tell my doctor that my condition has deteriorated, thinking he would either increase the dosage of my medication or add new ones. So, here I am, still stuck in my hole.

13th October 2006

Correlations

Excerpts from "The Green House by the Lake"

There was a lake behind the hospital.

A green house stood in a courtyard, not far from the other side of the lake. I had seen members of the medical staff going inside, carrying a stretcher with a corpse, stiff and wrapped up in dirty sheets.

When we die, our bodies are put in a mortuary. It is a transit passage between this world and the next. The first time I heard someone talk about a mortuary was when I was eight years old. A classmate whose mother had just died said: "Father and I rushed to the hospital, but when we arrived, Mother was already at the mortuary." I asked her what a mortuary was. She said that it was a place where dead people go while waiting to be burnt. Her father cried a lot, but three months later, my classmate had a new mother. Nobody talked about the dead woman anymore.

I often wondered about my classmate's mother: Was she afraid in the mortuary? Were there any lights? Did she have a blanket to keep her warm? Did it hurt when she was being burnt? Did she become a ghost and come back to see her children? These questions haunted me.

A story: An old woman died. They took her body to the mountain to be buried. On the way there, she came back to life and started banging on the lid of the coffin. But the people in the funeral procession were wailing so loudly and the cymbals and gongs were so deafening that no one heard her.

Another version of the story: The people heard the old woman banging on the lid of the coffin, but her son, pretending not to have heard, ordered the funeral procession not to stop. When they arrived at the mountain, they opened the coffin to find the shroud torn and the white bones of her fingers smeared with blood.

When I heard this story, I couldn't help but wonder what I would do if one day I were to be burnt alive.

I already had insomnia at the age of eight. At night, with the lights out, I had the sensation that I was lying in a mortuary or inside a coffin. I felt extremely lonely. I imagined that the wood of the coffin was infested with worms that would eat into my flesh and devour my decaying body. I was terrified of worms. Once, I saw fat white worms wriggling in the earth. I tried to imagine the agony of being burnt alive in an incinerator. I could see the fire spreading all around me and a sea of tongue-like flames licking my body, engulfing my flesh and skeleton. What happened to people when they die? What would happen to us afterwards? I couldn't believe there was nothing after death.

[...] Mrs Big Bear was much too fat. The upper part of her body was so bloated, and her buttocks so flabby that she looked like a rag doll. She had an enormous puffy face, and her eyes were so narrow that they had become mere slits. Every time she looked at me, I would feel a wave of panic. We both had hypothyroidism. In fact, I was her, when she was young; and she was me, when I grew old.

Of all the patients in the endocrinology ward, few looked like human beings. The patient with hyperthyroidism in the next bed, number 23, was skinnier than a monkey and her chest was flatter than a man's. She had a thin face, thick neck and high cheekbones, and a euphoric gleam in her bulging eyes.

I learnt that the girl in bed number 24 was only 16 years old, but she already looked like an old woman. She had a hunched back and thick waist. Her neck had almost disappeared, and she was covered in thick black body hair. Her face was red and puffy from taking too many hormones. I could smell her underarm odour from afar.

A nine-year-old boy was in bed number 10. He too had an endocrine disease. He had a swollen face, dry yellow hair and an abdomen as bloated as a woman who was seven months pregnant. He drank a lot of water and urinated often. He would wet his bed at night, and everywhere he went, his trousers would stink of urine. The other patients told him to take his meals elsewhere. The doctors ordered him to have a urine test once every 24 hours. Beneath his bed were jars of urine that looked like rice wine.

On the other side of the endocrinology ward was a ward for patients with severe renal impairment. Every time I crossed the corridor that led to this ward, I would be afraid to look inside. But the less I looked, the more I saw. A sickly smell emanated from the rooms. I saw empty beds, stripped of their sheets and blankets. The mattresses were soiled and repulsive and, lying there on the floor, they told in silence the end of a story. In the other beds, the expressionless faces of the living shone with the ghostly light of those approaching death. It made my flesh crawl to see how their cavernous eyes resembled those of the dead.

Every time I crossed this corridor, I couldn't help but steal a glance into the intensive care room. Alone, an emaciated old man was waiting for death. He had an eerie unearthly gleam in his black sunken eyes.

March 1987

Complementary Notes

Nine years after my stay at this hospital, I wrote about my experience in an article. But the editors weren't interested. At the time, people only looked outwards. They paid more attention to social conflicts than spirituality, life and death. When I wrote this narrative, I was going through a troubled period in my life. I was fighting hard against becoming a "Shenzhen citizen," meaning I refused to take on the identity of someone who belongs to the city of Shenzhen. I only saw uncertainty and turmoil ahead. Loneliness weighed on me. I took refuge in my memories of my stay at this hospital. The green house by the lake was a place of transition between life and death.

FORTY-EIGHT

Diary
Sunday, 22nd November 2003 10:40 am

My computer froze yesterday morning. No matter what I did, it wouldn't reboot. I got myself into such a state that I felt sick, had a sore throat and stomach pains. I gave up in the end. It's so stupid how little things get to me. The slightest problem is enough to make me physically ill. My morning is ruined, because I can't get any work done. I felt so demoralised at first, but then told myself to snap out of it and be positive. Since my computer won't restart, I might as well take a break.

It's rare that autumn is so pleasant and mild. The weather forecast announced a drop in temperature. A mild cold spell is on its way.

Had a most enjoyable lunch at the teachers' canteen. The *tangshi*[1] fish and rice casserole was good, but a bit salty.

Notes

In May, I worked at the second Shenzhen Cultural Congress. An event was held at the Shenzhen Opera on the day of the opening ceremony. That evening, I heard for the first time the Shenzhen Youth Choir.

It was an all-girls choir. The youngest singers were about eight or nine, and the eldest 12 or 13. It was funny seeing their little faces all made-up, making them look much more mature than their actual ages. Listening to their pure and angelic voices, I began to think about the lives of these young girls: What did their parents do for a living? How long had they been living in Shenzhen? Did they have a harmonious family life? Did their parents make sacrifices so they could sing on stage that night? Did they know anything about their family origins? Were they grateful to their parents? Were they proud of their city?

The Shenzhen Opera was part of the first series of cultural buildings to be constructed and is an emblem of the cultural life of the city. I saw how it was built from nothing. I remember seeing the flag of the first Cultural Festival floating at the main entrance of the building. But it was abandoned and there was talk of demolition to make way for a commercial centre. Fortunately, it was listed as a cultural heritage site of the Special Economic Region of Shenzhen. Subsequently, renovation and maintenance works were carried out. Today, it is an important cultural monument of the city.

Accepting that I am a citizen of Shenzhen was a long and difficult process for me. I didn't feel like I belonged and wanted to run away. But sitting in the concert hall that evening, I felt a sense of belonging for the first time. I was overwhelmed with both joy and sadness. I was proud to be part of the first generation of youth to settle in Shenzhen. And looking at the smiling faces of the second generation, I saw a bright future for this city.

Sometime after this, I was at the National Health Insurance Centre to inquire about claiming a refund of my medical expenses. I wasn't aware that the centre had been transformed into an open-space office. The counters, which resembled those in a pawn shop, no longer existed. I could now look at the clerks face-to-face. I don't know what other people think of this, but, personally, I welcome the change, which, to my mind, promotes equality. Now whenever I am at the Health Insurance Centre, sitting on a stool and waiting patiently for my turn, my heart is filled with gratitude. And when I am in the west wing lobby of the Citizens' Centre, waiting to complete my administrative formalities, I realise how fond I am of cities like Shenzhen. But I regret that many people have not lived to see this day. How many of them have dreamt of happiness in this city? The setbacks they encountered left them with psychological wounds. Believing in love and respect, they sought to be understood, to receive moral support and not to be looked down upon. But they lacked the strength to wait, and time was running out. With their dreams broken and carrying deep wounds inside, they left Shenzhen and revisited this city only in their nightmares. Others, who are less fortunate, died in various circumstances: pain, disasters, depression or dementia. How many broken and distressed souls are there in this city? Are there souls weeping in the night, lost under a nebulous sky?

14th October 2006

Correlations

Excerpts from *Life in Shenzhen*

At the beginning of the summer in 1983, I was on a training course to be a professional radio producer at the School of Radio Broadcast. One day, I went for an interview with the director of a newspaper, who was recruiting journalists. He had read my novel and wanted to meet me to see if I was suitable for the job.

At the time, Shenzhen's economic expansion was still in its early days and its future was uncertain. The director talked at length about various subjects: the Special Economic Zone being a window of China; the status of this city as a pioneer; the front page of his newspaper... I wanted to interrupt him to say that I had never worked on a newspaper before.

"Are you capable of facing hardships?" he asked me, suddenly changing the subject.

"Of course. That's my strong point, even," I answered, taken aback.

"Do you want to build a career?" he asked, a questioning look in his eyes.

What a question to ask. I was in my 20s and determined to succeed in life. I was only too happy to be offered the opportunity. He held out his hand and his thin face broke into a smile.

"I hope you'll accept the position as the editor of the cultural section," he said, shaking my hand. "Welcome to Shenzhen."

Was that it? I was surprised by the speed with which things were done in Shenzhen. The newspaper had, in total, eight members of staff, me included, with the average age being around 20. The director told me that the graphic artist and photographer were both self-taught artists. The others had recently graduated from the School of Journalism and had no experience.

"Wow...No one knows much about journalism. And we're publishing a weekly newspaper in three months' time," I said. "These people in Shenzhen, they have guts."

"There's a fashionable expression in Shenzhen: If you want to do something, just go!" the director said proudly.

So I left the School of Radio Broadcast without finishing my internship.

It was past midday when I arrived at Shenzhen station. The sun hit me as I was getting off the train. Its heat had the strength and energy of two suns combined. I was out in the sun for barely two minutes, and my skin was beginning to tan. I wasn't even sweating, but already I felt the heat burning its way into my bones. Not a single tree was in sight. The entire city was under construction. Looking at all this, a proverb came to mind: "The following generations harvest the fruits that the previous generations have sown." But in this case, it was the opposite that was true. My colleagues said to me: "You're lucky. Just before you arrived, we were still living in huts. It's only recently that we moved into a building." But the truth was, I was out of luck. For my first assignment was to steal electricity.

The newspaper's headquarters were divided into two sections. The first was made up of offices and the second was living accommodations. The headquarters were in the Yuan Ling residential district, which was under construction. The buildings wouldn't be supplied with water and electricity until three months later. But the construction site had access to electricity. Since the construction company refused to "lend" us any, we had no choice but to help ourselves. As Mao Zedong said: "A revolution is not an invitation to a banquet, nor the writing of an article, nor is it kindness or benevolence." All the members of staff at the newspaper were made to take part in this operation. We sneaked into the construction site. First, we collected all the Scotch tape and electric wires, which we then put neatly together. Then we carefully studied the layout of the wires, trying to find one that was well hidden, allowing us to divert the electric current without being found out.

The newspaper hadn't yet received any working capital and was short of money. Other than a small van, three bicycles and a few tables and chairs, it had no other possessions. We often went to the construction site to gather odd objects: bamboo poles to dry our washing on; planks of wood to make benches with; scraps of material to make mops. The workers took us for an organised gang of beggars. Sometimes I would ask the workers to give me a thermos bottle of hot water. Otherwise, we would drink water from the well.

The director lived in shared accommodations in another residential district called Tongxinling. The apartment was basic, but in the bathroom it had the most priceless luxury of all: running water. Every night after dinner, all the members of staff would sit in a row, each waiting his or her turn to bathe. We would be reviewing our work of the day and, from time to time, bang impatiently on the bathroom door.

Afterwards, we would stroll leisurely back to the headquarters. Nights are cool in Shenzhen. A soft light emanated from a sapphire blue sky that was like a piece of jade washed by the sea. Night and day in Shenzhen are like husband and wife, happy in love and living in perfect harmony. When the day is frantic, impetuous and passionate, the nights are mild, reserved and serene. The road was empty. Rice paddies and fields of vegetables ran along both sides. A faint smell of soap lingered in the air. In the pale light of the moon, on a road hazy with mist, a delicate sweet scent perfumed the air.

The newspaper's first edition had already been sent to the printing press. It was a four-page weekly newspaper. On the front cover of the literature and art supplement was a lovely photograph of a lotus bud. The newspaper was printed at the central printing plant of the Special Economic Zone. That night, we were in the printing room, checking the proofs and filling in the missing characters. Since the workers and our members of staff were all novices, progress was slow.

At midnight, the canteen served roast duck congee. In the editor's office, the printing room and on every floor of the building, everyone, tired and worn-out, stretched their limbs and grabbed a bowl, rushing to the canteen to queue up. Only our team stayed behind. With a blank expression on our faces, our eyes staring at the tips of our noses like monks in deep meditation, we were pretending we hadn't seen or heard anything. There would be no duck congee for us. Its exquisite smell rose and filled the air, wafting into every nook and cranny, up to the last floor. The sweet aroma of the duck mingled with the fragrance of the rice was tempting and made our mouths water. It was a torture. We could hardly sit still. And if we asked for a bowl of congee? Why not? We could beg like paupers at the foot of the rich. Or we could steal some. Let's go.

We arrived at the canteen, famished. Seeing there were a dozen people queuing at the counter, we hugged the walls, trying to make ourselves as small as possible, telling ourselves: "No, no. Wait a bit longer before asking." We waited until a kitchen staff shouted into the dining hall: "Anyone for more? We're closing." Like an arrow, we darted into the canteen, hands in our pockets, looking sheepishly around us, embarrassed.

"Hey, do you want more? Have you got meal tickets?" the kitchen help asked.

We climbed into the minivan with an empty stomach. And if we lay down for a while, maybe our hunger would go away. And if we took a nap, we wouldn't have to go back into the office and watch the others eat their roast duck congee. Just then, someone must have accidently touched a radio button, for disco music was suddenly blaring out. And like a violent tremor, it shattered our loneliness and annihilated our hunger, weakness, despondency and melancholy. We pulled ourselves together, jumped out of the van and started dancing to the rhythm of the music, laughing and shouting wildly. The first edition of our newspaper was published to the sounds of disco music. It fluttered into our hearts like a butterfly. At midnight, under a starry sky, the air was blue and clear. Light-headed and drunk on our feelings of youth, we wanted to fly up into the air. We wanted to live a beautiful and happy life.

Such were my feelings towards my life in Shenzhen.

Beginning of spring of 1995

Complementary Notes

I moved to Shenzhen in 1983. The first three years were particularly difficult, because I had nothing. I lived according to the proverb: "Have no regrets for yesterday; do not fret for tomorrow; and do what your heart tells you."

Between 1985 and 1987, I was among the first batch of students to attend an advanced training course at the Lu Xun Literary Institute in Beijing. In 1987, I returned to Shenzhen, diploma in hand. But the look in people's eyes didn't have the same expression of innocence as before. Students were drawn to the world of commerce and material possessions. The traditional notion of "attaching greater value to agriculture than to commerce" had been swept away. Pursuing a career in the civil service or setting up your own business was an end in itself. It was fashionable to say: "The ends justify the means," or: "To succeed in your enterprise, don't fret about the details." Once, I remember talking to a colleague who was a literary professional about how important it was to be sincere in life. He looked at me as if I were a Martian.

"Haha, sincerity, how much does an ounce of that cost?" he burst out laughing. "Who wants to know about sincerity? Don't even say that word. People will laugh in your face."

It left me speechless. I thought: "If everyone lacked sincerity, life would be awful."

The people of Shenzhen lack morals. In this city, the evil flowers of human nature spread like weeds. I spent my days in Beijing studying and attending lectures. Once back in Shenzhen, I found the city had changed. There was progress. Salary had increased from around 30 yuan to 70. People ate out more often in restaurants and partied more, but they also exploited each other more. Desire and envy was in the air. It's difficult to describe the atmosphere of this city. When I stayed at the endocrinology ward at Zhongshan Hospital, I remember seeing junior African doctors doing the rounds in the rooms. They smelt strongly of perfume. That was the first time I'd smelt perfume from a foreign country. But the scent mingled with a host of other hospital smells: alcohol, antiseptic, medicine, the smell of urine coming from chamber pots under the beds, the smell of blood coming from bed sheets with stains that repeated washings couldn't wash out. All this was blended with the sour taste in my mouth in such a way that I could no longer differentiate between the different kinds of smells.

Being away from Shenzhen helped me find peace.

I was constantly fleeing from the battlefield that was the city of Shenzhen in search of a place to hide. I attended courses in Beijing and Nanjing; I studied journalism in Guangzhou; I loafed around on the campus of Sun Yat-Sen University, pretending to do research; while writing scripts for a number of television series, I was a permanent resident at the hostel of the Guangzhou Television Centre.

1997 was a turning point in the life of Li Lanni, a citizen of Shenzhen. Once the speculative bubble was under control, Shenzhen successfully took its first blood-soaked step towards capitalism. We could now speak human language. At the dawn of the 21st century, a sense of belonging began to take root in me. The three stages of Li Lanni's spiritual journey can be summarised by the following three sentences:

> *I see a flower and it's a flower; I see a man and it's a man.*
> *I see a flower, but it's not a flower; I see a man, but it's not*
>   *a man.*
> *I see a flower and it's a flower; I see a man and it's a man.*

FORTY-NINE

Diary
Friday, 12th December 2003 10:45 am

I haven't written anything in my diary for a few days. I've slipped back into depression again. From the end of autumn/beginning of winter to spring, the symptoms usually become more severe. Must be careful.

   At the end of last month, a woman in a neighbouring building who suffered from depression committed suicide. She jumped from the seventh floor in the early hours of the morning. She was 38 years old. Her husband is a teacher at the Foreign Language Institute and her child is still in kindergarten. I was at the hairdresser's in the western district, and the hair stylist there told me that the woman didn't actually live in that building and couldn't understand why she had chosen to jump from there. I think it's because she didn't want to leave her child such blood-stained memories of her, because he or she would be living in that building for many years to come. She must have loved her child deeply and, in my opinion, made a mature and well thought out decision. She was suffering from severe depression and death was the only way out. Stop! Li Lanni, stop your morbid thoughts. That's your problem. Your way of thinking is toxic, terrifying and obsessive. Stop fuelling your monstrous thoughts of death, suffering and inner torments. A demon is lurking inside you. "Get behind me, Satan!"[1]

   I went back to Shenzhen a couple of times recently. The last time, it was to attend a literary and cultural seminar organised by Huang Liman, Party Secretary of the city. Apart from a few committee members and public officials, there were altogether 37 artists and literary professionals. Ten participants were supposed to make a speech. As I hadn't been chosen and had nothing to say, I felt relaxed and un-anxious. I ate an orange and a banana. I was bored and was about help myself to another banana, but I must have grabbed at it too suddenly, because it went flying off the table onto the carpet. Fortunately, it didn't land on the committee members, who were sitting on the front row.

   I got a good laugh out of it. It's wonderful to be calm and unworried.

   God watches over everything. He gives His blessings at the right time and according to His plans. He says: "Child, be serene and wait to see how things will turn out."

   Yesterday, Li Mei and Lao Fan paid me a visit at the Sun Yat-Sen University. They gave me 39 magnificent champagne-coloured roses. I haven't seen such splendid, delightful and romantic flowers in a long, long time. Even Lele, who was sniffing daintily at the flowers, seemed to appreciate their charm.

Notes

The sky is sunless. When I switched off the computer yesterday, I was shivering with cold and my hands and feet were frozen. I think the cold came from inside me. I had an urge to go outside into the sun, but the sky was overcast, and the morning sun was hiding behind the clouds. At 21 degrees, I shouldn't be shivering like that. I think I am going to fall sick.

I was waltzing around the apartment just now, holding Lele in my arms, and singing the song: "My Life is Full of Sunshine" non-stop. To understand myself better, I'm going to practise my cognitive therapy. It will drive the shadows from my mind and direct it towards the light. Lele was watching me warily. He didn't seem happy, nor unhappy. I have no idea what he was thinking, but there was a look of concern and understanding in his eyes. With Lele huddled against me, my body began to thaw and come back to life. I am grateful to emotional support animals, because they help us heal. Lele weighs 11 kilos. I whirled around the apartment a dozen times until I was out of breath. My shoulders were aching, but I felt much warmer. I put Lele on a chair, stood in front of him and jiggled my shoulders, as if I were conducting a choir. Then under a sudden impulse, I began to swing to the rhythm of the waltz, conduct my choir, dance around wildly and sing: "My Life is Full of Sunshine" at the top of my lungs. All at the same time. Lele was sitting and looking up at me, as if there was nothing unusual about my behaviour. Not wanting to frighten him, I changed posture and crouched down on a chair. I was looking, but couldn't see; I was listening, but couldn't hear. Agitated and edgy, I felt there was something hard in my belly. Maybe the meridians of my body were blocked, or maybe I suffered from Stagnation of Energy[2] and Stasis of Blood.[3] I had to find a way to disperse the blockage.

Recent discovery: It's much more comfortable hiding in the wardrobe than under the sofa.

The wardrobe calms my nerves. If I had a cat and it were locked up inside, it would wonder: "Is her behaviour normal?" Answer: "Yes." So, you see. I'm getting better. Inside the wardrobe, I can be in a sitting position. There is even enough space to move around a bit. It is dark, but the cracks around the door let in narrow threads of light. A thought: If I were lying inside a coffin that hadn't been sealed so that air could pass through, wouldn't it be more comfortable than being in a wardrobe? As a child, I often heard the villagers say how they should have a coffin prepared for when they die. Some elderly people kept their coffins at home, and some even slept inside them. And if I lay the wardrobe down on the ground in a horizontal position, wouldn't it be like a coffin then? The thing is, whenever I am inside the wardrobe, I feel nauseous and my head aches. The winter clothes give off a blend of smells: dry-cleaning chemicals, mothballs, dirt, dust and goodness knows what else. It makes me dizzy, and makes me want to come outside. Quick, a bottle of essential oil. I need a bout of aromatherapy.

Li Lanni, you're getting better. You'll find a new therapeutic method to cure yourself, whatever it may be. You have the willpower and determination. Don't give in to despair. Yesterday, you wanted to scream: "Don't despair. You keep everything bottled up inside. That's why you have something big, hard and painful in your belly. But you're pulling through. Well done. Look at what is bright. Go towards the light."

Li Lanni, you're upset with yourself. You blame yourself for relapsing into depression. During your moments of weakness, you think: "It's harder to live than to die." Control yourself and stay vigilant. You're teetering on the brink. Your soul is about to leap out of your body, screaming: "I'm going insane! Just let me fall to pieces!" And the demons and malevolent spirits are shrieking: "Let us out! Let us sing and dance. We're going to devour everything. Everything!"

Lanni, calm down. Don't be afraid. Have faith. You must believe that the sun will soon rise and dispel the malevolent spirits. And you will be saved.

2nd *December* 2006

Correlations

**Excerpts from a Colour Doppler Report
from a Medical Check-up in 2006**

Date: 13 December 2006

Place: Medical Examinations Department, Health Bureau, Shenzhen

Colour Doppler of the Thyroid

Report: The remaining thyroid is normal. Several superficial lymph nodes on both sides of the neck, the largest one measures 1.1 x 0.4 cm. The surrounding tissues and contours are blurred. An increased blood flow is observed.

Conclusion: Following surgery for cancer of the thyroid, an enlargement of the superficial lymph nodes on both sides of the neck is observed. A possible lymphatic metastasis on the right? Please compare with the clinical diagnosis.

(Further diagnosis is necessary in general surgery.)

Ms Li Lanni: Please make an appointment with general surgery and keep us informed.

Medical Examinations Department
19 December

Complementary Notes

It's the last twilight of 2006. We had a mild sunny winter's day with a clear sky.

Sunlight was streaming through the windows of the study and its glare on the LCD screen was dazzling my eyes. I drew the curtains but needed light to write, so I opened the curtains again. Although the light was hurting my eyes, it instilled a sense of calm and well-being in me.

I was planning to finish the first version of this book by the end of this year. I thought I could make it, that my willpower alone would have sufficient command over my computer to transcribe the words that have been buried in me all these years. But once again, my brain has ruined my plans. It really makes me wonder about myself.

I've been in a bad way these past three months. My initial intention was to write the "Diary" section from the point of view of someone suffering from depression. But I would be a person in good health for "Notes," "Correlations" and "Complementary Notes." But the reality is, if I am to pursue my writing career, I will always be a writer plagued by depression, meaning a sick person.

Worries are gnawing at my insides. When will my illness let me take up my writing again and finish this book? On the morning of 13th December, during a medical check-up at the Health Bureau, the doctor in charge of the colour Doppler imaging said that there were two active lymph nodes on my neck in the area where I had a lymph node dissection. He strongly advised me to undergo surgery as soon as possible. But I don't want to go through another surgical procedure, because it would be at least two more years before I regained the strength to write again. And who knows? Maybe I wouldn't even be alive. The problem is, cancer can still be active even after surgery. And if I undergo chemotherapy, I know I will spiral into depression. It's a vicious circle. And so pointless. I was so distressed that I screamed inside over and over again: "Enough, enough! Let's finish it once and for all!" But immediately afterwards,

I scolded myself: "Li Lanni, don't be so weak. I forbid you to think this way. You have no right. You must live. It's your duty. Your life doesn't belong to you. You say you've had enough. Your reason pushes you to do cognitive therapy. But the flesh is weak, it imprisons your soul and keeps on whining: 'Enough. I've had enough!' There is nothing I can do, except pray: 'Don't be afraid. Have faith.' Li Lanni, pardon your own weaknesses. You're only human."

When I see other people, I always try to smile. And people compliment me: "You're in better shape than the rest of us;" "You've got rosy cheeks;" "You've put on weight;" "You're fit as a fiddle." I laugh but I say to myself: "You know what? I've had enough. Up to here. I pretend to laugh and smile. Even when I breathe, I'm smiling. I hope my smile is warm enough for you."

The angel of death is a misunderstood being. People have the false notion that it is cold, repulsive, ugly and vicious. But not at all. To me, it is beautiful, warm, attentive, kind and always reliable. A gentleman and a prince charming, it has eternal youth and vigour. The angel of death is also an angel of love. We were born into its arms. We must love and not be afraid of it.

Li Lanni, 2006 is coming to a close. It is your duty to live and finish this book. You have a long life ahead of you. Those who search for longevity don't necessarily find it; and those who don't strive for it don't necessarily live a shorter life.

There is a time for everything in this universe.

Go on, smile. Even if it's fake. You must live.

FIFTY

Diary
Friday, 19th December 2003 11:40 am

I was away in Shenzhen for a few days, and Zhou Xiaobing attended several meetings in Shanghai and Meizhou, leaving poor Lele alone at home. Two part-time housekeepers took turns to look after him, feed him and keep him company. But he was alone and scared at night. Xiao He and Xiao Li, the two housekeepers, said he was well-behaved while we were absent. He did his business on the newspapers in the lavatory, like he is supposed to. He was afraid of the two women. Instead of jumping all over them like he usually does with people, he kept out of their way.

When I was 10 years old, my parents left without saying why. I didn't know if they were coming back and, if they were, when it would be. Before going to Shenzhen, I kept saying to Lele: "Big Sister and Big Brother are going away for work. We'll come back to play with Lele in a few days' time. Don't be scared. Be good."

I don't know if dogs understand our language, but it was my responsibility to let him know that we were leaving.

Lele caught cold when I gave him a bath. I took him to the Jinhui veterinary clinic where he had two chest X-rays. He has bronchitis, pneumonia and an enlarged heart. After a skin test for penicillin allergy, he had three injections to reduce inflammation and was prescribed anti-inflammatory medication. The head of the clinic showed me how to give Lele his medicine, but Lele bit him on the thumb and nail, which bled profusely. In the end, Lele only swallowed one tablet out of five. All this went on from midday until 2:50 pm, when I finally got home.

I bought a jumper and coat for Lele. He looks so handsome in them.

I do nothing but laze around house these days, letting myself go. God knows when I'll recover.

Waiting is a lesson to be learnt. Knowing how to wait with joy, serenity, and free from anxiety is a discipline of the highest order that has faith as its foundation. I am only a student, who still hasn't passed the test.

Notes

When I was having dinner with friends in Shenzhen, they told me about an attractive office worker who was suffering from severe depression. Every morning, dressed to the nines, she would sit and look out of a window in the reception hall of a high-rise building. She seemed to be reflecting on when would be the best moment to jump. My friends were saying how strange it was that it was always women office workers who descended into a state of depression.

Actually, this isn't quite true. The number of men and women suffering from depression is higher in Shenzhen than in other cities. Men often refuse to seek help and suffer in silence until they reach a breaking point. It's the reason why the rate of suicide is higher with men than with women. Some books even say that 70 percent of deaths related to cancer, cerebral apoplexy, cardiac arrest, etc. are, in fact, due to depression. I often recommend my friends to read specialised books on mental illness. Depression-related suicide is one of the reasons for the surge in emotional violence in a given society.

Once a friend asked me a naïve question: "Are there really lots of sick people in Shenzhen? How come I've never seen them?"

"Those who have died are dead," I answered. "Those who are still alive have shut themselves away. Then there're others who have left to settle in the countryside and no one knows if they're dead or alive. And those who aren't dead yet from depression...idiots like me...There's not a lot of them about. People in Shenzhen...aren't easy to live with. I've been saying this for the last twenty years: It's normal to be depressed, but it's not normal not to be depressed."

Another friend said: "A lot of artists and painters in foreign countries die from depression. Looks like creative people are more prone to depression than others."

"Shenzhen people are creative, there's no doubt about that," I said. "Look around you, do you see anyone who's depressed? Everybody looks happy. But if you look more closely, you'll see that everyone suffers from depression in one form or another. To a mild degree, of course."

Night. In Shenzhen. These dreams again.

I dreamt that I went to the countryside with some friends. I found myself alone, wandering along a winding pathway as sinuous as sheep intestines. I arrived at the foot of a hill, where I saw three or four men about to administer justice to a man who was obviously a criminal. He was on his knees, bare-chested, with his hands tied behind his back. Someone was holding down his head. I turned around and was about to leave when I heard the man screaming in agony. He was begging for a quick death. Then I was on a street, where a crowd was watching an old beggar dying.

Why did I have these dreams again?

I rarely dreamt during my first two years in Shenzhen. The first year, I worked as a journalist and editor. All day and every day, I would be out and about covering stories. It was exhausting. I went to bed most nights at 1 or 2 in the morning. I stayed up all night when the newspaper was printed and caught up on my sleep the next day. I was thin and pale but was never sick and slept like a baby.

I remember one day in 1983, at the height of summer, I was on my bicycle, on my way to cover a story in Luohu. I hadn't had a drop of water to drink all morning and, at midday, I was hurrying back to the newspaper's headquarters for lunch. When I reached what is now today's Shenzhen's Opera House, I felt dizzy because of the heat and sun. My lips tasted salty and the sweat on my face was literally beads of salt. Seeing a stand on the side of the road selling soft drinks, I realised that I needed one badly but had no money on me. I stopped to catch my breath. There were no trees along Hongling Road at the time, so I couldn't take refuge in the shade. The heat was stifling, and I said to myself: "When will there be trees along this road where I can cool off? When that day comes, I'll have enough money to buy soft drinks. I'll sit myself down nicely at the foot of a tree and drink two at one go." At that thought, my thirst subsided, and I regained the energy to continue on my way.

I was in the middle of writing this section when an episode of depression forced me to stop.

That was a month ago. Today, I forced myself to switch on my computer, in an effort to pick up the thread again. Headache and nausea. Impossible to think or write. I give up.

I can't win. Sitting in front of the computer makes me dizzy and nauseous. I fidget on my chair. All I want to do is to hide under the sofa, fully aware that it won't do much good. Last time, I hid under the sofa for 20 minutes, but it had no effect whatsoever. It's pathological. I shouldn't go under the couch. Pull yourself together. Do some therapy. Get out of the house. Relax. Go and sit in the sun. I'm falling apart at the seams.

It's a never-ending struggle.

Sometimes I hear noises inside me.

I want to throw up. Do you remember these sensations? The nausea doesn't come just from the stomach, but from the abdomen, chest, forehead, radiating from the inside of my body to the outside, from my brain tissues, blood and even my breath. It seethes outwards, slowly invading my whole body, eating me up, like a sticky lump seeping out of an extra-terrestrial organism.

Why do you pretend to be so calm and untroubled? How do you know your cells haven't become cancerous? You don't want to hear about the bad news. You're scared of doing more tests. You're scared of another surgical procedure. You're not scared of being killed by a bullet fired from a rifle, but of being skinned alive.

I am in no rush to have another operation. If it is my fate to die, then I could very well die even when I am being operated on for a cancer. If it is my destiny to live, then I'll live anyway. What terrifies me the most is switching on my computer and coming face to face with my own book, *A Crowded Silence*. Just standing next to my computer makes my brain start emitting interference signals, like the crackling sounds that loudspeakers make which grate on your nerves and hurt your ears.

Should I continue to write? Yes.

Are you capable of it? No.

Message from your conscious mind: Pull yourself together.

Message from your subconscious mind: Don't push me over the edge.

The message from my subconscious mind crept away and hid itself out of sight. As for my writing, I wrapped the idea up like a *zongzi*[1] and stuffed it into a corner so dark that I can't even see my own fingers. Then I covered it with straws and laid a big stone on top. Let sleeping dogs lie. Close your eyes and mouth. I'm taking a rest. Sleep, sleep.

My subconscious mind has curled up into a ball and closed its eyes, pretending to be asleep.

I must get out of the house.

Take it easy.

A Crowded Silence is lying on my grey desk in Guangzhou. My IBM portable computer is closed, its black lid covered in dust. I left the dust there on purpose to keep it sealed from the outside world.

Why are you always holding a box of cake? Do you have bulimia? You've just finished your meal, put down your chopsticks and now you're eating soda crackers, jujube paste cakes, nori seaweed cakes and bubble cakes. Your belly is so full that you can barely sit down. But, standing up, you keep stuffing your face with roasted peanuts, salt and pepper walnuts, dark chocolate, bananas and oranges. Your belly is bloated and aching. You rub it to ease the pain, but you can't stop eating. You pig out on all sorts of snacks until you are numb. It is to divert the blood circulation away from your brain to your intestines. It makes you feel better. This therapy is called "eat all you like."

Another person in my circle of friends has started taking antidepressants.

A neighbour said to me: "Ms Li, have you heard? The day before yesterday, someone jumped off a building. It was a woman in her early forties, a university teacher."

Antidepressants + bulimia + heavy dose of hormones + lack of oxygen in the brain = my self-styled technique for staying sane.

After the New Year holiday in 2007. Shenzhen. A sunny day at midday. Alone on Hongling Road. I was at the crossroads, waiting for the lights to turn green. Suddenly, in my mind, I saw the portable computer that was lying on my desk in Guangzhou. On its black surface was Einstein's face. That all-too-familiar face: tousled white hair, deep wrinkles, an enigmatic expression, eyes full of intelligence and a mischievous smile on his lips. Laughing, he said to me: "Why don't you come over?" The traffic, crowds of people, red and green lights, buildings and trees, they were all fading away into the background…My head was spinning. I took a step backwards. My soul was about to fly away. I grasped for something stable next to me, telling myself: "Hold on. Don't fall. Stay calm." Yes, it was Einstein, smiling at me from the edge of the sky. Light clouds passing. Tousled white hair. His cheeky eyes and smile were saying: "Why don't you come over?"

Sitting at my computer, I have this desperate urge to run out of my study.

Several days have gone by. I wanted to finish this section but am stuck. Writer's block. I make enormous efforts to control myself, and to stop myself from running away. Must talk about a thought that has obsessed me. It's been over a month now and my obsession is like a balloon that is blowing up bigger and bigger by the day. And it's extremely worrying. Why Einstein? Is it just a random mental image?

Einstein shouldn't even exist in my subconscious. I've always been useless at science. I never understood Einstein's theory and I am not interested in him either. So how come his face just appeared, sprouted even, on the lid of my computer, like a gigantic magic mushroom from a fairy tale? Over a month ago, while I was having afternoon tea at the Peninsula Hotel in Hong Kong, I suddenly thought of my computer and saw Einstein's face, cheerful and glowing, as if he were listening to a waltz.

Must get on with my writing, even if it doesn't go as planned. Otherwise I'll keep on seeing Einstein's face in the next few days, or the face of God knows who.

Can somebody tell me if it's just a mental image or a mental aberration?

12th February 2007

Correlations

Excerpts from "The Artist"

At the time, I was living in a dark and sunless room in a residence provided by my unit. I was on the ground floor and several bachelors, who worked in the arts, were on the first floor. One day, as I was coming home at dusk with my shopping, which consisted of green vegetables and a tin of pork meat, I noticed an unfamiliar face on the first floor balcony. The man had long tousled hair styled in an androgynous fashion. He was wearing a pair of loose grey trousers with braces. His small eyes with droopy lids and his round oily face gave him an arrogant look.

"Ah…Solitude," he cried out suddenly in a heavy regional accent.

Startled, I observed him more closely. He was facing west, admiring the last rays of the sunset. Later on, I learnt that he was a graduate of a prestigious art school, had won a national artistic exhibition award, and that his name figured on a list of celebrities. Fresh university graduates came to listen to his talks. Arrogant and solemn as an imam, he was pedantic and overbearing: Nietzsche said this, Fromm said that. He gave brilliant talks on Van Gogh, Dali and Kandinsky. Many young women, impressed by his talent, fell under his charm and wanted to marry him. But when his talks were over and the audience had gone home, the artists in the residence would tear him apart. They denigrated and poured scorn on him by saying he spewed nothing but rubbish; he left his dirty laundry soaking in a bucket for over a week; his talks weren't worth the rat poison you'd find in the streets; he only ate instant noodles. He listened in silence, smiling from time to time, as if he was about to cry.

There were composers, photographers and dancers living in the residence. They had all won an award of some kind and had had, at one time or another, their moment of fame. Even if they weren't listed as a celebrity, they were gifted with multiple skills. They could cook, do the gardening and make money on the stock market. From time to time, they would feel sorry for him and invite him to drink wine and eat meat. Wasn't meat much tastier than vegetables? He was sad, because he liked to eat fatty meat.

One day, I went up to the first floor to chat with him. He had three big bulky suitcases with his paintings inside, most of which were oil paintings. The painting technique of his first period was classical and precise, with fine brush strokes. Each character in his paintings told a sad story. His award-winning works belonged to this period. The portraits from his second period depicted shapes that were full of movements and changes, as if he wanted to blend the theme of madness into his work. They reminded me of Chinese burlesque theatre. You could tell from these paintings that he was striving to change his style but was struggling. Unable to go back to his first period or move forward into his next phase, he was stuck between the heavens and the earth.

"How come you haven't done any new paintings since you arrived in Shenzhen?" I asked him.

"I don't feel inspired," he answered. "My heart is both full and empty. It's really getting to me."

"Shenzhen is a peculiar place. A lot of artists and literary writers have come here…but we haven't heard of them since. You'd think they've disappeared into the Bermuda Triangle."

"Ah…that's the way it is," he said.

Then he looked up into the sky.

"Ah…Changjia…Come back," he shouted, tapping frantically on a photo album he was holding. "I want to eat fish, but there aren't any… I want to leave, but I have no car…no home…"

Soon after this, I moved into another district.

One time, I came across him in a bank. He was waiting in line and looked cold, haughty and imbued with a sense of superiority, like a stork standing above a clutch of chickens. When he saw me, his face softened. He joked and said that he was glad to see another poor person like him. I looked around me and saw people holding packets of money wrapped up in newspaper or brown kraft paper. A man who looked like a retired soldier was filling in a form. I glanced at it quickly and saw the numbers "10,000."

"What do you do to get rich?" I asked the artist, laughing.

He pointed to a counter, where there were wads of 10-yuan bills. The old woman, who was depositing the money, had a small face and yellow complexion.

"How many thousands are you going to deposit?" he asked me, lowering his voce.

"One hundred yuan. And you?"

"I'm going to withdraw fifty. For crying out loud, how long does it take to count all those bills? How about if I throw a grenade?"

I saw him again several years later. It was at some friends' place during the winter. People were talking, but he was quiet. His face had thinned, and his air of superiority had disappeared. He was wearing a stylish grey jumper. I talked to him about his work and he showed me an album of his paintings. But I couldn't make out what his paintings were about. Did they depict images or Chinese characters? Was the ink dark or light? Were the shapes moving or static? Did they express melancholy or joy? Were these people or spirits, earth or water, clouds or mist, sun or moon? His paintings reminded me of the ancient primordial world of earth, sky and wind. They made me think of mythical characters: Nü Wa,[2] Hou Yi,[3] Kua Fu,[4] Donghuang Taiyi,[5] Shan Gui[6] and Xiang Furen.[7] The souls of the ancient world were reincarnated in his paintings.

"They're splendid," I sighed to myself.

He had finally found his place in this city. Before, like an accursed artist, he was at odds with his environment. But he was more at peace with himself now, and this harmony came through in his paintings.

"You earn a good living now, right?" I asked.

"Not bad," he replied. "First, I sell myself, then I sell my paintings. I go and actively seek out the buyers and publish albums of my work. Every day… I learn how to be more thick-skinned and brash. But business is good…ah… Don't look at me like that. Money is a noble thing. The relationship between art and money is the same as that of a boat and the water that it sails in."

I haven't seen him these last two years. I heard that his business was flourishing, that he had made a fortune on the stock market and had bought several apartments and plots of land. But he had cut ties with the penniless acquaintances he had known in his previous life. Others said he was still painting, had taken up Zen meditation and was holding much publicised exhibitions abroad. Then there were others who said he was struggling and that he had gone to Nandao in the Shanghai region to seek his fortune.

Nothing surprises me anymore in this city. I believe only half of what I hear. Because what I hear doesn't make sense and what I see is unreal.

From time to time, at dusk, I remember that year, when a certain artist stood on a balcony and cried out in a heavy regional accent: "Ah… Solitude."

26th September 1990

Complementary Notes

That was a portrayal of a person with a certain level of culture living in Shenzhen at the end of the 1980s. The period between 1987 and 1997 corresponds to a time in my life when I felt demoralised and despondent as someone who had received a certain level of education. I was afraid of Shenzhen. My soul was lost. It was wandering from campus to campus and then curling up in a corner to rest. The Shenzhen economy was gaining momentum, but the city seemed so cold, and I felt more and more a stranger. I was a bee trapped in a sticky spider's web that was sucking out my life force.

The new housing policy that allowed individual citizens to buy apartments was first put on trial in Shenzhen. At the time, I had just finished my studies at the Lu Xun Literary Institute in Beijing. When I returned to Shenzhen, people were saying that the housing policy would soon be put into effect. But I lacked the financial means to buy an apartment, whereas most people were able to pay up in one go. Filled with shame, I thought: "Others can afford it, so why can't you? Those who arrived in Shenzhen several years after you can pay in instalments over a period of one to three years. And you, you'd still be paying after ten years. When did you become so feeble and substandard? You'll lose your footing in this city. It has no use for people like you."

What worried me was that I was only away in Beijing for two years. How come Shenzhen was now made up of middle- and high-income households? For the first time, I felt that Shenzhen was a threat to my survival. When I first arrived, I was considered quite talented. I was working as a journalist for a newspaper organisation. Although it was often short of funds, it was a place where I could grow professionally. When I was part of the arts and literature editorial team, I was like a handicapped orphan whose survival depended solely on myself. At the time, literature had no place in a city like Shenzhen. When I talked about the Writers' Union, people would ask me: "What kind of shoes do you make?" When I mentioned the Chinese Arts and Literature Federation, people would ask: "Is that a transport company?"

I heard that people with insufficient funds could apply for a mortgage at the Jianshe Bank. So I asked a former colleague, whom I trusted, to make enquiries for me. We came to Shenzhen together, and she chose to settle down here. She was competent and was full of romantic and revolutionary ideals. Much more so than I was. I needed to find out more about the mortgage: Was it possible to obtain a 15-year mortgage for people in my kind of financial situation? Was the interest rate high? I needed a trusted friend to help me find my way in this financial labyrinth and ease the pressure.

When she saw me, my friend waved her arms gaily in the air. Her voice was warm and clear.

"Lanni, what a coincidence! I was just thinking about you. Do you want to buy an apartment?"

I was touched by how thoughtful my friend was. Knowing I was in a difficult situation, she wanted to help.

"Yes, I lack sufficient..." I blurted.

Before I could finish, she cried out gleefully:

"Excellent! If you can't afford one, then can you relinquish your rights and transfer them to me?"

I was hoping to hear a sympathetic voice say to me: "Don't worry, we'll find a solution together." I was expecting her to say: "I hope you don't mind me saying this, but would you like me to lend you the money?" My friend's euphoria left me stunned and speechless. Then, getting hold of myself, I asked:

"And you...your apartment?"

"I've already bought it," she replied casually. "But I want to buy a second one."

I don't know how long I stayed in this state of shock, but I heard a small voice say: "And me, where am I going to live?" Obviously, my friend had thought out everything in advance, for she replied: "You could always go back to Guangzhou. Anyway, your job isn't nine to five." She had a good point there, but I was still numb. Then she proceeded to tell me the good news: Her husband had made enough money to buy two apartments. I forgot how I wriggled out of this situation, but knowing me, just to change the subject, I was probably blabbering the first thing that came to my mind and got myself tangled up in the process. After that, I probably ran away and hid myself in oblivion.

This was at the end of the 1980s. While writing this book, that incident floated up to the surface, after years of being buried in the underground layers of my mind, scattered among the debris of my memories.

In Shenzhen before 1990, if you said someone was educated, it was as if you were calling him or her mentally challenged.

One day, a neighbour from the floor above walked past my door. He saw me and asked:

"What are you doing?"

"I'm reading," I answered.

He looked at me, surprised, and studied me as a doctor would study a patient.

"Are you from outer space or what?" he said. "Who reads books these days?"

He used to be a well-known journalist. After having persuaded a woman millionaire to buy ancient manuscripts at the auctions, he gave up writing and became a businessman. He offered me advice with the utmost sincerity.

"You really have to change your way of life," he said. Then, pointing to himself, he continued: "Look at me, was I well-known? Yes, but that wasn't enough. I could have died, and no one would have been sorry. They'd just say I was loser. I had to change my bloody career. I had to make money. I had to show these bastards and myself that I could afford a car and an apartment. These nouveaux riches are peasants and their days are numbered. It's somebody else's turn now. It's time for us writers to get rich."

He finished by saying:

"I'll be frank with you. Being a public servant isn't difficult. Doing business isn't either. The most difficult job is writing. You shut yourself away, alone, slogging and sweating blood over every single word. You get calluses on your fingers. Stupid. I was really stupid. I changed my career late in life. Look around you, opportunities are everywhere. What're you doing, holed up at home with your nose in your books? Don't wait until your hair turns grey. You'll regret it."

When my neighbour left, I stared at the books on my shelves, agonising over what he had said. I was reading *Songs of the Yuan Dynasty* that day. I had chosen it not to gain knowledge, but to pass the time. I like songs from that period. As I read them silently to myself, their rhythm and cadence usually create a theatrical ambience that puts me in good spirits. I had no other reasons for reading them.

I felt a rush of anxiety and heaped reproaches on myself: "Shenzhen people want to become rich before anything else. Time is money. Reading is a waste of time. Its sole purpose is to kill time. You'll never change. Aren't you ashamed of yourself? You're sick. Apart from reading books, what else can you do? What *can* you do in Shenzhen?"

Overcome with dismay, I didn't know what to say to myself.

A man leaves his native village. He goes into the world to learn a trade. He wants to learn: "the technique to kill a dragon," as the old saying goes, which means gaining mastery of an extremely difficult skill. He pays for a master to teach him. After several years of hard training, he returns to his village. He gives a demonstration of his "technique to kill a dragon" to his family and the entire village. But instead of applauding him, they laugh in his face and scoff: "Dragons don't exist."

I was such a fool. My life was a modern version of this story. In such difficult times, I couldn't afford to be proud, nor think I was better than others. I was no longer the mistress of my life, nor of this city. When I asked myself what I could do with my life, I looked up into the sky, filled with shame. I was roaming aimlessly in search of my place in life. This city didn't need me anymore. There was nothing I could do.

But what did I want to do?

It was no longer a question of what I wanted. I had been eliminated from this city. I no longer knew what I wanted to do.

The irony of it was that my first novella was called "What Do They Want to Do?" It is a story about a group of young journalists who come to Shenzhen to live their ideals. It was hailed by the critics as a breakthrough in literature that addresses the theme of population migration. That was two or three years before the incident with my neighbour. My decline had been spectacular. I no longer knew what I wanted to do. That was how I came to be eliminated.

Go on, smile. Even if it's just a wince. Life goes on.

FIFTY-ONE

Diary
Saturday, 20th December 2003 10:15 am

I am in good shape today. None of the usual aches and pains like dizziness, headache, stomach ache, or dry mouth. Urine is normal. Although I have a slight cold and runny nose, I feel relaxed and in high spirits.

I am both happy and puzzled that I should feel so good.

What's happening? Is it because of the weather? I slept well last night and didn't have any nightmares. I feel refreshed and in top form. If only every day were like this.

Today, while reading the Bible, I came across Psalm 103 "Praise the Lord" of David, Verse 3: "[...] Who forgives all your sins / and heals all your diseases [...]." The blessings of God are upon me. Here's the last verse: "Praise the Lord, my soul." Yes, yes, praise the Lord! Always.

Notes

I was flipping through *Searching For Memory: The Brain, the Mind, and the Past*[1] by Daniel Schacter.

In writing *A Crowded Silence*, I try to explore the connection between the mind and memory. And I came across Professor Schacter's book. Although he is harsh on those who suffer from depression, his book deserves to be read closely. But at the moment, my mind finds it hard to take in and digest what I read, let alone put his theories into practice.

When I read, my brain goes into slow motion. It's its way of showing displeasure. I use highlighters in red, green, purple and blue to help me. I highlight entire sentences and paragraphs until the page is splashed with different colours. But afterwards, I don't remember a single sentence I marked out. Going back over the main points, all I see are stripes of florescent colours that hurt my eyes.

Purple highlighter: "Memories that are repressed in the subconscious and which are associated with painful experiences are expressed through strange and perplexing behaviour. This serves to call our attention to the fact that these memories exist in us. We call this implicit memory."

I struggle to grasp the meaning of this.

Yellow highlighter: "In order to have a better understanding of ourselves, we should make an effort to look for clues that would otherwise be forgotten or lost forever in our memory."

Is it the translation that is ambiguous and obscure? Or is it the style of this Harvard professor that makes it incomprehensible?

Blue highlighter: "Since our implicit memory functions independently of our will, most of us are unaware that it exists. However, it has a far-reaching impact on our lives."

I am intrigued by the notion of a memory of the brain, of the mind and of the past.

Why are my memories of Shenzhen so "weak?" And how can a "weak memory" become "strong" enough to trigger depression?

Professor Schacter says: "According to research, those who suffer from major depression [...] have the ability to remember the dominant emotional tones of their experiences. However, their memory for specific details are only slightly better than normal people. [...] They tend to remember the negative aspects of their experiences more than the positive ones, thus perpetuating their depressive state of mind. [...] Their memory is extremely accurate when it comes to words that express all that is sad and tragic [...]."

When I try to write about my experience in Shenzhen, my memory becomes a blank. I see nothing but a hazy mist before me: grey fog, shadowy lakes.

Li Lanni, you still can't see straight, right? Why? What are you afraid of? You can't use depression as an excuse to run away anymore.

I'm not running away. Not for now. The truth is, I can't think straight. My mind is foggy, and I can't see...see anything. I am terrified of having hallucinations, of being tricked by my own memory and getting the confidential code wrong, unleashing the dragons and demons into my world.

I have never been close to my family. I have no roots, no native homeland, no ties.

I only have a few memories before the age of five. They say I was born on a military base in Zhanjiang. I had just started primary school when my father was transferred to the island of Neilingding. Then my mother followed my father onto the island, taking me with her.

I remember vaguely that one day, my mother, whose belly had grown big and round, left the island on a boat. She came back a few days later with a flat tummy, holding a bundle in her arms. I had no idea what was inside. I only remember people coming over to our house and making a lot of noise. They said my mother was holding a little brother and that this "bundle" was called Fanding, named after the island of Neilingding, where we were living. The adults wouldn't let me touch the "bundle" and I felt left out of the joy that filled our home. I went outside and walked into a hut on the side of the road.

There was a wardrobe inside. I leant against it, watching the soldiers go by. Some of them asked me:

"Xiao Lan, what did your mother give birth to?"

"A kitten," I said casually.

"Haha, what does that make you?"

Annoyed, I answered back:

"A puppy."

It made them laugh even more.

"What's his name, your little brother?"

"He's called 'He Bugs Me,'" I snapped.

The following year, I started my first year of primary school and lived with my grandmother in Pingxiang. As my father was transferred several times after that, I changed schools a few times the second year.

When I was in sixth year, I had already been to five or six different schools: one year in the province, the following year on the island and the year after that in town. It was the same in secondary school: one year in the mountains of the island of Hainan; the following year on the plateau of Hainan; and the year after that in Jiangsu.

I had no roots. During my entire childhood, I had no friends and lacked the affection of my loved ones.

I was left to my own devices during my adolescence and spent my youth in various hospitals. My sense of family is virtually non-existent.

When I was living in Shenzhen, I refused my family's help. I didn't miss my parents. I was working as a journalist and focused all my energy on my job. I was under tremendous stress and then, one fine day, my parents arrived unannounced, which annoyed me to no end.

"I told you not to come. You did it on purpose."

They stayed one day and returned to Maoming the next day. Before leaving, my mother said to me, half-jokingly:

"When you were five years old and we were living on the island of Neilingding, every month I used to take you to the town Baoan to buy books. The first time you came to Shenzhen, it was your mother who accompanied you. Don't you ever forget that!"

But it left me indifferent.

The above entry was dated the 30th day of the 12th month of the lunar calendar. It was unfinished. Depression stopped me from writing.

Correlations

Excerpts from *"Stories of Old, Stories of New"*

"Do you remember the island of Neilingding?" Father asked. "Wild grass, the height of a man, grew in front of the military barracks. There was a lovely beach not far away."

Father wanted to visit the island again. He had spent the best years of his life on the islands of the southern seas of China under the slogan: "Stay vigilant, protect our fatherland." Sometimes, I think that during his youth, or later when he was no longer young, he only thought of himself as a warrior, forgetting that he was also a father. If, before joining the army, he had been less interested in literature, his revolutionary ideals would certainly have been much stronger. He was assigned to his post on the island of Neilingding in the prime of his life. There is a photograph of him together with a dozen or more soldiers. Everyone was looking at the camera, except for him. He loved classical poetry and, above all, the poem "Crossing of the Lingding Sea" by Wen Tianxiang.[2] I wonder if he confided in his wife, who had a sensitive temperament, or if he talked to her about his fears and what Lingding meant to him. As a child, I often heard him recite these two verses from his favourite poem: "Since the dawn of time, who has never seen death / I keep my loyal heart for the glory of my country." But he left out the following verses: "Standing on the sands of terror, I speak of my fears / Watching the Sea of Lingding, I sigh with loneliness." I suspect he knew this poem by heart.

When I arrived on the island of Neilingding, my predecessor was preparing to leave. He faced the island, bowed three times, patted me on the shoulder and said:

"Don't worry. You won't spend the rest of your life here."

Then he burst out laughing, making no effort to hide his joy at leaving. After the boat had left, I spent a long time on the beach. My father also loved the beach, where he often spent evenings walking by himself. Whenever he was tired, he would sit among the thin and sparsely-grown wild grass, looking silently out at the sea.

"Do you remember what happened that year?" Mother asked. "A boy pointed a pistol at his sister's head and shouted: 'Surrender or I'll fire.' But the little girl didn't surrender and there was a loud bang…"

The little girl was four years old. She had dark eyes with long lashes, a pony tail and a green ribbon in her hair. She liked to say that a dragonfly was really an aeroplane and that she wanted to be a military pilot when she grew up. She transformed into a red dragonfly a long time ago and has flown away.

My mother was the only doctor on the island. She pressed her hand down on the gun wound, but blood was spurting out and running between her fingers. Bright red sticky blood. Her hands were trembling. Not even when she was a nurse in the Korean War did her hands tremble so much. Holding the gun in his hand, the father threatened to kill his son. The boy ran away, hid inside a cave and descended into insanity.

A child of seven doesn't deserve divine punishment. Adults make war. They are trained to fight on the battlefields and be on high alert, always ready to fire. They even sleep in their uniforms. It is only natural that a child would follow their example. At that time, which child had never played with a pistol?

"The little girl lost so much blood," my mother said. "I think she was buried on the island. But I can't remember if she was buried or cremated. I don't even know if her grave is still there…"

She was going on and on.

It was getting on my nerves.

I had told my parents that I would make inquiries about the boat. But I was overloaded with work: attending meetings; compiling dossiers; listening to recordings; writing summaries and organising conferences. With my head buried in work, I had forgotten that I was my parents' daughter and didn't make inquiries about the boat.

In 1984, I returned to Neilingding with a group of tourists. The trees were a magnificent green. My heart was beating away, as if something were about to happen. Two hours later, this feeling of expectation had gradually subsided. Numbness began to take hold of me and boredom set in. Everything around me seemed strange: the blades of grass, stones, bricks, military barracks and uniforms. I didn't have the feeling that I had come back to something warm and familiar. The beach was dull and uninspiring. There were crowds of people, but the mood was flat and insipid. The sand was littered with coloured food packages and drink cans. The tall wild grass was still there. From afar, I could vaguely see the yellow, run-down military barracks.

I didn't feel the need to go back to see my old house. Not wanting to move, I sat on a tree stump by the wild grass. I was tired and drowsy, and my head ached from the sun. My eyes were squinting from the wind blowing in my face.

Don't look back on this island. Don't think about this beach anymore with nostalgia.

Don't leave. But the boats are infrequent, and you don't know when you can catch the next one.

What we have is time.

In reality…there is nothing there anymore. Don't go back. You won't find anything there. Better to try to know the Shenzhen of today. Really, it would be better.

Alright, but what does all it have to do with me? Nothing.
I don't understand anything anymore.
You will, when you're old.

June 1990

Complementary Notes

Three years have gone by in a flash, and I still haven't picked up the thread of my writing. Stories and narratives float through my mind, but I am unable to put them down on paper. It's agony. Every day, I go through the memories of when I was trapped in the bottomless pit of my depression, but the details keep fading away. Out of my grasp. Sadness and melancholy weigh on my heart. I try to drive out torturous and morbid thoughts that consume my mind, but in vain. Like grasping dust in the air, it slips through my fingers; like fog that I can't dispel. I am powerless.

Every day, I wait for something to happen to take me away from this world. Every day, I think: "If I have an accident, I don't want to be saved. Please respect my wishes and let me go." Maybe I should leave a note in my bag saying: "I, Li Lanni, the undersigned, solemnly declare that I refuse all attempts to resuscitate me. Please let me go."

I wish to leave this life. I am prepared for this eventuality.

FIFTY-TWO

Diary
Thursday, 25th December 2003 4:30 pm

It's Christmas Day and also my birthday. Mother called me this morning and sang "Happy Birthday" over the phone. Around 10 o'clock, Fanding and Liu He came over with Li Jiean. Fanding gave me two musical Santa Clauses – one big and one small. One plays an electric guitar and the other carries a golden sack. It just so happens that I wanted a Santa Claus that would bring me a bag filled with happiness.

As they said on *Hour of Power*: Christmas is a season of joy, beauty and love. It's also a time of revelation and wonder. The Holy Spirit is real and all-powerful and He loves us. These days, I keep thinking how my life is full of blessings. In his sermon, the Reverend Robert A. Schuller reminded us of this: "When we talk, we must say what is on our minds. If we believe in success, it will come to us and wonderful things will happen. The Holy Spirit grants us His blessings and we should say: 'I am grateful to the Holy Spirit for His benedictions and I can say that I am truly blessed!'"

I switched my mobile on at midday and found several birthday messages. Then we ate at Kangle Hongmei Restaurant.

Li Jiean is a happy and well-behaved little girl. She looks more and more like Fanding when he was little. She is cute, mischievous and as fit as a flea. I am happy for my brother. To my surprise, Lele is jealous of Li Jiean. He started barking at her as soon as she entered the apartment. It's as if he knows that this child is going to share the love that he receives. He was irritable and agitated. Unable to calm him down, I put him out on the balcony. When I went to see him later, he was whining like a little doll that had suffered a thousand wrongs. Poor thing. But he's been behaving himself today. He did his business on the newspaper and finished his kibbles and snacks.

I am blessed, and I give thanks to God. Praise the Lord.

Notes

My mind is elsewhere, and I just keep staring at the computer. Hours have passed and I've only typed one character. I read it and delete it. I type, read and delete. It's been one hour. Is it my right or left brain that has a short-circuit? Li Lanni, what do you mean by that?

An incident just came to mind.

Once, Mother and I were talking about the time when we lived in the small courtyard.

"The hidings I gave you," Mother said, "they were just to frighten you. The other parents used the belt and military whip, you know."

"But you beat us with a bamboo cane," I said. "They left red bumpy marks on our arms and legs. And they stung."

"Nonsense. I never hurt you."

"What? When you were in a temper, you had no idea how frightening you were. You always hit where it hurt the most and never on the tendons."

At this point of the conversation, Mother refused to listen.

"How's that?" I continued. "You never hurt us? Once I had a sty in one eye. You took a plastic toothbrush, heated it up and burnt my eyelid with it, saying it was a tip that such-and-such friend gave you. I said it really hurt, that I couldn't stand it. But you wouldn't have any of it and wouldn't let me move until the skin of my eyelid was burnt. Only then did you believe me and stop."

"I never did such a thing. You made it up. I've never heard of such a tip."

"Oh yes, you did, I remember it as if it were yesterday."

"I have no recollections of it whatsoever," said Mother, annoyed. "Don't blame all your unhappiness on me."

"Blame you for what?" I asked, not knowing whether to laugh or cry.

The conversation stopped there. I wanted to go back to the past in an effort to understand my mother's state of mind at the time. But people have selective memories. And our memories are fragile. I think the uppermost layer of our memory has a defensive role. Our reason filters all the incoming information. For we need to eliminate the negative thoughts and prevent harmful elements from entering our data bank. Although I don't understand how our memory functions as a system, I think that, at a certain level, there is a "recovery plant." Its function is to recuperate all the "files" containing toxic substances. But as the waste material accumulates, the "recovery plant" becomes more and more cluttered and congested. And if we don't clean out our minds, then our brain functions will slow down until the machine "breaks down." We may think that the toxic waste has been eliminated, because we are unaware of its existence. But, on a mental level, the waste is giving off toxic gas and a stench of decay. It seriously damages our minds. And one fine day, our psyche just breaks down and we sink into insanity.

I brought up the subject of the past with Mother not because of the painful hidings she gave us, which I will always remember, but because of her peculiar behaviour. Whenever she disciplined us, she would forbid us to run away and stopped others from coming to our aid. Her thin white face became red and blotchy. She held a bamboo cane in her hand, and her eyes, usually devoid of expression, gleamed with anger. Sometimes, she would even tell my brother and I to fetch the cane and give it to her. Then she ordered us to lock the door and windows, so that no one could hear her shouting and us crying. She liked to keep everything secret.

She had an unusual way of punishing us. We had to stay and bear the brunt of her anger until she started to laugh. I was only in my fourth or fifth year of primary school, but, deep inside, I knew inflicting such a humiliation on someone else was despicable. She wanted us to beg her for forgiveness and make her laugh, but I refused to give her that satisfaction. My brother was the shrewder of us two. He would meekly close the doors and windows and fetch the bamboo cane for Mother. Sometimes, he would even roll himself inside a straw mat that was lying on the bed. And then from inside the mat, he would shout: "You can beat me now, Mother!" He even took the initiative of showing his buttocks and said: "Go on, hit me!" He would think of all sorts of ways to make her laugh. For he knew that as soon as she started to laugh, his torture would be over. Although he was too young to be in primary school at the time, he was already a docile and obedient child. When I wanted to open the door and run, he would shout: "Big sister, don't leave. If Mother can't beat you, she'll be sick. If you don't let her punish you, she'll be angry." His pleas would remind me that if I didn't let Mother have her way, there would be no end to our torture. So I let Mother vent her anger on me. Following the example of the heroine Liu Hulan,[1] I would take on a defiant expression and look down haughtily at my torturer. This infuriated Mother and she would thrash me even harder, yelling: "How dare you look at me like that. I'm going to tear your eyes out. If you don't bow down in front of me, I'll beat the living daylights out of you. I'm going to break you." Sometimes, when Father was home, even he dared not intervene. I was hoping he would protect us, but nine times out of ten, we would be left disappointed. When he saw that Mother had worn herself out, he would say: "Stop, stop...That's enough." But Mother would say: "No, not until I laugh." Beside myself with rage, I would say: "Why should I make you laugh? You give me a thrashing and I have to make you laugh? Go on then, if you're not afraid of going to prison, beat me to death. I'll never bow down to you!"

Many years later, I was talking to my friends in Shenzhen about the hidings we endured as children. They had all been through it. They ran and hid until their parents calmed down. I said it didn't happen that way in my family and that my mother would beat us until she laughed. My friends were stunned. After a moment of silence, someone said: "But...it must have been awful, mustn't it?" Only then did I realise how appalling it truly was.

Talking about this aspect of my childhood allows me to clean up my "recovery plant."

I can bring myself to talk about it today, because the hate inside me has dissipated. I'm beginning to understand and respect my mother and even love my parents. Others who have had a more normal life might think this trivial.

They must think: "Li Lanni is hypersensitive, she's overreacting. She and her mother are both a pain in the neck. They're sick." And for those who have mental illnesses, this kind of story is just the tip of the iceberg. We are all sick, and psychotherapy has just begun. Li Lanni, you're such a bird brain. You don't think. You haven't a clue what it is to be sick.

I am angry at myself. Li Lanni, you have a memory problem, choosing only to recall the unhappy memories. Where others see a sesame seed, you see a watermelon. It's you who goes searching for things that bring you pain. There is a destructive virus loaded in your computer.

Correlations

Excerpts from *Depression: An Undiagnosed Illness*

Those who suffer from depression have inherited "organic scars" in their brain. When a child rebels, it is to express his or her pain and anger. It is a way of freeing him or herself from the injustices that he or she has suffered. The consequences of such an act are minimal. However, if the parents forbid the child to express his or her instinctive reactions (tears, sadness, anger) and resort to educational methods to exert control over him or her, whereby stripping his or her own means of expression, then the child will psychologically shut him or herself up. This behaviour is an expression of despair. Most people would then find themselves in a psychological dead-end. A child who has learnt to repress his or her emotions is incapable of developing a healthy sense of self-worth.

Ursula Nuber (Germany)

Complementary Notes

Psychologists and psychiatrists alike warn us of the following: In everything that has a connection to our memories, we are able to discern signs of depression in the same way we perceive a young shoot, a pistil or a bitter fruit growing on a stem.

Those of my generation carry "scars" inside them. As children, we lacked unconditional love. Who could have protected these children? If we can't trust our parents, then who can we trust? If our parents were incapable of accepting our instinctive reactions, then in whom could we have placed our hopes? How could we have lived, except locked up within ourselves, repressing our emotions or even inflicting self-harm?

FIFTY-THREE

Diary
Sunday, 29th December 2003 1 pm

Went for my medical check-up at the Health Bureau early this morning.

Notes

On the evening of 1st April, around 10:20 pm, I went up with Lele to the rooftop of this building on the 16th floor. I sat on the safety rail. Its stone base was 12 inches high and was decorated with mosaic tiles. A cool breeze was blowing. Bending forward to look down, I saw someone dressed in white walking with a comical gait. The big round patch of flowers on the patio resembled a face with no features. Suddenly, Zhang Guorong's face appeared in my mind's eye. I asked myself what day it was. The 28th or 29th March? No, it was 1st April. I must be careful. Then I sat astride the security rail, one bare foot dangling on the outside. The cool breeze gave me a sensation of wellbeing and I thought of freedom. I stood up on the edge of the rooftop, looking at the void around me. I was now closer to the sky than I had ever been before. Go on, rise up. An image often seen in films came to mind: Someone is standing on the rooftop of a building, about to jump off, because he could see no way out. It was exactly where I was at that very moment. I only needed to move forward, just a tiny little bit, not even one step, and I would fly into the sky.

Lele was lying beside the stone base. He was looking up at me with his little black eyes. I climbed up onto the stone base. No other building around me was taller than the one I was on. Emptiness stretched out into infinity before me. I felt a pain on the left of my navel. My nerves were acting up again. My thighs were aching, but my heartbeat was normal.

I had no intention of committing suicide. I wanted to stand on the edge of the rooftop. Just to see. But I didn't want to think too much about it, otherwise I would lose my self-control. I began to feel dizzy and queasy. It meant that I was normal, and that I didn't want to die. It was a perfectly normal reaction.

I could see through the bay windows of a balcony in the building opposite. Inside the apartment, a television was switched on, but no one was watching. Luxuriant plants were growing on a balcony slightly further away - a sign that the people living there were strongly attached to life. Several households had put their washing out on the balcony to dry. Many of the windows were unlit. I told myself to stop looking into other people's homes, because it was an invasion of their privacy. Not far below me, I saw a light coming from a window that looked into a sitting room, where there was a cabinet with an indoor potted plant on top. The pot was decorated with colourful floral patterns. I was afraid someone might see me and take me for a burglar or a voyeur or think that I was about to commit suicide. I shouldn't frighten people for no reason and, what's more, it would be embarrassing if someone called the police.

I wanted to walk along the edge of the rooftop, keeping my balance, like a tightrope walker or a ballerina dancing on the tip of her toes. Would I be able to stop myself from falling? All of a sudden, I felt tired and drowsy. I yawned. I felt my chest, but my heartbeat was still normal. My brain was working in slow-motion and again I wanted to yawn. It struck me that feeling sleepy in the dark meant I could easily lose my footing and fall off. The irony of it was that I had no intention of killing myself, but it would have all the appearance of a suicide. Perhaps there were other people like me, who simply wanted to walk on the edge of the roof without intending to jump. In stifling a yawn, a bubble popped out of the corner of my mouth. My eyes were watery and sticky from lack of sleep. Lele, knowing that I wasn't going to jump, no longer paid me any attention. He wasn't worried and was looking elsewhere. My reason was telling me that 1st April was a day full of risks. It must have been around 11 o'clock at night. Midnight wasn't a favourable time to be up in the heights.

Sleepiness was creeping up on me. If I stayed sitting on the security rail, I would probably end up falling into the void. Go, leave. Go home. Take the lift. Pick up Lele and take the lift. Home. Go home.

The orchids are dead. Six of them. In spring, I ran on a rampage and cut off all their leaves. If I hadn't done it, I would have hurt myself. But I think they'll survive. The leaves will grow again in two months' time. Their primitive energy might have been damaged, but not to the point of being irreparable. In hindsight, I realise that my subconscious mind knew that my behaviour was destructive and that the orchids could die. But my ego and selfishness wouldn't let my subconscious take control. During my outburst, I picked on something outside of myself. In order to protect myself, I had hurt these orchids - beautiful, innocent, defenceless and filled with vitality.

At the end of last year, the media was talking about a young man who came from the province to Guangzhou in search of work. As soon as he stepped off the train, he was robbed of his luggage, papers and money. He grabbed hold of a little girl, who was on her way to the market with her mother. She was only an infant and a complete stranger to him. He threw her over a bridge into a river and jumped in after her, ending his own life.

Although this incident made the headlines for a while, it failed to draw attention to the fact that depression, anger, resentment and aggression are alarm bells for mental illnesses.

Violent impulses lurk deep inside every one of us, and this is especially true when we find ourselves in threatening situations or when we are confused. It is an animal instinct. We live in threatening and insecure times, and our souls have no safe place in which to take shelter. Even if our economy continues to expand, material wealth would be incapable of lowering crime rates.

I believe in what the Bible says: We are all guilty. We all need to repent, ask for forgiveness and have a clear conscience.

I've reduced my intake of antidepressants, except for Seroxat and alprazolam, which I am afraid to reduce without the doctor's permission. But I wonder if I could decrease the extra dose of buspirone. If only I could.

Apparently, many suicide cases are the result of stopping medication. I have no intention of stopping, just reducing my intake. Do other people who are also on antidepressants all want to stop or consume less? I don't hold out any hope that the doctors will decrease the dosage. In fact, I won't even mention it, in case they increase my intake. These days, I only see doctors whom I have never consulted before. The purpose is to get hold of prescriptions, and I never go back afterwards. Several times, I skulked around a medical department like a thief, trying to avoid doctors who knew me.

With a smile on my lips, I would say jovially to the doctor: "I've come to see you for some medication. I've been prescribed the same medicine for many years now. They're written in my medical file."

"How do you feel?" the doctor asked.

"I feel good," I replied with enthusiasm. "I'm a lot better. Everything is fine."

After spouting my lies, I would hurriedly get up, a smile still plastered all over my face, thank him politely and back out the door. As soon as I was out of his office, I would scarper out of the psychiatric department. At the payment counter, I was on high alert, constantly looking around me, in case a doctor I know might spot me. I couldn't stop thinking: "What if such and such a doctor saw me here or at the dispensary? Or in the lift? Get out of here, quick!" Like a patient fleeing from a mental asylum, unwilling to stay one minute more, I scuttled out of the hospital like a mouse. Aware that I shouldn't work myself up, I was nonetheless incapable of controlling my agitation and nervousness.

I like it when the doctors say: "You're normal." Once, I talked to a doctor who I was consulting for the first time about that one rainy night on 1st April. I was on the rooftop on the 16th floor of my building. Standing on the security rail, I had an urge to fly up into the sky.

"It's positive to want to fly up high into the sky," the doctor said. "It's good to have high ideals."

Pleased that he was so encouraging, I blurted:

"Yes, yes, that's right. I wasn't really going to jump off the roof. I just thought how beautiful it'd be to open my arms wide open and fly into the sky."

"You're a very unusual person."

"Do you think so? Even when I was up on the roof earlier that day, I felt the impulse to fly or go near the security rail."

"Yes, it was the night, rain and solitude. You needed to feel the melancholic atmosphere."

This doctor left me puzzled. Was my state of mind positive or negative? I should shut up, in case he decided to increase my medicine dosage. Quick, get out of there. But I needed him to reduce the dosage, because my concentration was becoming poorer by the day. Even though the new generation of antidepressants have fewer side effects, I could feel their toxicity in my brain.

In my previous entry, I talked about how I would stand in front of the public toilets, struggling to tell the difference between the signs for men and women. This has gone downhill since the beginning of the year. Once, my brain had a malfunction in front of the toilets in a restaurant. I stood there for God knows how long, staring into space. My brain had seized up. Noticing that something was amiss, a waiter asked me: "Can I help you?" I looked at him, incapable of answering. He was smart and said: "If you're looking for the toilets, the 'Ladies' are here and the 'Gentlemen' are over there."

An even more ridiculous incident took place recently. I was convinced that I had worked out the difference between the signs for men and women. But, as I was leaving the toilets and going down the stairs, I saw a 10-year-old boy coming in. He looked at me and I glared at him, thinking: "He's well past the age of going into the women's. A right mummy's boy, he is!" A middle-aged man was walking behind him. He stared at me and I gave him a dirty look, thinking: "Honestly, it's a bit much, following your son into the ladies' room. Why don't you go to the men's? Some example this father is!" Then a young man came in. Thinking he must have made a mistake and had just followed the man in front of him, I was about to point out his error when it dawned on me that maybe it was me who had it wrong. I rushed to the door and looked at the sign. My brain couldn't register it. I forced myself to focus hard. Look at it. Look. It says: 'Gentlemen.'

Don't blame me. Put it down to the antidepressants.

9th June 2007

Correlations

Excerpts from a doctor's letter to my father

[...] Your daughter, Li Lanni, has been discharged from hospital following a surgical procedure. Everything went smoothly. After removing the thyroid tumour, we have made the following diagnosis: papillary thyroid carcinoma. Even though I had already received the report before discharging her from hospital, I waited until she had left before putting it in her medical file. We must do our utmost to protect Li Lanni. On the question of whether it would be necessary to tell your daughter the truth, it is my opinion that the word "cancer" would cause unnecessary fears and anxieties in a young married couple, placing an immense burden on their shoulders. I strongly recommend not letting her know of the diagnosis at this point in time. My impression is that she is not mentally strong enough to take the news. This is the reason for which I wrote 'papillary thyroid carcinoma' in the report.

(doctor's signature)
14th February 1988

Complementary Notes

I found the doctor's letter at the bottom of the bookshelf. I copied an excerpt. It's my way of purging out painful memories and exploring the latent wounds that have accumulated in me.

My eyes are puffy from looking at the computer for so long. They sting. I want to close them but can't. I am a nervous wreck. It's only when I lean my head against the computer that I can close them and give them some rest. I hate the memories of my past. Hate, hate, hate them.

The contents of this book are disorganised. It's a mess. The "Diary," "Notes" and "Correlations" sections are disconnected. How did it happen? It's because I'm going to pieces. I feel agitated and edgy, as if my blood is burning. Impossible to sit still. I need to do some bloodletting, but the pharmacies nearby don't sell needles or syringes. I have to go to the ones on Beijing Road, where they stock them.

I go through phases where I need to do bloodletting on myself to calm my agitation. The first time it happened was in Shenzhen. There were no single-use needles or syringes at the time. At the pharmacy, I bought needles, syringes and tin boxes to sterilise the needles in. I put them in a pan and steamed them for 15 minutes. I can't for the life of me remember where the idea of bloodletting came from. But I must admit, it's become a favourite little vice of mine. It makes me feel so much better afterwards. I usually do it several days in a row and a certain inner calm is restored.

Blood tests are always part of my annual medical check-up. I like to focus my attention on the needle, so as to catch the moment when the blood spurts into the syringe. I also like to watch the barrel slowly filling up with my own blood. I derive a certain pleasure from trying to make out if my blood is a dark or light red, or if there are any tiny air bubbles.

I wonder if my auto-destructive impulses have anything to do with my depression.

How did I get here? Performing phlebotomy on myself and getting a thrill out of seeing fresh blood spurt into a white basin. I'll come to that in the next few days, when I can think straight.

I'm going to talk about the first time I was operated on for cancer. It was in February 1988. I am still alive after all these years, so does that mean I have won the battle? The chemotherapy that followed my third surgical procedure was particularly trying on the nerves. A physician in Traditional Chinese Medicine prescribed me some medicine to counter the secondary effects. In an effort to reassure me, he said: "The survival rate is high for this type of cancer. Around forty percent of patients live for up to ten, even fifteen years after the operation." Feeling encouraged, I laughed: "We're in 2000. Twelve years have passed since 1988, and I'm still alive. Fifteen years isn't all that far off from now." Taken aback that my history of cancer went back such a long way, he said with sympathy and sincerity: "Eh...some even live longer than that. You have every chance of living up to twenty years with your positive attitude."

While going through chemotherapy, I felt profound anger towards my parents. Once, I said to Ququ: "Have you ever seen parents that stupid? If they hadn't made such a mess of my therapeutic protocol, I wouldn't have to go through so much pain." It wasn't until February 2000 that they showed me the biopsy report from 1988, which indicated a metastasis of my cancer. They had hidden the results from my husband, my brother and me. My mother had worked at the department that dealt with military secrets. Several years before my father retired, he belonged to the army's regulations department. My parents specialised in state secrets.

They had sent me to a local hospital, saying that I had a swollen lymph node on my neck that had to be removed immediately and that everything would be fine after a few stiches. To keep it secret, they had contacted a retired head surgeon at a hospital in the city. He came to the local hospital to perform the operation. Once again, they falsified the results of the pathological analysis. True, the operation was over quickly and only several stiches were needed. It took place in the afternoon, and in the evening I took a stroll in a park before eating out in a restaurant.

It was written in black and white in the report that it was a "metastatic follicular thyroid carcinoma," which is more serious than the "papillary carcinoma" of the first surgical intervention. According to the therapeutic protocol, in order to avoid serious sequellae, a lymph node dissection should have been done 24 hours following the operation. But my parents hid the report in a drawer, while waiting to decide if they should tell me the truth.

My father was against telling me, and my mother was undecided. The retired surgeon, whom she trusted, was abroad, and she had no one to discuss it with. My parents aren't illiterate. They are high school graduates and are considered to be intellectuals. But they were unaware that a patient with cancer should be treated by oncologists in a hospital and that a patient with metastatic cancer should be operated on in a hospital specialising in oncology. They knew about the metastatic cancer cells in my neck but did their utmost to keep it under wraps. That was why whenever we saw each other, they would eye me, looking concerned. They took to behaving in an almost neurotic way, always granting me preferential treatment. When I was at their place or at my brother's, I was never allowed to wash the dishes or sweep the floor. As soon as I started doing something around the house, they would worry and tell me to stop. They would order my brother to finish whatever I was doing. I had no idea of what was going on and protested in vain.

"Let me do it. I'm just the adopted son around here," my brother said, laughing at himself.

I was completely overloaded with work throughout 1998. I had assignments in Beijing once every two months. I had numerous writing projects going on at the same time: essays, scripts for television series, film scripts, creative writing courses at the Lu Xun Literary Institute. That year went by in a flash. My brain was clogged up with words and I had no idea that something was amiss. I thought my parents' strange behaviour was because they wanted to make up for their failings during my childhood. I was oblivious to the fact that the cancer cells in my neck were thriving and spreading. Like a merry-go-round, they were spinning round and round my lymph nodes, gaily encircling one before attacking another, invading one site after another until all of them have been vanquished.

Before starting chemotherapy in 2000, the oncologist said:

"Regarding the metastatic cancer cells that were discovered in December 1998, the hospital at the time was wrong not to have performed a lymph node dissection. You have the right to file a complaint."

"It won't be necessary," I said. "All this is thanks to my parents. It's not the hospital's fault. If, by a stroke of bad luck, I am dead, it's my parents who will have dug my grave."

FIFTY-FOUR

Diary
Monday, 12th January 2004 10:40 am

I haven't written in my diary for over 10 days. Been in good spirits.

Had an ultrasound on the morning of 29th April. The head physician, suspecting that there might be a tumour in the liver, recommended that I pay a supplement of 23 yuan for an ultrasound to set my mind at ease. A professional with a strong sense of responsibility, he asked an older and more experienced head of the department to look at the images with him. Neither of them thinks it's a cyst, but probably a solid tumour, and the chances are that it's benign. The swollen lymph node in my neck has disappeared. Has it moved to the liver? I hate the idea that what was vague up until now has suddenly become crystal clear, and that what was weak has suddenly become strong and inevitable. Further tests are needed.

Too exhausted to write at length about my mental state. I'll stick to the facts.

On 1st January 2004, I left Guangzhou and arrived in Shenzhen at midday. As it was the first day of the New Year, I couldn't do any major medical examinations at the hospital. I had no choice but wait. The 3rd and 4th fell on a weekend. I wanted to consult Dr Zeng, the head physician, who was working the following Monday (the 5th) and Tuesday (the 6th), so I made an appointment by phone and was third on the waiting list.

On the morning of 6th, Dr Zeng, prescribed me screening tests for "cancerisation of the liver." I voiced my concern to the secretary, who was sympathetic and understanding, and she gave me an appointment that same afternoon. At lunch time, I had Chaozhou cuisine in the Song Xuan Room at Hua Tai Restaurant. I took a rest after that. For two hours (from 3 pm to 5 pm), I kept on praying while waiting to do my medical tests. I felt calm but fainted as I was coming out of the room after the tests. The nurse told me to lie down on a bed and put me under observation for half an hour.

The results wouldn't be ready until the morning of 8th. I kept imagining all sorts of things. The Hong Kong singer, Mei Yanfang, died of pulmonary failure at 2 am on 31st December 2003. She had cervical cancer, which had spread to her liver, lungs, etc. They say she couldn't tolerate the pain and had asked to be euthanised. She had fallen sick two years earlier. Normally the cure rate for this type of cancer is 100%, but she refused to be treated. Apparently, she was devastated by her elder sister's death, as well as the deaths of Zhang Guorong and Luo Wen.[1] The media talks about it non-stop and it gets me down.

I picked up the results on the morning of 8th. It turned out to be a cyst of 0.5 centimetres. Fanding called me. Unaware of the stress that I had just been through, he offered to accompany me to the hospital, which touched me. In the afternoon, I hurried back to Shenzhen for an evening gala. I was tired, but in good spirits. On the morning of 9th, I went to the National Health Insurance Centre to claim a refund of my medical expenses. Then I saw a doctor for my cold. All is well.

Notes

To give my book some kind of structure, I drew up a rough plan for a narrative:

5th March: Had a discussion with Dr Li, a specialist in psychiatry at North Shenzhen Hospital.

4th March: On the 15th night of the first moon, went alone to Yuan Ling, where I destroyed two diaries I kept from 1991 to 1992.

3rd March: Dreamt that Lele ran away from the hotel and I couldn't find him.

2nd March: Dreamt that Lele was dead. I was digging in the ground at the spot where he was buried and found white bones and a lump of dried-up meat.

1st March: Dreamt that Lele had drowned in a washbasin and I was giving him mouth-to-mouth resuscitation.

I can feel myself sliding into depression but am too apathetic to ask for help. I'm coming apart at the seams. Even the computer is having a nervous breakdown. I wanted to copy "Correlations" into the computer, but every time I typed in a *pinyin* letter, it blinked twice and refused to register, as if it had feelings and a life its own. As if it were terrified of the words and were spitting them out. I totally sympathise with it. To make things worse, the LCD screen kept blinking and the words wouldn't show up on the screen. When I forced it, it would freeze. It'll give up the ghost any time soon.

I might as well stop writing.

Have an urge to shave my head, but people would think I'm out of my mind.

Cut. Cut. Cut. I've cut off all the leaves of the two boat orchids on the balcony. Stripping them of their leaves made me feel lighter afterwards. I went on a rampage. I also cut off all the leaves of the cattleya and crab cactus. The floor of the balcony was covered with leaves of all shapes and sizes. And I still wanted to cut some more. You would think there was a tacit complicity between the pair of scissors and I. Cut, cut. Chop them all off. I cut the leaves of the moth orchid, aloe vera and goodness knows what other species. The aloe vera had an unpleasant smell. And I cut off the leaves and stems of the magnolia. Its leaves smelt lovely. Lele was whining and wagging his tail behind the bay windows. I put down the scissors and let him out. He sniffed at the leaves and looked at me with a worried expression on his face. He sniffed at the jade green magnolia leaves and scratched at them with his paws. The way he looked at me made me uncomfortable. I stopped, gathered up all the leaves and threw them outside. Feeling much lighter, I sat down in front of the computer. But wait. Where was Lele? He should still be on the balcony. I had to let him in. But he wasn't on the balcony, nor in the sitting-room, nor under the television stand in the dining-room. Unable to remember where I had left him, a wave of panic swelled inside me. As I was walking past the study, I saw him sitting on the window sill beside the computer. He was looking at me quizzically: Were you looking for me? I ran over to him and took him into my arms. Lele, I am sorry. Forgive me, I am sick. You must help me.

16th March 2007

Correlations

Excerpts from "*Red, Red, Red...*"

At night, when I think of someone, and it could be anyone, his or her face would start to change. I would then try to focus my mind on a family member, someone with a beautiful, round and happy face... but it, too, would change after a few seconds: The head is squashed; there is only one eye and a big black hole instead of a mouth. Go away. Scram. Wipe this picture from my head. Quick. Think of another image. I concentrate on a colleague's plain oval face, but...ah...It is changing too... Many tiny faces are mushrooming out, like balls of cacti. God, even these have eyes and mouths. Quick. Think of something else. A pretty oval face... It is changing...into a squashed watermelon. Watermelon was everywhere.

I will do some *qigong*. And if I focus my energy on my *dantian*?[2] Quick, the *dantian*. It is below the navel. I press down on the *dantian* with the palm of my hand. It will help me to concentrate. *Dantian*. One, two, three, four, five, six, seven, eight... Sleep. Go to sleep. I could do with some light in the room. Then my imagination wouldn't run amok.

There is a gaping blood-coloured hole in the sky.

Cars. Cars. Cars. Seventy-four of them passed in front of me within the space of one minute. My head is spinning. I have been waiting for the connecting bus for 25 minutes and it still hasn't arrived. I am angry, very, very... very...*very*... *an..gry*... "*Mama de*..." I like this swear word that Ah Q invented in Lu Xun's novel. Every time I am about to blow my top, I repeat it over and over again in my head.

A container lorry just roared past. I lowered my head to look beneath the vehicle, wondering how many wheels it had. As it was speeding past, inside me I could feel bones being crushed beneath its wheels, and I had visions of pulps of bleeding flesh, splintered skulls and bits of milk-coloured brains flying into the air... A thick, nauseating stench of blood hit me.

I have been reduced to just a bundle of nerves in this city. Whenever I come back from an assignment, as I leave Shenzhen station I become, for no apparent reason, excited, anxious and irritable. My head aches and my chest feels tight and heavy. People say it is because of the frantic pace of life. But I ask myself which aspect of life here is so frenetic. Is it because of the people rushing around on the streets? Are their schedules always full? Is it because of the new faces constantly popping out in front of you? Could it be the speed with which the city is expanding? I cannot say for certain. I like this flourishing and bustling city. But I am also afraid of it.

"When you have nightmares, do you also have hallucinations?" the old man with red puffy eyes asked me.

The psychiatrist was a pitiful sight to behold. He had been seeing patient after patient all morning, and when my turn came, it was already half past midday. He was sweating, had lacklustre eyes and pale lips, and his big nose was the only part of him that still had a hint of life. Exhausted from hunger, thirst and the heat, he rubbed his weary eyes vigorously. I was tempted to say to him: "Go home and get some rest. I'm fine." He was meticulous and thorough and certainly gave me my money's worth in consultation fees. He tapped me several times on the elbow and knee with his little rubber hammer; examined me with a little torch; and after he had been through all the instruments on the table, he sat down and listened to me talking about my hallucinations.

Metamorphosis. Have you heard of it? I am talking about the metamorphosis of a human being. When I think of a person, for example, I am here talking to you, and when I go home, I try to picture you. In my mind, I see your face, but a few minutes later, it changes. It doesn't matter who it is. It could be anyone I have come across and, in my mind's eye, his or her face would change: gaping skull, mouthless, crushed face, smelling of death. Also, when I am under a flyover and I hear the noise of traffic above me, in my mind I see cars falling off, or the bridge cracking, and slabs of concrete crushing down on people. Heads scattered everywhere on the road. A total massacre. Or, sometimes, I would wonder if there was a road accident somewhere, and the scene of a disaster would come to mind: A bicycle is crushed under the wheels of an enormous container lorry. Dismembered body parts here and there, and bright red sticky blood splattered all over the tarmac.

The doctor listened closely and then asked:

"Tell me, when you do the laundry, after washing and hanging it out to dry, do you wash and hang it out to dry again a second time soon afterwards?"

What did he mean by that? Did he think I was a nutcase and was tricking me into confessing? He looked a bit cuckoo himself with his dishevelled white hair, grubby old white coat and his trousers with braces that seemed to have come straight out of the 60s. It wouldn't surprise me in the least bit if he had a screw loose somewhere. Birds of a feather flock together. He saw lunatics all day long. If he didn't die from exhaustion, he would certainly go stark raving mad himself. He looked more unhinged than most of his patients.

The doctor was smiling at me kindly and was taking his time discussing my daily life. I was reluctant at first, but he encouraged me to open up.

"Are the hallucinations more frequent at night?"

He was right. That is why whenever I was alone at home, I always kept the colour television switched on, just to have some background noise. I had no social interactions with my neighbours. I don't even know by sight the neighbours who had been living next door to me for two years. I was afraid of looking at myself in the mirror at night. Because it gave me the impression that it wasn't me, but a lost ghost. It hid behind me, and when I looked in the mirror it would jump out with a sly smile on its face.

The doctor wrote me a prescription for an electroencephalogram and a rheoencephalogram. He didn't make a diagnosis and had only one question: Was it an obsessive notion? In psychiatry, there are three major types of obsessions: obsessive notions, obsessive thoughts and obsessive behaviour. I made no effort to understand what it all meant.

The nurse was as thin as a rake. She couldn't believe that the electroencephalogram was for me. She said I looked perfectly normal and was a picture of health. No, I am not normal. She gave me a peculiar look. Was it because of what was written on my prescription: "Obsessive notion?"

In the procedure room, a young woman wearing a loose white coat was scolding another woman, who was old enough to be her mother:

"I told you to close your eyes, so why are you still looking at me? Are you deaf? If you're not, close your eyes."

The nurse was still looking at me strangely. She showed me a long silver needle and then proceeded to put the sphenoidal electrodes on me. She looked for the entry points and pricked me several times here and there on my cheeks, which made me yell out in pain: "Ouch! That hurt!" I was protesting loudly when the doctor rushed over to calm me down. Then he inserted the needles in the right places on both sides of my face. It had a numbing effect, and following the doctor's instructions, I closed my eyes and took deep breaths. Then I lost track of time. I was waiting for the doctor to tell me to stop. I had a maddening impulse to smash the machine, rip out the needles from my face and blow up the whole building. One, two, three…Seven, eight, nine… But I was terrified of these people. Because they would tie me up, send me to a lunatic asylum and force me to drink medicine that would prevent me from sleeping. They would put me in a chair to torture me, give me electroshocks until I am twisted up in convulsions, until my eyes roll back into my head, and until I drool or pee in my pants.

I understand that when you are in a bad way, you start imagining all sorts of things and your mind becomes confused. But if you feel poorly most of the time, then what do you do?

A young woman with freckles is peeling an apple for her little boy. I want to… take the knife and cut the woman's thumb into slices as thin as the blade of my knife. I want to see the white bones and the wound filling up with watery blood. I will cut the tip of the woman's nose and her lips, painted red with lipstick. The shiny blade would be dripping with blood. I would then put the knife under the little boy's eyes. Quick. Think of something else. What can I think about? It is a beautiful sunny day, the green grass… And if I jump from the third floor, will I die? I see a rusty razor blade on the lawn. The quickest method to die is to cut your throat. The blood will spurt out from under the blade. A blade can cut a thumb into razor-thin slices. Slices so thin that they will turn your stomach.

Enough. Stop thinking about it.

I dream a lot both night and day. Nine times out of ten, they are dream fragments.

Two thin planks of wood were laid across a wide latrine. I pressed my foot down to test their resistance, but they weren't solid enough. I trampled on the ground next to the latrine to make the earth firmer. Suddenly, the ground beneath me collapsed and I fell into the latrine. It turned into a muddy swamp, which heaved up and spat out a huge shipping container and two thieves covered in mud. They looked like hippopotamuses. One of them turned around and when he saw me, his big eyes sprang out of their sockets and were dangling like lit-up light bulbs. He let out an enraged scream and lunged at me with his muddy arms outstretched. I knew my hour was up and that I was going to drown in this mud swamp. I screamed: "Help!"

War. And more war. I had no idea how long the war had been going on. I have forgotten the events leading up to it and can only recall the last part. I was standing in front of a vast expanse of paddy fields. Harvest had taken place, leaving only water three inches deep and arable land covered with straw. The fields were strewn with big square pieces of human flesh, glistening with oil. I don't know if human flesh is supposed to be pink or not, but the pieces I saw in front of me were whitish, which could have been fat. The water in the paddy fields was red and a film of oil was floating on the surface.

28th July 1986

Complementary Notes

I came across the draft of the entry above as I was tidying my bookshelf on the 15th night of the first moon. I was too tired to even flip through it. I had already destroyed two diaries. I found them one evening and immediately threw them in the bin.

Today, I was reading through a diary that dates back to the summer of 1986. In it I talked about a therapeutic session with a psychiatrist, and an electroencephalogram and rheoencephalogram that I'd had. My memory has deceived me. I thought my depression began after 1987. I remember the consultation with the psychiatrist. We were chatting away and I even showed him some chiromancy and physiognomy techniques. He prescribed me a couple of neurological tests. The rheoencephalogram report indicated the presence of opaque areas in the right temporal region. I was put on medication, but don't know which ones, because their names were written in Latin and I don't understand Latin. At that point, I stopped reading my diary. There was no brain tumour and I was relieved that an operation wouldn't be necessary.

Today, I realise that I nearly lost my mind in 1986. Nearly went over the edge. I thought it was later. By a stroke of luck, I didn't destroy my diary that night, otherwise I would never know the extent to which my behaviour was obsessive.

Rereading my diary made me feel morose. I got up from my computer and went out of the study a few times. I couldn't breathe and was in such a state of agitation that I wanted to tear out my heart to cool it down in front of the fan. I jumped around in the sitting-room, waving my arms around, kicking and punching violently in the air. Zhou Lele was lying on the sofa, watching me from the corner of his eye, as if there were nothing unusual. I picked him up and buried my face in the soft fur of his neck. He smelt faintly of dog and even though it was slightly unpleasant, it was mingled with the fragrance of my shampoo and gave me the sensation of still being present among humans.

The consultation with the psychiatrist in 1986 reminded me of another one that took place on the morning of 1st April 2003. There are similarities between the two: I was the last patient on the waiting-list; for reasons which I don't even want to understand, I had made the appointments against my will; it was also in this provincial hospital that, in the summer of 1986, the head physician of the psychiatric department had observed an obsessive-compulsive tendency in me. At the time, this major provincial hospital was the first to have a psychiatric department.

I eventually stopped undergoing psychotherapy. As little research had been done on mental illnesses in China at the time, even doctors had limited knowledge on the subject. In hindsight, I think I was already showing pathological symptoms.

I am disappointed in Li Lanni: You are one of the first patients in Shenzhen to have a mental illness.

My nightmares became more frequent from 1986 onwards. I realise now that it was my subconscious trying to show me the real and underlying situation of my life. My subconscious was crying for help. It saw Shenzhen as a latrine, a muddy swamp with thieves and terrifying industrial machines and equipment, like the shipping containers in my dream. Shenzhen was not a place where humans could live. My subconscious was trying to tell me that this city was a battlefield in a permanent state of war, where no one would emerge from it victorious. Only corpses crushed by the societal machine and then transformed into pieces of meat would emerge, homogenous and identical. This is a truthful representation of the psychological reality of an ordinary Shenzhen citizen.

FIFTY-FIVE

Diary
Thursday, 15th January 2004 10:35 am

Mentally exhausted. Had another dream that completely drained me of my energy.

I was on an assignment in Beijing, I think, and wanted to see my friends Wang Yun, Xiao Wei, Li Ding and Tian Huiping, but they were on assignment elsewhere. Disappointed that I had come for nothing, I went into a coffee shop to kill time. Inside, I found a couple that was about to commit suicide. The other customers tried to stop them but ended up retreating into a corner so the couple could blow themselves up. I tried to take away their explosives and we struggled for a while, which left me exhausted. They thanked me sincerely and explained to me the reason why they had chosen to end their lives. There was a tacit understanding between us and we became friends. The man was holding a football and the woman a white Pekinese dog. I said to her: "Give me the dog. Don't hurt an innocent life." She shook her head, holding her dog even tighter against her. I understood her feelings and motivations and didn't insist. The man wanted to give me his football. It had great sentimental value for him and he wanted me to keep it as a souvenir. But I refused to accept an object that meant so much to him. They kept on insisting, saying it was to thank me for empathising with them and that it was a gift to remember them by. They gave me the ball, and I took a few steps backwards, asking myself: "Are you going to just stand by and watch them blow themselves up in front of a crowd?" Feeling helpless and anxious, but in full sympathy with them, I watched them pull the pin out of the grenade. I closed my eyes when it detonated. Lacking the courage and the stomach to look, I hurried out of there.

Night had fallen, and the surrounding streets were empty. I was thinking how strange it was that I didn't feel any sadness, only relief for the couple that a weight had been lifted off their shoulders. Bone-tired, I looked for a taxi but without much success. It was dark, the streets were poorly lit, and pedestrians were few and far between. I carried on walking, afraid to stop, even to take a rest. I wanted to leave these dark shadowy streets and go to a vibrant place full of light. But I didn't know anywhere that was safe or lively. Holding onto the hope that I might find such a place, I was praying silently to give myself courage. Although I was exhausted, I was walking briskly. My fear was subsiding, and I was confident that I would soon arrive at a place filled with life and light.

Lord, grant me the wisdom and will to live.

I am blessed. Yes, I am blessed. Every day, every hour. In all things and in all places.

Notes

We had two sunny days in a row. The dreadful "depression season" is coming to an end. I don't remember having any nightmares for the entire month of April. I love May. The weather is splendid, and I feel light.

Current events: The shooter in the state of Virginia suffered from depression; 32 workers were burnt alive in a steel factory accident in Liaoning; the Hong Kong billionaire Xiao Tiantian, aka Gong Ruxin, has died of cancer and her heirs are fighting over the will; the mayor of Nagasaki was shot dead. Is the "depression season" (March and April) a world-wide phenomenon?

Yesterday morning around 8 o'clock, I was doing my mental health exercises in the sun when Lele's new nanny came back from their walk together.

"Hi baby, you're back," I said happily to my dog.

Lele looked up at me, his mouth opened as if in a smile, but the nanny, looking sheepish and uneasy, threw a quick glance behind her. My eyes followed the direction of her glance and fell on a pair of white sneakers. Apparently, the nanny was chatting with some people on the rooftop of this building when Lele came off his leash. He dashed over to White Sneakers, who was doing her exercises, and gave her two scratches on her leg through her tracksuit trousers. White Sneakers nearly jumped out of her skin and yelled: "Help! Someone! Quick! Help!"

My heart was pounding away, and the sun disappeared from my vision. Hitching up her trousers, White Sneakers showed me her calf, turning it left and right, back to front. Repressing a shiver, I inspected her calf. She had two wounds. You could see paw scratches in one area, but the skin was intact and there was no blood; in another area, the skin was abraded. I felt relieved, but tension was still in the air.

Li Lanni fell over with apologies. She looked for her purse and Lele's vaccination certificate, telling the woman that Lele was healthy and was vaccinated every year. She offered to compensate her immediately and accompany her for a rabies vaccine.

Dressed in her blue tracksuit, White Sneakers said:

"Alright, let's go to the vaccination centre together!"

"Okay, okay. Give me a minute. I have to change."

"Don't bother. Hurry up or I might die."

This is so upsetting that I must stop writing. It's only a summary of the incident. I'll pick up the thread of the story once I am feeling better.

So, there I was, rushing to the vaccination centre in my pyjamas with White Sneakers. The doctor alarmed us when he suggested giving a rabies immunoglobin injection. I brought up the risks involving an anti-rabies serum. Although I was prepared to assume all the medical expenses, nonetheless, I asked White Sneakers to talk it over with her family before deciding. We went out to catch a taxi, but White Sneakers insisted on going back to the centre. She wanted the nanny to come over to apologise to her in person. In total, I paid 6,000 yuan for a rabies vaccine, a rabies immunoglobin shot and other miscellaneous medical expenses. But White Sneakers demanded 2,000 yuan more in compensation for psychological trauma, sick leave and food. The nanny accused her of blackmail. White Sneakers threw a fit and immediately called the police, who obviously had better things to do. But White Sneakers wasn't having any of it. I explained to her that I was suffering from cancer and depression and that I must go home to take my medicine after every meal and that I wouldn't do a runner. She studied me, a shrewd light in her eyes, and saw that I was in distress. As a goodwill gesture, she let me go home.

By coincidence, my parents came to see me at the Sun Yat-San University that day. Not wanting to alarm them, I put on a bright and chirpy face. After taking my medicine, I grabbed a wad of bank notes without even counting them, because I was worried White Sneakers would turn up on my doorstep and give my parents a fright. I rushed downstairs just in time to see White Sneakers about to ring the doorbell. Worried she might trigger an episode of depression in my mother, I talked to her calmly and politely, caving in to all her demands. She wanted to file a complaint at the police station. Her sister-in-law and her sister-in-law's elder sister arrived and acted as her advisors. The nanny refused to come with us. So the three women and I left the university campus to look for a taxi.

White Sneakers demanded 6,000 yuan in compensation for psychological trauma. I asked her why it had gone up from 2,000. Her sister-in-law said it was just an advance and that this case was far from over. Wanting to put an end to this at all cost, I agreed to all their demands. The whole thing lasted from 8 o'clock in the morning until 1 o'clock in the afternoon. Depressed and feeling sick to my stomach, I could barely stand up straight or breathe. I just wanted to hide myself in a corner, my head in my arms. I wanted to scream but had to hang on. I quickly paid the 3,000 yuan in cash, leaving me 20 for the taxi.

Back at home, my parents were worried that I had been detained at the police station.

"Nonsense. Everything is fine," I laughed, not saying a word about what had just happened.

Later that afternoon, as I was talking and laughing with my parents, I could hear my own laughter, which sounded far away and unreal. My mind drifted off and I thought of Virginia Woolf. I understood why she had ended her life and why she was afraid of her own domestic servants. I was asking myself why she had chosen death by drowning. Weren't there any tall buildings from which where she could have jumped? Was it because of the pristine water? When she came to the deep end of the river, maybe she yearned to let herself glide into the cool limpid water. The angel of death took her gently into its arms.

After my parents had left, I was alone at home. Hugging Lele in my arms, I said to him again and again: "Lele, Big Sister is sad. Do you know that? Lele, Lele, Big Sister is sad, very sad." It wasn't the incident itself that had saddened me, it was human nature. My sadness was tinged with melancholy.

White Sneakers represents a certain category of society. They aren't bad people. They are educated, have social experience and know the difference between good and evil. But they have psychological problems; in other words, they are sick. In any given situation, they imagine the worst to scare themselves. Their self-preservation mechanism is overdeveloped, creating a rift in their personality, a breakdown in their mental cohesion. Their lives are a constant battle between good and evil. Unaware that they are sick and unwilling to lose out in life, they become shrewd and calculating.

A 19-year-old girl from a neighbouring building has taken her own life. At 11 o'clock in the evening, I was on the rooftop talking with some neighbours, who are also dog-owners. One of them said:

"My colleague's daughter jumped to her death this morning."

"It's dreadful. The girl had more than six hundred points in her exams, but her mother wasn't happy," the neighbour's husband said.

"I was on my way out to do the shopping when I saw a crowd standing in front of the building. There were over a hundred people," another neighbour said. "Someone said to me: 'The girl jumped off the building, but the mother didn't know. She left for work and when she saw the crowd, she went over to see. It was only then that she knew her daughter had committed suicide.'"

I often pass that building on my walks with Lele. Sometimes, I would come across high school students. They love dogs and would kneel down, a big smile on their faces, and stroke Lele on the head.

Nineteen years old. Such a brutal way to leave this world. The building where she lived only had eight storeys. How many nights did she spend walking up and down along the rooftop beside the security rail? Did she hear spirits telling her to take one step forward? Did she see a shadowy face in the middle of the flowerbed that was in front of the building? Like me, did she yawn while standing on the edge of the rooftop? Did her heart cry out when she jumped into the void? Nineteen years old. Tomorrow, the day after tomorrow and the day after that, there will be more adolescents of 15, 16, 17 or 18 years old who, in a state of depression and despair, will embrace with open arms the angel of death. Who will comfort these children? Or their mothers?

On the afternoon of 7th June 2007

Correlations

Excerpts from *The Noonday Demon*[1]

People are unaware that depression poses a major public health risk. One person dies by suicide every 17 minutes in the United States [...] According to a WHO survey, nearly two percent of deaths in 1998 were due to suicide. The suicide mortality rate, which is constantly on the rise, is higher than the mortality rate from war and homicide [...] I read in a document that we are 500 times more susceptible to having suicidal thoughts during a depression and that the suicide mortality rate is 25 times higher among people who suffer from depression.

Andrew Solomon (United States)

Complementary Notes

The Chinese edition of *The Noonday Demon* was published in 2006. The statistics for suicide rates are from 1995. However, since the beginning of the new millennium, 9/11 and the Iraq War, I wonder to what extent the suicide rate has gone up in America. What is most worrying is the public health risk that it poses in China. What is the percentage of Chinese who die by suicide? What is the suicide mortality rate among students under the age of 20? Are we burying our heads in the sand, pretending to see nothing and hear nothing? Is the suicide mortality rate higher than that from cancer, cardiac arrest, AIDS or renal impairment? Who can give us precise and truthful figures? Who will treat the psychological trauma inflicted on parents, friends, family, colleagues and even on the neighbours of those who committed suicide? We can continue to bury our heads in the sand, but our subconscious mind sees clearly. It registers everything at lightning speed. Our memories "ferment" in our subconscious and mutate into a Trojan horse virus that destroys our psyche.

FIFTY-SIX

Diary
Tuesday, 3rd February 2004 11 am

Why do I remember the dreams I have in the early hours of the morning so clearly? Maybe it's because I spend most of the night in a state of slumber, which most likely affects the quality of my sleep. But look on the bright side of things: Feelings of fear, sadness and sorrow have diminished in my dreams. I even argue with people, which almost never happens. I can evacuate my anger that way.

Over the years, I've developed a reflex to repress my anger and have lost the ability to express it through normal channels. Mental anguish is built up inside, pushing me into depression. Fear, anxiety and pain joined the fray to form different layers in my psyche that are inextricably interconnected. My intrinsic nature and the substance of these emotions began to undergo changes. In trying to liberate myself from these negative emotions, I resorted to force; but it was a force without faith, which transformed this negativity into cancer and other illnesses.

I wonder how many sick people like me there are in China.

Over the last few years, I've come to believe that our society desperately needs to be governed by moral rules. It has been three generations now since our nation has established the absence of faith as its guiding principle.

Notes

I saw my parents last weekend. My father suggested that I should do some medical tests at the hospital, as well as a CT-scan to see if my cancer cells have spread. But I'm not going to. Whether I do it or not, the results will be the same. What would I do if there was a metastasis? I don't want to go through another operation, because it can make the cancer spread even more. I'd rather stay with chemotherapy. Anyway, I don't have the strength to drag myself to a hospital. Father didn't insist, but he looked concerned.

In February 1988, Father received a letter from the doctor informing him that I had cancer. After discussing it with Mother, they both decided not to tell me, worried that the shock would send me spiralling into depression. My paternal grandfather died of stomach cancer six months after his diagnosis. Father hid the truth from him until his death, telling him that it was a stomach ulcer. Grandfather stayed in a military hospital in Guangzhou for a while.

Then the doctor advised him to go home because he was already in the terminal stage and had three to five months to live. Father was deeply distressed by the news. He had enrolled in the military forces at the age of 17 and had never been able to fulfil his filial duties towards his parents. After my grandmother passed away, for more than 10 years, Grandfather lived by himself in a village in the Heilongjiang Province. He would eat the same dish of food he had cooked himself for several days in a row, and his meal times were irregular. That was one of the reasons why he developed stomach cancer. He sold his house to come down to the south to spend his old age with his children and grandchildren. But he was diagnosed with advanced cancer during a medical examination at a hospital in Guangzhou. Even though Father never talked much about Grandfather's illness and death, I know that his conscience isn't clear and that, deep inside, he is plagued by remorse. His feelings of guilt and sorrow are impossible to soothe. But he never talks about it. After all, what can he say?

People of the same generation as my father carry within them feelings of guilt and sorrow. They don't talk about it and don't want to, either. They are unable to look inwards into themselves, and some even deny having these feelings at all by eradicating them from their conscience. They have built their lives on the pride they derive from being at the service of the Revolution and the people. This is the milestone to which their lives are attached. They have strong characters, and their private and family lives are relegated to the background. They entrust their parents and children to the Party, which, in turn, loves and protects them. They don't know how to give love to their family. I wonder if they suffer from some kind of personality disorder. Are they mentally balanced? Does this pose a threat to the physical and mental health of an entire generation?

I think my father loved my grandfather but was unable to show it. He has hidden his love in the depths of his heart, dormant and invisible. People of his generation despise family ties.

I also think my father loves my brother and me. At the age of 14, I was operated on for a venous angioma. He dropped me off at the entrance of the hospital on his way to a meeting and then drove off. When my brother was nine years old, he was bitten by a poisonous snake. He was admitted into the emergency service at a hospital tens of kilometres away from home. But Father was too busy attending a meeting and didn't go to the hospital. The meeting wasn't held in response to a natural catastrophe or other disasters. It was to study the impact of deforestation and the development of rubber plantations. The slogan of that era was: "A drop of rubber, a blow to imperialism!" He was incapable of spending time with his children, even if their lives were in danger, preferring to attend meetings instead. He was a loyal soldier.

When I had my first cancer operation, I was on a creative writing course at

Nanjing University during the winter holidays. They told me it was a benign tumour, that it was a minor operation that only needed four stiches. However, I was put under general anaesthesia and a horizontal incision was made across my neck from left to right. The expression "to cut one's throat" probably comes from this horizontal hand gesture.

Not suspecting that anything was wrong, I asked the doctor:

"Why was I put under general anaesthesia? I was told it'd be local."

"You were very nervous. We were worried that you wouldn't be able to go through with it," he answered.

I was about to explain to him that I wasn't at all nervous, but felt uncomfortable at having to justify myself. He said that due to the length of the surgical incision, many stitches were made as a precautionary measure. But what he said next took me by surprise:

"You have to take one month of sick leave."

I asked him why.

"As you were put under general anaesthesia, you should take some time off to rest and eat properly."

It was true that after being under general anaesthesia, my brain wasn't functioning the way it should. I couldn't remember the names of people I knew well. With my head in the clouds, I was an easy target for the next swindler who came along.

The day I was discharged from hospital, a friend's cousin came to fetch me. She took me to a quiet spot to talk. Having worked as a doctor at the hospital, it was she who had advised me to go there. During our conversation, she hinted that my operation wasn't a minor one and that I should eat American ginseng and be extremely careful about my intake of nourishment during my convalescence. She seemed ill at ease and unable to say what was on her mind. It wasn't until the spring of 2000 that I understood. She had wanted to tell me the truth, to warn me. If I had all my wits at the time, I could have asked her the right questions, and she could have told me the truth about my biological test results. Often I can't help thinking: If only I'd known in February 1988 that I had cancer, I would have lived my life differently. I wouldn't be the Li Lanni that I am today.

"If you knew you had cancer in 1988, you wouldn't be alive today," my father said.

"I wouldn't have been so confused. I would have suffered less and lived my life with more freedom," I retorted.

"Even today we aren't sure we should have told you the truth," my mother said, in an attempt to justify herself. "You shouldn't blame your parents. You know what, this secret has been like a time bomb for us. Not a day goes by without it weighing on our minds."

Poor things.

I recoil from my own memories. There is so much agitation inside that something is going to give. I'm going to explode. Quick, I must let out some blood. I need a phlebotomy.

I bought some single-use syringes: five 10 millilitre syringes, and ten 5 millilitre ones.

"This is a self-destructing model," the sales girl explained to me.

The word 'self-destructing' struck a chord in me.

"What do you mean by self-destructing?" I asked.

"Once you've pushed the plunger down, it's locked inside the barrel and you can't use it again."

I understand. It means I have to get it right the first time.

I didn't buy a rubber tourniquet because I dislike its texture. Buoyed by a kind of joy, light-heartedness and impatience, I wanted to hold my arm out right there and then at the pharmacy and stick a needle into my vein. This thought was racing around in my head, and a film sequence rolled out in my mind's eye: A drug addict gets hold of his drugs, looks desperately for somewhere to hide and jabs a needle into his arms and thighs. Every time I saw scenes like this in films, I would say to myself: "Doesn't it hurt? What idiots!" But now I understand, a pin prickle is nothing to a drug addict.

After buying the syringes came the waiting. I waited to be alone at home to do the bloodletting.

Yesterday at 6 o'clock in the afternoon, I was alone at home with Lele. Quick, action! But I was in a quandary because I didn't have a tourniquet and was dying to start. It would be a waste of precious time to go looking for a piece of string. So I grabbed the first thing I could find: a dog leash. But it was too thin and dirty, so wasn't suitable. Then I tried using the cable of my mobile phone charger, but it didn't make my vein stand out enough. I felt a rush of panic and thought of those who are about to hang themselves. They must go through similar panic-stricken moments, when they can't find the tools they need to carry out their act. What an utter waste of time! In the end, I made do with a plastic flexible hose. With my right hand, I tied the hose around my left arm, even using my toes to keep it in place. Too impatient to go looking for a cushion, I rested my arm on the portable computer. After disinfecting the skin with balls of alcohol-soaked cotton wool, I took a 10 millilitre syringe. But its needle was twice as thick as a 5 millilitre one. I picked the most prominent vein in my arm and inserted the needle, bevel up, into the vein. But it was thick and went in extremely slowly. I managed to push in two-thirds of the needle but couldn't pull up the plunger. The 10 ml syringes were more difficult to handle than the 5 ml ones. The three fingers of my one hand didn't have the strength to pull up the plunger, so it was blocked inside the barrel. Lele came moseying over. Worried that he might get up to some mischief, I quickly pulled out the needle, drawing a few drops of blood in the process. The bloodletting was a failure. Lele tilted his head and looked at me inquisitively. I said to him softly: "It's alright. Everything is fine." He kept staring at me, so I put him behind the sofa. I don't like being stared at, not even by Lele.

Let's get cracking. The second bloodletting was with a 5 ml syringe. The needle was finer and more manageable. Tying the hose around my wrist, I tried to prick the vein on the back of my hand, but, once again, it was a failure. The vein was too fine and slippery and moved whenever the needle pressed down on it. So disappointing. It had been several years since I last performed a phlebotomy on myself, and I had lost the knack. Calm down. Don't get worked up. Don't be so hard on yourself. You're doing nothing wrong. You're simply doing self-therapy. In the past, people in the west performed bloodletting to relieve agitation. *Guasha* in Traditional Chinese Medicine serves a similar purpose. Outside, it was dark and raining. Thunder was rumbling in the distance. It had been humid and stormy for the past few days. I switched on the ceiling light and desk lamp. Start again. The needle was extremely fine and glided into the vein. It was going smoothly. Blood slowly filled the barrel. As soon as it was full, I pulled out the needle, but blood was trickling out on the back of my hand. Not wanting to stop the bleeding, I let it flow for a while. But it left big blobs of fresh red blood on my desk. It was unsightly. I dashed to the washbasin, switched on the incandescent lamp and started emptying the barrel into the snow-white porcelain washbasin. Blood was spurting everywhere inside. It was like I was doing spray paint art. I made circles, little ones inside big ones, like the whorls of a snail shell. Unfortunately, there was too little blood, because the syringe was small. I would have liked to play around a little longer. Red blood on a white background was pretty. I had to hurry and clean up, otherwise the blood would dry and stick to the washbasin. I turned on the tap, and the clear water was quickly tainted red. So red. But not red enough for my taste. Blood was splattered all over the edge of the washbasin, on the bathroom tiles, the parquet floor in the sitting-room and study, and on the desk. It looked like a red work of art that was rather pleasing to the eye. I was almost sorry to have to wash it off. But it had to be done quickly, because blood leaves stains, and you have to rub hard to remove them. That is why in movies, police detectives must find traces of the victim's blood in order to solve crimes. And it doesn't matter if the victim has been dead for a long time or that the murderer tried to make the blood stains disappear. Suddenly, I noticed there was blood on my calf near the back of my knee. It must have trickled down from the hose. What an airhead. So clumsy. I wiped my calf and examined the blood closely. No, it was bad quality blood. Too runny, as if it had been half diluted with water. And what's more, it smelt unpleasant. In the future, I must do my sessions of bloodletting earlier on in the day. The blood would be thicker then.

Yesterday's bloodletting didn't count, because there were no therapeutic benefits, as if there hadn't been a session at all. The needle must have pierced through a vein, because there is a bruise next to the puncture site.

This morning at 10 o'clock, I was alone at home. I have more practice now in bloodletting. This time, I used a pair of silk stockings as a tourniquet. It was tight, but comfortable. I see why the writer San Mao used a pair of silk stockings to hang herself with. In historic films, emperors order their concubines to hang themselves with a white silk ribbon, because silk ribbons are tight but soft. This time round, I used a 10 millilitre syringe and Lele's small cushion. And I got it right at the first go. The barrel filled up with warm blood. Even though the blood was a tad darker than yesterday, it was still too light and watery for me. As I was pulling the needle out, blood nearly spurted onto my computer. The bloodletting made me dizzy, but the sensations it gave me weren't strong enough. The purpose of this therapy hasn't been fulfilled. There were no bruises at the puncture site, only a slight discoloration of the skin. I'm finally getting the hang of it.

Be sensible. Enough for today. Tomorrow. Practice makes perfect. But I do wonder if bloodletting isn't a waste of blood.

I often want to donate blood. It is a way of helping others and myself. Whenever I see a blood donation mobile centre in Shenzhen or after watching programs on students who give their blood for free on their birthdays, I have an urge to roll up my sleeves and donate my blood. But will the blood of someone like me with cancer and depression save someone's life? Is my blood unhealthy, or of low quality? I'm afraid my blood won't be of much good to anyone.

Is my secret little vice of doing phlebotomy on myself a positive or negative behaviour? Is it therapeutic or self-destructive? Are there any answers to my questions?

Normally I can't stand the sight of blood – both animal and human. It makes me want to throw up, and I start shivering. In fact, I am terrified of it. I feel nauseous just seeing blood on sanitary towels in the public toilets, or when I have a sudden discharge of menstrual blood. I feel weak, dizzy, and start quivering inside. Blood-smeared images rush into my mind and I have to exert enormous control on myself not to scream. The strange thing is, when my inner turmoil and restlessness reach a boiling point, and I have no choice but to do a phlebotomy on myself, the sight of fresh blood flowing from my vein brings me such relief and pleasure that I don't want my blood to stop splurging into the washbasin. It gives me such a thrill, and I feel invigorated and much lighter afterwards.

After my bloodletting session this morning, I had a long nap in the afternoon. I feel much less agitated.

I will carry on tomorrow, the day after tomorrow and the day after that.

12th June 2007

Correlations

Excerpts from *"Buddhist Affinities"*

I was dog-tired after my visit to Mount Huangshan. When we arrived at Mount Jiuhua,[1] I already had had enough of sight-seeing. The other tourists were asleep on their feet. The night in Mount Jiuhua was dark, thick, serene and cool.

At 6 o'clock in the morning, I suddenly sat up in bed.

"Go and burn some incense as a sign of offering," I said to myself.

Troubled by this thought, I left hurriedly.

[...] I stood in front of the lamp to light my incense sticks. I told myself to hurry up, otherwise I would miss the 7 o'clock bus that would take me back down the mountain. But the incense sticks wouldn't light. That was odd. I kept on trying for a while but became irritated when they still wouldn't light.

The bus was leaving soon, and I was worried that my fellow travellers would be looking for me.

"Why are you cross?" asked a voice impatiently. I was startled. A monk wearing a black robe was standing behind me.

"I bought a ticket for the seven o'clock bus," I answered, surprised.

"Do you want to make an offering or catch the bus?" he asked, his voice hardening.

I was speechless. Heavens, it was exactly the question that was bothering me every day: What did I want? I searched desperately for an answer without finding one.

"You want to catch the bus," the monk said, as a matter of fact.

I was stunned, as if struck by lightning. What the monk said gave me goose pimples and I was rooted to the spot.

"I...I'd like to make an offering... of course..." I stammered.

At that moment, the incense lit up.

Faint smoke rose up in spirals and a sense of restfulness and serenity came over me.

6th November 1990

Complementary Notes

This story goes back to 1988. I became a vegetarian in 1990, but my body lacked the strength to continue. In 1989, I developed symptoms of anorexia. I felt hunger in my stomach, but not in my head. I didn't want to eat, drink, talk or move. I lost so much weight that I had to take medication to regain weight, which worked for a while. From that period on, I became increasingly tired. As time went by, my energy became more and more scattered. Unaware that I had cancer, I loathed my physical condition, which was deteriorating. In my mind, I often saw images of disasters: fatal car accidents, drownings at sea, plane explosions, skulls being split open by an axe, executions by hanging, etc. I didn't know what was causing my physical and mental fatigue. I asked a friend of mine, who was studying Buddhism:

"Could it be that in a past life I was someone bad who harmed a lot of people? And that I've committed many sins throughout the ages? I don't know how many past lives I've had, but maybe each time I met a violent death."

"No, it's highly unlikely," my friend said. "What makes you think that?"

"I feel that these images that appear in my mind are déjà-vu. It's like they've come from a previous life a long, long time ago, that they are part of a reincarnated foetal memory that is trying to tell me something."

For several years, I regularly read Buddhist sutras. Even though I didn't have an in-depth understanding of these texts, the act of reading them made my mind more lucid. I vaguely felt that a force was driving away the negative thoughts and malevolent spirits that were plaguing me. But in 1993, my connection with this mysterious force was abruptly broken. I talked about it to people who were studying Buddhism and they gave me this explanation: "You have taken a life." Once, twice, three times. I was afraid of facing up to the truth. It was unforgiveable. Between 1987 and 1993, I had three abortions. My friends tried to make me change my mind, but I refused to listen to them. It is karma, the law of cause and effect.

In 1996, I received a letter from a monk from Mount Jiuhua, asking me to convert to Buddhism. I thought about it for a long time and after much hesitation, I gave up on the idea. I particularly like this Buddhist saying: "If one has an affinity with something, one must try to keep the connection, otherwise one must let it go."

That was how I severed my affinity with Buddhism.

FIFTY-SEVEN

Diary
Monday, 16th February 2004 11 am

In the early hours of the morning, I dreamt that I was sitting for a maths exam. Again.

I was in an examination hall. The other candidates had their heads bent over their papers and were scribbling away. But I had copied the wrong questions from the blackboard. Panic-stricken, I was too embarrassed to ask the classmate next to me for help. I stared at the blackboard, and after giving it some thought, it dawned on me that I hadn't been taught the subject and was therefore unable to answer the questions. I had a bright idea: What if someone took the exam for me? But I chided myself: "No, you can't do that. You're not going to cheat!" I explained to the teacher that I hadn't been taught the subject and asked her to make an exception and allow me to hand in my exam paper a day later. The teacher, who looked like the television actress Pan Xia, was kind and polite. Tactfully, she told me that she couldn't break the rules. I left the examination hall with a clear conscience. I told myself: "Since I haven't studied the subject, there's no point in fretting over it. I'm better off taking a breath of fresh air outside." But as I was walking, I couldn't help thinking: "My classmates are all taking the exam and here I am, strolling around outside and enjoying myself. Will my teachers and classmates think badly of me? And if they think I am just a drop-out, how can I stay on at the university and have any hopes of graduating?" Disheartened by this thought, I carried on walking. Suddenly, it all became clear: "Don't I already have a Bachelor's degree from Nanjing University? I am in post-graduate studies, so why do I need a basic degree? I haven't been taught the subject, so I won't need to sit for the exam, nor ask for an exemption. Why don't I leave instead of wasting my time here?" I was standing in the middle of the sports ground, mulling over my future: "Will I have the courage to tell the university office that I'm leaving? I am in a bit of a quandary. On the one hand, leaving college will come as a relief, but on the other hand, if the university isn't going to expel me, what reason will I have to leave? Li Lanni, why are you pussyfooting around?" As I was chastising myself, my anxiety began to subside.

Upon waking, I realised how telling my dream was about my current situation. I patted myself on the back, for I was slowly getting back on my feet again. In my dream, I was practising self-therapy, which helped to alleviate the anxiety that was preying on my subconscious. I must strive for the better and give myself hope.

Notes

I remember a story from a few years ago.

One day, a neighbour from downstairs came up to see me.

"Ms Li, my daughter is taking her father to court," she said. "She has contacted a lawyer without my knowledge. She is suing her father for child support. Can you try to talk her out of it?"

I was taken aback. Her daughter was a high school student – shy, fearful almost, reserved and soft-spoken. The essays she wrote for school were penetrating and sensitive, and her style was refreshing. Gifted in art and music, she had been accepted by a fine arts and music school. But reluctant to leave her mother, she refused to go. When she was three years old, she came home one day from kindergarten to find her father in bed with her school mistress. She was so upset that she cried herself sick. Then her parents divorced. For her daughter's sake, the mother didn't remarry. Between a well-to-do father and a poor mother, the girl chose to stay with her mother. The court ruled that the father should pay a monthly alimony. I don't know what had gone on in this family for the last 10 years, except that the mother was teaching in a secondary school. At the time, teachers were looked down upon; they were poorly paid and lacked social recognition. Life was harsh. The child, introverted by nature and mature for her age, was worried for her mother.

The social assistance apartment in which they lived had been obtained under extremely difficult conditions. Single divorcee mothers were not qualified to apply for social housing. Every year, the mother would apply for housing assistance, which was systematically rejected. She had received an award of excellence in teaching, as well as a best teacher award. She was desperate. Flouting the rules of propriety and unafraid of losing face, she resorted to means not unlike those of a private detective and managed to obtain the mayor's license plate number. She waited for the right moment, threw herself in front of his car and presented him with her application letter, just like in ancient times when the common people would throw themselves in front of a public official's palanquin to air their grievances.

The gardener of our residence was small, puny, pan-faced and timid to the point of being fearful. The front door of the mother's apartment was made of solid wood. The outer folding door was made of steel and the third door of stainless steel. At the bottom of the stairs was a wrought iron door. Several times, the mother came up to ask me:

"Ms Li, there's only my daughter and me in the apartment. I'm always afraid that we might come to some harm. Do you mind taking down my phone number, or if something ever happens to us, call for help?"

This mother, who is capable of throwing herself in front of the mayor's car, wasn't afraid to die. The daughter, who had been brought up in a disadvantaged family, had a good character and was a brilliant student. But what about the psychological wounds and pain that had been inflicted on her? Would it make her vulnerable to depression? In the end, she dropped her lawsuit against her father. The lawyer was of the same opinion as the mother and I: The trial would cause her a lot of unnecessary attention and, therefore, trouble. The situation could easily get out of hand. Even if she did win the case, she would always be looked down upon as the victim. To protect her child, the mother did everything in her power to stop her from being caught up in legal proceedings.

How many broken homes are there in Shenzhen? How many girls suffer from psychological trauma? So many scars and shadows are sketched upon the backdrop of this beautiful city. The more opportunities there are, the bigger the temptations. Be it for a family or a city, prosperity has a price attached to it. How could there be a rainbow without a storm or rain? How can one attain paradise without first navigating the seas of desire?

I have heard numerous stories about the unhappy lives of the women in Shenzhen. I have heard how these women curse and love this city at the same time. Here, they have learnt this truth: "If one can obtain things in this world, it is by intelligence, but if one can become detached from this world, it is wisdom." Desire is emptiness; emptiness is desire; and hell is paradise. The process of learning is like the intrinsic nature of water. One should learn to love oneself and others.

Correlations

Excerpts from *"The Old Man's Beautiful House"*

One year, I was part of a delegation of Chinese writers on a visit to the United States. Our last stop was in the city of Buffalo [...].

"Are you Chinese?" the old man asked and, bubbling with enthusiasm, pointed to his red T-shirt with a picture of the Great Wall of China.

Looking tired, Little Wang, the interpreter of the delegation, was talking cheerfully with him. Even though I didn't understand English, judging from the expressions and gestures of the old man, I could tell that he was speaking highly of China. Indeed, he had visited China several times, a country he was particularly fond of.

"I can eat with chopsticks. I like Chinese tea, and Beijing roast duck is excellent!" he said with the excitement of a child.

He invited us to his home.

"It's a beautiful house, you'll really like it," he said warmly.

Getting out of the car, I saw four small houses.

"It's that one there. It's beautiful, isn't it?" asked the old man, pointing to one of them.

There were no trees nor flowers in front of the house; the façade was undecorated and plain to the point of being ugly. Unable to say yes and not having the heart to say no, I smiled awkwardly. He ushered us eagerly inside and gave us a tour of the house. He drew our attention to the ceiling light, table cloth and curtains in the sitting-room.

"They're lovely, aren't they?" he asked gaily and confidently.

The ceiling light was original; the table cloth had an antiquated simplicity; and the curtains had an oriental touch to them. But in comparison with the houses of writers I had visited in Los Angeles, it was banal and colourless. The home interiors of some of my colleagues in Shenzhen were more interesting. However, the basement was filled with collections of books so rich that it was worthy of a university library in China. There were numerous bound editions that were thick and exquisitely crafted with beautiful paper. It must have been a treasure trove for the old man.

The old man's son had psychological problems. He was in his 30s but behaved like a child. Unemployed, he spent all day at home researching information on the helmets worn by the comic strip characters "Transformers" and the arrows used by Mongolian archers. Seeing there were visitors in the house, he wouldn't stop talking. The air inside the house was stuffy and stale, as if the house hadn't been cleaned for a long time. The floor was covered with clothes, newspapers and daily objects. I asked myself: "Is this what you call a beautiful house?" At that moment, a plain and ugly woman came out of the bedroom. She was unsteady on her feet and was leaning against the wall. The skin on her expressionless face was loose and saggy. It was the old man's wife. Suffering from a muscular disease in her whole body, she could only utter a few sounds. A thread of saliva was dangling from the corner of her mouth, and she looked at us with resignation and helplessness in her eyes. Putting his arm around his wife, the old man proudly introduced her, saying that she was a beautiful and courageous woman who had brought up four daughters. They had also adopted a black orphan, who was now an expert in computers and had her own happy little family. Looking at this old couple, I could see that under the tender gaze of her husband, the woman had a kind of pride and bashfulness in her veiled eyes that came from her happiness. It struck me as inconceivable that the old man could have found her beautiful, his son well-mannered and his house opulent. But he was happy and serene, cherishing everything he possessed. Pointing at a window in a bedroom, he told me to look outside. But I could only see vacant land.

"What is there to see?" I asked.

"Don't you see the sun setting? It's beautiful," he answered.

I followed his gaze and saw that the ground of the vacant land was lit up with the golden rays of the setting sun. A fine misty rain was floating in the soft light. It was like a veil in the air. A breeze was blowing. In the distance, I heard music, laughter and footsteps, as if a fairy tale were about to come to life before my eyes. Again, I was left astounded. It was as if the old man had magical eyes. Everything he saw became infused with light and warmth. I walked out of the sitting-room and onto a lawn just behind the house. Seeing me sitting on the wooden steps, the old man suggested that I walk barefoot on the grass. Out of curiosity, I did as he said. The grass gave way beneath my feet. The blades of grass were small but hard, and their roots were deeply embedded in the soil, drawing in all the quintessence of the earth, sun and moon. Suddenly, I was in communication with the earth and sky.

Looking up into the sky, the wind in his white hair, the old man said:

"Every day I give thanks to God. My life is complete."

Through the eyes of the old man, I saw a world filled with happiness. Even though I am not of the Protestant faith, during that split second, I glimpsed a heaven where those who know how to show gratitude reside.

September 1995

Complementary Notes

When I was writing this travel narrative, I didn't understand why this American old man felt happy and grateful. For me, his car, house, wife and son were all flawed. This family was burdened with heavy responsibilities, and their lives were hard and full of worries. Today, I realise that if the old man is so happy and grateful, it is because his heart is filled with love. Compared to him, our lives lack beauty, gratitude and a sense of appreciation.

It is impossible not to think of money in Shenzhen. Without money, you can't eat, drink or even do your business. The people of Shenzhen understand only too well how miserable life is without money, because being poor in Shenzhen is more wretched than anywhere else in China. The body and soul are in agony. Even if you do have some money in your pocket, you can't help but imagine the panic and desperation of being penniless. The more you think about it, the more you feel that you are the poorest and most miserable person in Shenzhen. Imagination, much more so than reality, is a purgatory. It is as if we were ripping our own guts out, chopping them up into thousands of tiny pieces, sprinkling them with salt, marinating them in vinegar, basting them with oil and then roasting them over the fire at the most ideal temperature.

I had a colleague who is originally from Shenzhen. She is kind and attractive. Many of the migrant workers in our team had benefitted from her help and selfless actions. She advised me to rent out my apartment, because she could find a reliable tenant who could pay the rent in advance. I had borrowed money from my brother and this would mean I could pay my debt. But for security reasons, my brother refused to rent out the apartment. What if the tenant were a con woman or a prostitute? Or a murderer who hides corpses in the apartment? What if she cleaned out the apartment and disappeared into the wilderness? Maybe she is a psychopath or has an infectious disease? And if she refuses to leave? What if she were a drug dealer or involved in other criminal activities that could implicate me? And if she is murdered by a jilted lover? Or if she were a loan shark from the mafia, a drug addict or a compulsive gambler? Or a murderess who kills in her sleep? Everything was possible.

After much hesitation, I decided to rent out the apartment. I was afraid the housing policy might change, and I would end up losing my apartment for good. And I would have nowhere to hide. I had also considered another option: becoming a Buddhist nun. Seriously. I had often toyed with the idea. But, deep down, I knew that I would never find paradise in a temple and that I should stay in Shenzhen a bit longer.

Resistance is a trait that is deeply engrained in the genes of the Li family. My paternal grandfather didn't hesitate a second before braving the guns of bandits. He was taken prisoner by the Japanese. In liaising with the resistance movement, he risked being executed by firing squad. His motto was: "What is there to be afraid of? There is nowhere to hide. Such is life."

The tenant moved into the apartment. She stayed for one year, but during this time, I never did manage to make out which category of women she belonged to. Was she a…good person? But this adjective didn't suit her. You couldn't judge her using the usual criteria of good and bad. My brother and I weren't afraid of her. She didn't fit into a specific category. I never knew her real name. The one on her identity card was nothing like the one I knew her by. And when her family called from the province, they called her by another name. She liked talking to me about the people she knew in Shenzhen. She was pretty, had a good character, was optimistic and easy-going and never meddled with other people's business. She told me she was learning English at an adult education centre. She'd gotten married recently and was waiting for the green light to emigrate abroad. She belonged to a group of friends who were in the same situation. Living carefree lives, they often accompanied their bosses' friends to restaurants. After dinner, they would be out having fun with these men, whom they called *malalao*,[1] and the games they played were called "pressing the fish down into the water."[2] They didn't need to sell their bodies, but their roles in this setup were clear and unambiguous. Young and attractive, they knew how to play with these men. Through my tenant, I had a glimpse into the lives of women living on the fringes of society. These women were neither moral nor immoral, were neither kept mistresses, nor prostitutes. They didn't do fake marriages and were simply earning a living by using their youth to its full advantage. It is a phenomenon unique to Shenzhen at a given time in history. Before moving abroad to a life as a homemaker, these women chose to live for themselves, have fun and get the most out of what the material world has to offer.

It was in Shenzhen that I spent a long time studying the new interpretation of *Five Short Stories of the Ming Dynasty*. It made me reflect upon the practice of male and female castration. A lecturer at Nanjing University once talked about the five main methods of torture in ancient China. He casually wrote the word *fuxing* – the word for male castration - on the blackboard. Female castration was called *youbi*. Some say that the latter consisted of banishing a concubine to an isolated part of the palace for a period of a few years, or for life. Others say that concubines were imprisoned in an underground dungeon until they died. Then there are others who say that *youbi* was to drive a wooden stake into a woman's intimate parts...A practice too barbaric for words.

Psychologically, we have all been through male or female castration in one form or another.

FIFTY-EIGHT

Diary
Thursday, 19th February 2004 10:05 am

I am reading, or rather leafing through, a biography entitled *The Ephemeral Past*. Since my relapse into depression, reading has become a difficult exercise. As soon as I start, I am besieged by a host of aches and pains: dizziness, nausea, bloated belly, dull pain in my stomach, tightness in my chest, a pulse so faint that it's barely perceptible. My primordial energy is already weakened and reading drains it even more. What's more, I suffer from a Deficiency of Blood and Energy. But old habits die hard. I pick up a book, I am back on the sick list again. I force myself to carry on reading as long as possible, but in the end, I just give up. I can't concentrate; it's frustrating and bogs me down even more. It isn't worth the effort. These days, I just flip through my books, skimming the pages. Not being able to read is so annoying. For a sick person like me, it's a torture.

Does this mean all those who suffer from depression can't read as well? I don't think so. I force myself, but my efforts are fruitless, and I end up feeling even worse than before.

A list of things I can't do: read, listen to music, watch films, travel, talk to people, do the shopping. I lie there in a daze, waiting for my strength to come back...slowly, slowly... *very slowly*... I am so envious of others who are sick like me but strong enough to read or listen to music.

I am writing this on my computer. But my condition isn't stable enough for me to do it on a daily basis. And when I do have the strength, it's just to jot down a few notes. Sometimes I manage to muster up the willpower to write a bit more, even if I can barely sit up in my chair. Or I write hanging onto the table, half falling off my chair. Each word sucks the life force out of me, but the results are mediocre. Sometimes I don't even know what I'm writing, but it brings me some comfort. I'm wiped out afterwards. The price of this small comfort is physical and mental exhaustion.

There is a persistent tightness in my chest. Get a grip of yourself. Li Lanni, buck up and take a deep breath...again... and again. Be strong. Are you tired already? Did the deep breathing make you tired? Breathe slowly then. Be happy. Think of happy things. That's good. Go and find Lele and give him a cuddle.

Notes

While going through chemotherapy, I was bored and agitated and didn't know what to do with myself. I was always looking at the clock, staring at the minute and second hands crawling slowly. I asked Li Lanni: "If you hadn't gone to Shenzhen and worked in the arts and literature field, would cancer have struck so soon?" They say our bodies possess a limited number of cancerous cells. But as for how long the illness lasts; at which point in time the cancer manifests itself; and to what degree it deteriorates or spreads, the following factors play a vital role in how cancer develops: living environment, state of mind, genes, hardships, misfortunes, emotional and psychological trauma, etc. Hereditary factors aside, it is possible that living in Shenzhen could have caused the illness to break out earlier. Literature as a profession remains relatively marginal in a city like Shenzhen. The social framework and ecological environment can significantly increase the risk of the cancer being triggered. But then, I have never experienced major setbacks in my life. I only half consider myself a Shenzhen citizen, because I'm always running away and hiding in Beijing, Nanjing, Guangzhou, etc.

Does this mean that I am weak? It is true that the moral weaknesses that characterise Chinese intellectuals are in my genes coming from my mother's side, whereas, on my father's side, the hereditary traits are strong work values, courage, endurance and the ability to face up to the hardships that migrants encounter. Also, the Li family has an innate tendency for revolution. I wasn't born weak.

The only explanation possible: fate.

I was told that the Li family didn't arrive in Heilongjiang Province by chance. According to my paternal grandfather, our branch of the family left Yunnan Province and crossed Hebei Province before settling in Heilongjiang. Our family originally came from Shanxi Province. What did they do in the provinces of Yunnan and Hebei? Grandfather never said anything about this, except that one of our ancestors was a public official in the imperial court. He liked to say: "We arrived in Manchuria like nomads." "The place where we lived was called 'The Big Ash Mound of the Li Family,' because our family was large and had many mouths to feed, and the ashes from the cooking stove piled up into a huge mound." My grandfather passed away in 1975. When he was alive, it was forbidden to boast of our ancestor, who was an imperial court official. On the few occasions when Grandfather did mention him, he never said much, and it was accompanied invariably by a note of caution. Even my father knows very little about our family history.

The continuity of an individual's family history is a major problem in

China. Many families are unable to trace their family trees because they cannot go back more than three generations. Many aspects of their ancestors' lives are lost: their beliefs and dreams, moral conduct, fortunes and misfortunes, illnesses, level of talent and intelligence, and their destinies. I know very little about the Li family, but through my research into my own personal history relating to cancer, I've also been searching for the motivations behind my decision to settle in Shenzhen. It led me to explore my paternal lineage.

The Li family left Yunnan, crossed Hebei and settled in the northeast of China. From there, the family descended south to Guangzhou and Shenzhen. This journey is a testimony to the intelligence and inventiveness of agricultural people. If today's peasants dare to dream, strive for happiness, and have strong ideals, whether they choose to settle in a city or elsewhere, they should follow in the footsteps of the Li family. They would then have the hope that would enable them to one day live like human beings.

Stop. Enough for today. I am tired.

This morning, I did some bloodletting with a 10 millilitre syringe. It was on a vein on my left wrist and left a few bruises on the back of my hand, around the wrist, and in the fold of my arm. Tomorrow I'll do it on the vein on the right side of my left hand, or on the top of my foot. Afterwards, I collapsed onto a chair, my head spinning and unable to sit up. I was too agitated and edgy to take a nap. I have an excessive thirst, which can't be quenched no matter how much water I guzzle down. Today, I pulled the needle out of my hand over the washbasin, so there wouldn't be blood on the cushion or table. Because the needle was thick, some blood came out of the vein. I get a thrill from watching the blood trickle out like a stream. It imparts a sense of warmth and well-being in me. But the blood had a faint smell that made me queasy. It'd be perfect if it didn't smell at all. As I was untying the silk stocking from my hand, I noticed a bruise beside the puncture site. The vein is so fine that a needle can easily pierce through it. I turned on the tap and watched the water slowly diluting the blood. I got such a kick out of it that I wanted to let the blood flow for a little longer, but it was beginning to coagulate. The body's ability to heal itself is so powerful. The puncture site stopped bleeding and I cleaned it with balls of cotton wool. But I think they were dirty. I had bought them for Lele. They were to be used with oxygenated water and hadn't been sterilised. It would have been more hygienic not to have used them at all.

I've always thought that slitting one's wrist was stupid way to go, because the time it takes for blood to coagulate is different for everyone. I've toyed with this idea, but decided it wasn't for me, because my blood coagulates quickly. I am half a peasant, you see. There is peasant's blood flowing in my veins. It coagulates much more quickly than that of students, artisans or merchants. Today's bloodletting session confirmed this hypothesis that I formulated many years ago.

What's the point of talking about all this? None.

Let me get on with Li Lanni's family history.

From the time when they left Hebei to when they settled down in Manchuria, the Li family never stopped growing. The tree was planted on fertile soil and sprouted branch after branch until one of them moved from the Mulan district to the Bin district. My father's knowledge of our family history begins only with his grandfather's generation. The fortune belonging to this branch of the family was squandered by Grandfather's elder brother. At the time, we were the wealthiest family in the village. Most of the land, cattle, workers and commerce belonged to his grandfather and his brothers. The Jia family in the neighbouring village was extremely jealous and was vying to outdo the Li family, who came first in terms of wealth and numbers. But our family suffered a dramatic reversal of fortune. The daughter-in-law of my great-grandfather's eldest brother had a physical disability in her legs. Her husband, that is the eldest son of my great-grandfather's eldest brother, was angry at his own misfortune and ruined the family through drinking, gambling and prostitutes. His father had worked hard all his life, and the son squandered the family wealth that had been built up over several generations. There was a custom in Manchuria: When a family is unable to pay its debts, the creditors had the right to seize the assets of the entire family without leaving them a single grain of rice or blade of grass. Our family was bankrupt, and its reputation ruined.

I was told that my great-grandfather was an honest man, but had no skills. He was willing to work as a coolie, but no one wanted to employ him. In order to provide for his family, my grandfather began working very hard from a young age. He was courageous and rose to the challenge. When he approached middle age, his income was sufficient enough for him to acquire lands. His goal was to buy back every plot of land that had been seized from the Li family. At the time, bandits were rampant in the northeast. They looted the villages, sowing terror among the villagers, who were afraid to retaliate. But my grandfather wasn't to be intimidated and defended the village, rifle in hand. When night fell, the bandits would fire shots into the air as a show of force. Inside the village, my grandfather would fire shots back and shout at the top of his lungs. He put up a resistance all night, and the bandits, seeing that they didn't have the upper hand, would make a hasty retreat. When the village was plundered by Japanese soldiers, the men, women, children and the elderly were terrified and defenceless. Afraid that the entire village would be burnt to the ground, the villagers chose my grandfather to be on the front line to resist the Japanese, thereby saving the day. When my grandfather eventually bought back all the family land, the Jia family refused to hand over the title deeds. My grandfather resorted to crafty means in order to recover the deeds, but the Jia family bribed the public officials, who accused him of liaising with the anti-Japanese resistance movement. By a stroke of luck, he was given a heads-up and told to flee.

"What will I do hiding in a Buddhist temple?" Grandfather said when he heard the news. "No, I'm staying. I'm not afraid to die."

He was arrested by the district police and sentenced to death. He was to be executed by firing squad a few days later. Against all odds, the town fell to the Communist Army, and Grandfather's life was saved.

"Money and fate are tied up together," he said. "If it's your destiny to have money, then it will come to you. But if it isn't, then obtaining it by force will only bring misfortune. The Jia family had lots of land, but they were shot during the agrarian reform.

"Your grandmother liked to hoard things. Women loved fabrics of all kinds. She had a huge collection that she kept stored away. During the agrarian reform, all her fabrics were confiscated and distributed among the peasants. She became bitter, short-tempered, moody and cantankerous. If her family hadn't been in the military, she would have been arrested.

"The Jia family were bullies. They were cruel, and, in turn, the peasants showed them no mercy. Wealth doesn't last forever. A family can't stay prosperous eternally. A family won't stay poor for more than two or three generations and, likewise, a family can't be rich for more than two or three generations. Money, it comes and it goes. When it comes, it doesn't necessarily bring happiness; and when it goes, it doesn't necessarily mean unhappiness. That's what I came to understand. There's no point in hoarding things. Everything belongs to the commune."

At this moment, sitting in front of my computer, I am filled with pride for my grandfather and for his peasant origins. Thanks to the genes of the Li family, I have chosen to settle in Shenzhen. Thanks to my family's peasant's blood, I am bold enough to live half my time in Shenzhen and the other half elsewhere. It enables me to become, for better or for worse, a Shenzhen citizen, but only part-time. If I didn't have the intellectual genes of the Zhang family, I would never have had the confidence to stay in Shenzhen for so long. I would have ended up singing and dancing in a mental asylum.

18th June 2007

Correlations

Excerpts from *Searching for Memory: The Brain, The Mind, and The Past*

Emotional memory: the power of the past.

We try to understand the recording mechanism of the brain. Is it activated in a passive way or is it triggered off by a flash? Its implications on a given thing vary [...]. As soon as the flashbulb memory is activated, the negative of this instant will be preserved in us forever [...]. When researchers asked the volunteers to produce their three most vivid memories, hardly any of the recollections involved events of national importance; they tended to be highly personal events with great emotional significance.

Compared to normal people, those who suffer from depression have a tendency to recall negative memories rather than positive ones. This has the effect of maintaining the depression sufferers in a depressed state.

Daniel Schacter (United States)

Complementary Notes

In tracing the development of Li Lanni's depression, I am often confronted with the blanks in her memory, especially when it comes to Shenzhen. She is unable to talk with clarity about this flourishing economic zone that has such a far-reaching influence on the rest of China.

I can't write anymore. What kind of life do I want for myself? Why live in Shenzhen when my mind is elsewhere? What's the use of having a body when it has no eyes nor ears? I hate my life.

Reading *Searching for Memory* has cheered me up. It has given me a fuller understanding of my illness. My flashbulb memory is malfunctioning. It is triggered by just about anything. When it comes to national events, the flashbulb breaks down and the images are lost forever. And when it comes to the negative aspects of my personal life, the flashbulb keeps going off, and all the data is registered inside me permanently.

Every day on television, you hear about the euphoria that is sweeping across the stock markets. People give you all sorts of advice on how to play the stock market. At the same time as finding all this rather amusing, I realise that I don't have any vivid memories of the financial markets since 1990.

When the stock market crashed in 1987, I was in Shenzhen. There is a bank three minutes on foot from my home. At the time, I heard that people were borrowing identity cards from others so they could buy more stock market shares; some were even queuing up at the bank with jute bags full of identity cards. Twice, I toyed with this idea: "Shall I borrow my husband, brother and parents' identity cards to take part in the random draw? You never know, I might get lucky and be selected, winning the right to acquire stocks." But I ruled it out immediately. Too complicated. And I'd probably have no luck. Just before the market crashed in 1987, I was thinking: "So many of my acquaintances are enthusiastic and hopeful about buying shares. A lot of people have come to Shenzhen for this. So how come I, a Shenzhen citizen, can't rouse myself out of my apathy and indifference? Why not have a go? They say that the chances of being chosen in a drawing lot is high, and it'd be a good way to make some money." But I only had a few thousand yuan in my bank account. Families were raising funds or borrowing money for the purpose of acquiring stocks. As for me, I couldn't be bothered. Just like Xiaotao's maternal grandfather, who refused to borrow money to travel to Beijing for the imperial examinations. Apathy was indeed in my genes.

On the morning of the stock market crash, I went to the bank near my home out of curiosity. People looking dishevelled and unkempt were waiting in line. They were pressed up so closely to one another that they gave the impression of belonging to the same body. Some kept others in check who were trying to jump the queue. An unpleasant smell permeated the air. I kept my distance, wondering if the foul odour came from their mouths. As they had started queuing up a few days ago, they probably hadn't brushed their teeth or washed their faces. Was it a fecal or urine smell? Or was it nauseating body odour? Was the stench chemical or organic? Or did the stink come from rotting garbage? I hadn't the faintest idea. At that very moment, it struck me that desire was something material and palpable. The air was so heavily saturated with it that I thought it was going to explode. Suddenly, a wave of anxiousness hit me. These people's spiritual malaise was so strong that it was infectious. It had contaminated me. I left hurriedly, went home and lay on the sofa. I couldn't help thinking how, by some happy coincidence, I couldn't stay. I would have passed out on the streets. This goes to prove that I lack the physical and mental ability to make money. Since I became a Shenzhen citizen in 1983, I haven't taken advantage of a bull market to make a fortune, but nor did I go bankrupt in a bear market either. I watched from the side-lines and entertained the idea of playing the stock market but was too apathetic to do anything about it. Here are eight reasons why I didn't buy shares:

1. I've never been desperate financially. At the time, I had just rented out my apartment, which helped me overcome any temporary financial difficulties. Although I could barely make ends meet, I was happy with just a bowl of congee and salted egg.
2. I went through a phase of being a vegetarian and had studied Buddhism. But I was malnourished. How could I have had enough

physical strength and mental stamina to convert to Buddhism and become a nun? Not eating animal protein for a long time had diminished my worldly desires. If I had entertained the idea of becoming a nun, why would I want to play the stock market?
3. Coming from a poor branch of the family and with laziness running in my blood, I am accustomed to being penniless. I've resigned myself to the fact that I will never be rich.
4. The Li family are middle-class peasants through and through. Their blood runs in my veins, which means I am wary and unenterprising. I'll never make anything of myself, nor keep up with the revolutionary movement, nor have the willpower to change my destiny.
5. I have no children to whom I can leave my family assets. So what would be the point of owning shares? There's nobody to leave them to.
6. My subconscious mind knows that my cancer can spread and that I can 'kick the bucket' any time.
7. I come from a family of middle-class peasants and village school teachers. These people lead lives of idleness and reverie. They wait for everything to fall from the sky and into their hands.
8. No one in my immediate family plays the stock market, so I have no one to show me the ropes.

Someone once said to me: "You've lived in Shenzhen for a long time, but you've never played the stock market. Are you normal?" I have no answer to that.

FIFTY-NINE

Diary
Friday, 20th February 2004 5:58 pm

I saw the doctor this morning and bought some medicine. I told Dr Gong, the head physician, that I had taken up my social activities again, but still couldn't read or write properly because I tired easily. He suggested I should increase alprazolam to two or three tablets if necessary, and reassured me that the side effects would be minimal. I am wary of taking too much medication, and people talk so much about their adverse effects. But it's better to listen to the doctors. Progress is made in the medical field every day, and we must be positive. Mutual trust between a doctor and his/her patient is essential.

I read a report in a newspaper on the shame Chinese doctors felt when they saw how American doctors treated their patients. The Americans had come to China to perform operations that were part of an educational program. When they arrived at the hospital, the first thing they did was to go and talk to the patients. Their disinfection procedures were thorough and meticulous. I read this report twice. Too few doctors in China question their working methods, let alone the lack of attention and reassurance they give to patients before the operation.

I was traumatised by my lymph node dissection. In the operating theatre, the doctors and nurses were laughing and joking when they talked about my cancer metastasis. They were completely oblivious to the fact that there was a human being lying in front of them on the operating table. Same in Beijing. After announcing that the surgical procedure was a failure, the doctor asked someone to bring him a camera to take pictures of my botched operation. To them, we are no more than guinea pigs.

Throughout the centuries, the deep wounds that the Chinese people carry in them have gradually eroded their ethical and moral values. Nowadays, doctors lack compassion, and intellectuals no longer have the noble spirit of ancient times. The elite contributes almost nothing to this country. And its people have lost their moral compass. China must find a way to regenerate itself and restore a more compassionate and ethical society. Only in this way can the people become strong and show the rest of the world the noble ideals of the Chinese civilisation.

Words fail me. It's so disheartening.

Notes

Extra strong tea - coffee - bloodletting - write. Not exactly a healthy routine. But lately, it's the only way for me to sit down at my computer and get some work done. Before, I would drink regular tea followed by a cup of extra strong tea. If this wasn't enough to get me going, I would have coffee. Half an hour later, my mind would be functioning at full speed, focused on my work. But these days, my brain refuses to switch itself on even with strong tea and coffee, forcing me to resort to bloodletting. This makes me think of war horses. They say that in the past, when the war horses were tired after having travelled long distances, the riders would jab the horses' ribs with the points of their knives. The pain made the horses keep on running, sometimes even until they dropped dead.

This morning, I performed bloodletting on a vein on the top of my left foot. That was after I had downed two cups of extra strong tea. I used a dark grey silk stocking and a 5 millilitre single-use syringe I had kept hidden away in the wardrobe. I disinfected the skin with a ball of cotton wool soaked with alcohol. Then I tied the silk stocking tightly around my left ankle. I positioned the needle on the vein, but no matter how hard I tried, I just couldn't put my left foot in a comfortable enough position. I tried sitting on the desk, on the arm rest of the sofa and on the floor. In the end, I just put my left foot on my right thigh. It was the only way. It hurt when the needle pierced into the vein, but I felt nothing after that. It's like playing tennis. When the racket hits the ball, sending it flying into the distance, we feel a sense of relief as the tension in our muscles subsides and our arms relax. Unfortunately, the bloodletting didn't go well today. At first, the blood wouldn't flow, and a bruise appeared at the puncture site. Then I pulled so hard on the plunger that the muscles of my hand were aching. I wanted to start again on another puncture site, but since there aren't many areas on the body where you can perform venipuncture, I can't afford to keep on changing. Finally the barrel began to fill up with blood, but slowly and in spurts. While waiting for it to finish, I looked up and saw Lele watching me from the window sill. It made me edgy. His big eyes were staring at the needle, blinking from time to time. I smiled at him.

"It's... alright. Everything's fine," I said, trying to reassure him.

I emptied the barrel into the washbasin, but there was too little blood. I tested a drop between my thumb and forefinger, but it was too watery and not viscous enough. As I was washing away the blood with water, I noticed that, instead of being a nice bright red, it had a yellow tinge to it. This was far from satisfactory. Maybe the quality of the blood in the foot is different from the hand's. It's tepid and lacks warmth. To cover up any traces of my phlebotomy session, I stuffed the syringe at the bottom of the dustbin and covered it up with paper and paper bags for bread.

Lele was curled up in a ball, his head buried in his chest. Did I frighten him? I sat on the window sill, took him into my arms and stroked his back. Nuzzling my head against his, I could feel the softness of his golden fur. It was so soothing. I had been feeling tense and uneasy, as if a hand was pressing down hard on my heart. But now this hand was letting go... One finger...Two... Like a flower unfolding.

"Thank you, Lele," I said.

Lele was licking his lips. I watched his tongue making small darting movements, like he was licking the air. I had read in a magazine that this was a stress signal in pets. Was he sensitive to the smell of fresh blood?

"Don't be scared," I said to him softly. "Look outside. The sun is out."

Holding him against me, I looked outside the window. I could see the classrooms and playground of the primary and secondary schools opposite. Drawn by the sound of children playing, he stopped licking his lips. All was well. A cup of extra strong coffee. Take a deep breath. And I was back at work in front of the computer.

These last few days, big purplish bruises have appeared on the back of my hand, wrist and in the fold of my elbow. One evening, as I was playing with Lele under the lamp on the coffee table, my family suddenly asked me:

"What's that you've got on the back of your hand?"

Luckily, the light was dim. I quickly pulled my hand away and said:

"I must have knocked it against something by accident."

Then, pretending to pick up the newspapers, I quietly slipped away. I watched some television before going to bed. As I was changing channels, I came across the old Hong Kong movie *Ghost Fever*. The actress Guan Zhilin played a vampire who had bitten into the actor Wang Jing's neck to suck his blood. The actress Xia Wenxi, who plays Wang Jing's wife, noticed a purplish teeth-shaped wound on her husband's neck. Vampires drink blood without taking life. They feed on human blood. A bite and a mouthful of blood is enough to last a vampire for a good while. Suddenly, an association of ideas led me to reflect on my own situation. I quickly switched channels. I felt sick. It was night and I was scared. Were there malevolent forces inside me? And if so, were they in any way related to vampires? A syringe full of blood every day. Blood, that's life force. Was the washbasin equivalent to a vampire's mouth? No, it's the throat.

The other day, as I was drawing blood from a vein on top of my right foot, I was thinking how I had gotten the hang of it. But there was nonetheless a slight hitch. My knee was bent, and the sole of my foot was dangling in mid-air. The veins were small and tight, and blood wasn't flowing out. The whole length of the needle was inside the vein and it was hurting me. There was a slight skin abrasion at the puncture site. It felt as if the needle was about to pierce through the vein, tearing away the skin and tendons. Holding my breath, I carefully turned the needle left and right. The vein was slippery, tough and rubbery. I slowly pulled out the needle until the tip was almost visible. Blood began to flow. Feeling much lighter after the phlebotomy session, I said to myself: "Don't worry. There are no vampires. Malevolent spirits can't stand the sight of blood." But I didn't disinfect the skin properly because the puncture site was stinging and had a greyish tinge. I felt slightly feverish. But I wasn't sure if the sensation of heat came from my head or my throat. And I felt dizzy.

I can count with one hand the family members most suited to living in Shenzhen. The best-suited would have been my paternal grandfather. If he had been born 60 years later, he would have settled here in 1983. More than anyone else in the Li or Zhang family, he would have made a success of his life. With his intelligence, talent and determination, he would certainly have been one of the first migrants to make a fortune. He would have started a business, played the stock market and become a millionaire in no time. Then, as soon as he had made some money, he would have invested in real estate. For this is the preferred terrain of the Li family. And after that? He would have moved abroad. There is no place on earth where the people of the northeast wouldn't dare to go. Or he would have travelled to Yunnan Province to trace his family roots. Yes, he would have retreated from the world to go into a kind of hibernation. In Shenzhen, he wouldn't have become a university professor or worked in the high-technology sector. Because it is written in his genes. And he certainly wouldn't have suffered from depression. That is also written in his genes.

Correlations

Excerpts from "Chauffeurs Extraordinaires"

A chauffeur of around 20 years old was standing in front of me. He was sporting a crew cut with a tuft of hair sticking out over his forehead; a Montagut suit worth more than a thousand yuan; and a pair of Trumppipe shoes worth a couple of hundred. He was drenched from the rain.

Before working at the airport, he'd been a driver with a private transport company in Shenzhen. He started in this profession at the age of 15. He worked hard, earned a decent living and liked to play cards in his spare time. He earned money easily and spent it just as easily.

I admired the young chauffeur's casual attitude. After going through the job offers in the newspaper, he'd lost no time in applying.

"I like working at the airport. It's honest work and it's legal. I'm an entrepreneur now," he said, rubbing his hands together.

Time flew by and summer came. On the airport tarmac, the temperature was over 50 degrees. Put a thermometer on the ground and the mercury would shoot to the top of the scale. Before leaving the airport to go to my interview, I drank some extra strong ginseng tea and a cup of Wang Laoji.[1] This time, the taxi chauffeur was a woman, the only one on her team. Unlike her colleagues, she looked vigorous and healthy. She had a round face, small eyes, a soft chin and a round curvaceous body. Ten years ago, she'd gotten married and left the mountains to settle down in Baoan. Her husband made a comfortable living, so she stopped working to enjoy family life.

For many years, her two goals in life were sleeping and playing mahjong.

"I have everything I need at home," she said. "Even my Mitsubishi car that I drive to go play mah-jong with my friends is in better shape than this old banger."

She became bored with sleeping and playing mah-jong, and she quickly became tired of travelling on planes and going on sight-seeing holidays. She began to put on weight, often fell ill, and had headaches and chest pressure.

"When I'm at the airport, I feel good," she said loudly, her face beaming. "I don't mind working hard," she enthused. "What matters is that I'm happy."

She looked beautiful and radiant.

June 1992

Complementary Notes

Between 1991 and 1992, I was on assignment at the new airport in Shenzhen. My job was to write scripts for television series. As creative writing cannot be rushed, my work was still unfinished when I was released from my assignment a year later. The two characters in the extract above represent the emergence of a new state of mind among the people of Shenzhen. This new generation chose their professions with care and refused jobs that were unsuitable for them. They liked to say: "This is what I like doing," or: "This job suits me." At the time, people's determination to make money was stronger than it had ever been, and opportunities were plentiful. But a certain category of people preferred freedom and personal fulfilment. This change in attitude, represented by these two chauffeurs, is in contrast to the attitudes of previous generations, and is a valid and genuine foundation upon which a society can be built. At a time when I thought the people in Shenzhen only cared about making money and the values of this city were stifling me, I felt a breath of fresh air caressing my face.

SIXTY

Diary
Monday, 1ˢᵗ March 2004 11:08 am

The dreams I had these last three nights were filled with anxiety, fear, disappointment and resentment. Need to jot down some of the fragments.

A dream from three nights ago:

I was crossing a river with some friends. The river wasn't wide and had some stones in the middle. The water was shallow and came up to my knees. By the riverbank was a rock, which was probably used as an observation point. My friends were waiting for me on the other side. I started crossing and was standing on the second stone when I noticed that there were three dead bodies in the water. One of them was next to the stone I was standing on. The body was curved and belonged to someone around 30 years of age. It was well-groomed, and its face was expressionless. I panicked and screamed, too scared to look at the other two corpses to find out if they were male or female. I wanted to go back, but my friends shouted: "Hurry up! There are more behind you!" I turned around. Heavens, the river was filled with dead bodies. The corpses of young men and women were stacked on top of one another, piling up into a big heap that stood out from the water. It made my blood run cold. I asked myself: "Why didn't I see them? Where did they come from all of a sudden? I can't go back now. It'd be too gruesome. And it's impossible to gain a foothold with all these corpses." On the opposite bank, my friends were holding their hands out to me and shouting: "Quick, hurry up! Don't look down!" I plucked up my courage, and keeping my eyes on my friends or on the stones, hurriedly crossed the river. I arrived on the other side feeling pleased with myself. It wasn't that difficult after all. I felt encouraged that I was able to overcome my fear and apprehensions.

There was more to the dream but I was unable to recall it when I woke up in the morning.

I gave Lele a hiding yesterday. It was a lovely spring day and we had a positive start. I was spending the afternoon on the campus of Sun Yat-Sen University. A woman was playing with her three children on the lawn at the bottom of the stone steps that led up to a stele with the names of scholars who were successful at imperial examinations engraved on it. An old woman of around 70 years old was doing her exercises next to a flower bed. Lovers were strolling along the paths. Some people were taking photographs; others were enjoying the spring air. I was sitting on the steps, using my velvet green cardigan as a cushion. I was reading *50 Ways to Fight Depression Without Drugs*.[1] Lele was running around on the lawn. When I looked up, I saw that he was holding something black in his mouth. My gut feeling told me that he was up to no good. As I was dashing towards him, I realised that it was something dirty. In fact, it was a dead dried-up rat. I yelled at him to let go. Not only did he not listen to me, but he held it even tighter between his teeth and started racing around. I chucked my book and cardigan at him but missed. I finally caught him in front of the bushes, but he still wouldn't let go of the rat. Grabbing him by the scruff of the neck, I threw him down on the lawn, sending him flying into a double somersault. I picked him up and smacked him six or seven times.

I was livid. It reminded me of the hidings my mother gave me when we were living in the big courtyard at number 403.

Notes

According to the weather forecast, the next few days will be hot and sunny and the temperature will be over 35 degrees. Guangzhou is on yellow alert for a heatwave. Everywhere in the media, people are giving advice on how to fight the heat. For example: Eat congee made with haricot beans or lotus leaves or green soya beans. The light has a strong glare and the sun sets much later on in the day. All this is beneficial for those who suffer from depression. I will make good use of this opportunity and get on with the writing of this book.

Yesterday around 7 o'clock in the evening, I took Lele out for a walk. He was bright and bouncy as usual. On seeing a female French bulldog, he wanted to go up to her. But she had been in a fight with a cat, which left her with a scratched nose, and her owner was wiping the blood off her face. To show his support and sympathy, Lele wanted to go up and sniff at her. But I was worried that it might cause trouble by bringing up painful memories in the poor dog, or make the wound bleed again. So I yelled at Lele, pulled hard on his leash and scolded him. Finally I managed to get away.

Lele is a nosey old soul and likes to poke his nose into everything. When he saw a two-year-old child being told off by his mother because he was throwing a temper tantrum, he started barking at her. When he saw some school children running and screaming, he looked excitedly around him, hoping to join in their games. A German shepherd walked past close by. It wasn't interested in small dogs and ignored him completely. Lele, feeling snubbed, snarled at it and wanted to pounce. I yelled: "Stop! I'm angry now!"

When I left home earlier, the sun was still out, so I put a cap on. I had with me a black soya milk drink for myself and a feeding bottle of water for Lele. Twenty minutes into our walk, he was stretched out on the grass, drooling and refusing to move. The searing heat made me dizzy, and my stomach was hurting. I picked up Lele and went home. His body was burning, and he was drooling all over the floor. To lower his body temperature, I put a wet towel on his belly and soaked his paws in water. He was lying on the parquet floor. I switched on the air conditioner, and while waiting for the temperature to drop in the room, I used a handheld fan to keep him cool. His breathing was rapid and heavy. He was suffering from heat exhaustion. The ground outside was hot. I am tall but could still feel the rising heat. It had affected Lele much more than me. Of the 10 species of dogs most affected by the heat, Pekinese dogs are sixth on the list. For they have a snub nose, stubby legs, and their thick, dense coat prevents their body heat from evaporating quickly. The room was now cooler, and Lele's breathing was slower and less heavy. But an hour later, it was my turn. I had stomach pains and diarrhea; my eyes were watering; my nose was runny, and I kept wanting to sneeze. I took some *huanglian*[2] tablets. I had difficulty walking and was slouching with my head bent over my knees. My breathing was shallow; my forehead was covered in sweat; and my head ached.

As I've been rushing through my writing these last few days, the quality of my work is mediocre, leaving me unsatisfied. Almost all my friends who know I'm writing this book tell me to take my time. Some of them even tell me to stop. They're all worried about me. But I can't stop. I feel it's my duty to leave a testimony of someone struggling with depression. Sometimes I ask myself if my book is worth the paper it's written on. Should I bother at all? Is it capable of giving moral support to those in the same plight?

My mind drifts, and I forget what I want to say. When I am like this, I am neither a sick person, nor a writer. The "Diary" section was already finished when I fell ill, so that's that out of the way. But the "Notes" and "Complementary Notes" sections still bother me. Inserting excerpts into the "Correlations" section has given an internal structure to each chapter. I am scared that my health will deteriorate and affect my brain, ruining any chance I might have of finishing this book.

One thought haunts me. As soon as it erupts in my mind, I try to erase it, but it keeps coming back to torture me. When it happens, I use cognitive therapy to help blank it out. But this thought has a life of its own. It becomes uncontrollable and slips from my grasp. It springs out of the blue, leaps in front of me, shouting: "Li Lanni, are you capable of finishing this book? I doubt it very much. If you relapse into depression, it'll finish you off, won't it? And if you dropped dead? If you were given the choice, would you let yourself die? Don't think, just answer me! Li Lanni, if your cancer spreads to your brain, you'll never finish this book. Face up to reality. The chance of not finishing your book is 50/50. And that's being optimistic. I'm telling you the truth and the truth isn't nice to hear, but you have to look it in the face. You're scared of going back to the hospital for a check-up. You can't bear the thought of going through another operation. It's all very well, praying and singing hymns in church. But I'm not Satan. You're wasting your time, banging on the keyboard and making such a din. You're overdoing it. Do you want to drown me with your noise? Stop. Take a deep breath. That's good. And now, breathe out. Relax. I'm not a malevolent spirit, but a voice coming from inside of you. Let me out, so I can breathe. Are you tired? Get some rest then. That's good. I'll shut up. Just now, your mind was confused. Your hands weren't doing what you wanted them to do. Ah... a force bearing down on me. I was about to pour scorn on your stupidity and your mumbo-jumbo prayers, but the Holy Spirit is on your side. He changed the words I was going to say. The Holy Spirit is coming, I'm leaving... I'm leaving..."

A malevolent force was here. It's gone, leaving me weak and drained. I need to lie down on the sofa.

I was lying on the sofa, exhausted, as if I had been doing strenuous exercises. I tried breathing through my abdomen but with no results whatsoever. I stopped after a while. I closed my eyes to rest but felt burnt out. My brain had broken down. How could I make it function again?

Quick, where's Lele? He's my personal doctor. I found him lying on the floor in the sitting-room beside the coffee table, where I had put four porcelain tiles with Snoopy painted on them. He has a habit of lounging around there in the summer. He was lying on the floor, so calm, his eyes half closed. I took him in my arms and sat on the sofa in my study.

"Lele, you must help me," I said to him.

There was a bamboo mat on the sofa. I lay down on my side, hugging Lele against me. His head was snuggled against my chest, like a doctor listening to my breathing and heartbeat. He looked up at me and yawned, opening wide his mouth, as if to say: "Everything is fine." He stretched himself, exposing his belly, then sat up and sniffed at me. He was looking at me with an expression in his eyes that resembled that of a ... little genie. I don't know how to describe it. He looked relaxed, as if he wasn't worried about me anymore. Then, squinting his eyes, he yawned again and snuggled against my arm, wagging his tail. A month ago, I had taken him to a dog groomer, who cut all his hair except for the fur around the neck. A neighbour, who is a teacher, said he looked like the lion in the logo for the anti-virus software, Ruixing. Others said he was like the small lion in *The Lion King*. I jumped up from the sofa and ran barefoot to Lele's box of snacks. Rummaging around inside, I found some Yili milk snacks. I shared them with Lele, with the two of us sitting on the sofa.

Zhou Lele is a wonderful doctor.

21st June 2007

Correlations

Excerpts from "Women Who Drink"

When I was 10 years old, the older pupils in my school were busy writing *dazibao*[3] and denouncing their teachers. We, the younger ones, were stuck at home and spent all day playing "soldiers and bandits" and "what time is it, big bad wolf?" One day, bored out of my skull, I began rummaging around the house and found, hidden inside a wooden trunk, a book that seemed to make no sense at all. It was the story of a young woman called Xiuxiu. She ran away from a prince's palace and met a young man by the name of Cui. They drank wine, and after two cups the young woman suggested that they elope together. The book said: "The wine played the role of a go-between for the desires of the flesh." At the time, I didn't understand the meaning of "desires of the flesh." I only knew that in a feudal society, a go-between was bad person who held superstitious beliefs. And as for wine, it was certainly nothing good. I imagined it to be black, like the ink you wrote *dazibao* with. And one mouthful would turn your insides black. It wasn't until later, at my maternal grandmother's home in Jiangsu Province, that I saw wine for the first time. It was wine that she had made herself from glutinous rice. She said young girls should drink a cup of rice wine before going to bed at night, because it was good for the skin and gave a rosy complexion. The wine had a sweet and perfumed aroma, but I was afraid to drink it. Because, deep down, I felt a repulsion for it.

In secondary school, I would read poetry of the Tang and Song dynasties and *Dream of the Red Chamber* in secret. Through poets and writers, I discovered that wine was good. Without wine, how could Li Bai[4] have become an "immortal poet?" If the poetess Li Qingzhao[5] had not "drunk wine at dusk beside the fence facing east," then how could she have had her "sleeves soaked with the delicate fragrance of wine?"[6] Or how could the beautiful women in *Dream of the Red Chamber* have taken delight in playing in the gardens of Daiguan?

When I was studying at Nanjing University, all my fellow students, whether they were men or women, could drink a glass or two. When we greeted each other, instead of saying: "Have you eaten yet?" as was the custom, we would say: "How about a glass?" And we would answer: "Okay, let's go." I would never get myself into a state of inebriation, because the wine had a low alcohol content.

I enjoy watching other people drink, especially women. Men drink, and it sets a convivial atmosphere for a dinner party. But when women drink, the evening becomes more interesting, because women are polite, reserved and gracious. At the start of the evening, the women are quiet, sipping calmly and elegantly on their orange juice. As the men continue to drink, their faces turn red, and their voices grow increasingly louder. But the women just smile and carry on eating, savouring the dishes, their lips shiny with oil from the food. When the men get tipsy, they start rambling, and the air becomes tense, as if a fight could break out any moment; the women signal to the waiter to bring them a glass. Then, with a gleam in their eyes, each woman fills her glass, stopping well before it's full, and they propose a toast. The tension in the air immediately dies down, and the men courteously drink with the women with great gallantry.

A woman rarely becomes drunk. Even when she is tipsy, she remains quiet and polite. Sometimes, with her bright and rosy complexion, she looks like an innocent and delicate doll; sometimes, weeping silently, she resembles from afar a jade statuette of a beautiful woman, melancholic and moving.

Men are particular about the surroundings in which they drink. In spring, they like to drink under a pavilion, and in the summer, outdoors in the countryside. But women are selective about their drinking partners. For she would never drink with someone she hates, nor with someone she loves. And when she is enjoying herself and gets a man into a state of inebriation, he would be neither her enemy nor her lover.

I like women who drink without being inebriated. I admire them. For they are capable of facing hardships and trials with men. Women who drink are the gentlest and the tenderest of them all.

March 1993

Complementary Notes

My mother forbade my father to drink. To her, it was evil. She thought that all was well, until the day she found out that her son and daughter drank.

At Nanjing University, the wine we drank was low in alcohol. The reasons why I drink in Shenzhen are many: social obligation; to relieve stress; and to share a convivial moment with friends.

I once knew a woman in Shenzhen who would drink wine at 52 degrees on an empty stomach while rereading her personal diary. Then, at midnight, she would call me and cry over the phone. She was a competent career woman, strong and authoritarian, even. But when she had a few drinks, her personality would change. She became soft and gentle and would think about her children and all the mistakes she had made in her life. She would blame herself for being a bad and inadequate mother.

I knew a man in Shenzhen who was stern, taciturn and chauvinistic. But one time, he became intoxicated and was running around in a hotel corridor. He was about to undo his fly to urinate when his friends stopped him, held him by the arms and dragged him onto the bed. Roaring drunk and laughing like hyena, he was bashing on the pillow and hitting the bed and walls.

"I'm not drunk," he said. "I know what I'm doing. Let me tell you a secret. It's been a long time since I can't get it up anymore. If you don't believe me, I'll show you."

He was about to lower his trousers when his friends quickly threw a blanket over him. He cried like a baby. Many people in Shenzhen don't cry. But tears have the power to heal.

For years, many women in Shenzhen often confided in me. They were in their 30s and all had some kind of emotional problems in their lives. None of them trusted their husbands or lovers, and they felt insecure in their marriages or relationships. Even those under 30 confessed that they didn't believe in love and felt confused and helpless.

A friend once told me that her husband hadn't made love to her in a year. When he came home in the evening, he said he was tired and went straight to bed. In the morning, he would leave without eating breakfast or saying a word to his wife. He never talked about divorce, but he never showed her any affection, either. Thinking he had a lover, she hired a private detective to follow him around for a couple of months, but didn't find any woman that might rouse suspicion.

"All the men in Shenzhen are trash," she said bitterly.

Then she continued with utmost honesty:

"People say we're made for each other, that we have the same social status and that we're perfect together. But what they don't know is that I can't take it anymore. I can't stand the sight of him. I hate him so much that I wish he'd get run over by a car. I'd rather he be dead than leave him to those little sluts."

Another friend told me that she knew her husband inside out and that he was a perfect bastard. If he wasn't running after young, pretty women, then he'd be panting after attentive, affectionate widows.

"Nowadays we talk about sexual equality. I have no intention of staying all by myself in my little corner," she said. "My lovers are all rich and good-looking and are doing just as well as my husband. He wants to compete with me. Well, he's not worthy enough to be my rival."

A close acquaintance, who was 30 years old and had already been divorced three times, told me that she couldn't see herself getting married again.

"It's simpler being a mistress," she laughed. "Anyway, being married isn't economically viable. There will always be a mistress number two or three threatening to oust you."

"Times have changed," she said confidently. "The family model is no longer in fashion."

She worked as a hairdresser and masseuse, because this line of work provided more openings. When I saw her the second time at the hairdresser's, I was left speechless.

"You belong to the Writers' Association," she said to me. "I know one of your members, a Mr X. I met him at the hairdresser's where I used to work. He fancied me, but he was too old. In the end, he hooked up with the ugliest girl there, a girl from Sichuan. Haha, he even showed us a letter he wrote to her. But who wants to read his stupid letter? The idiot read it out loud and we nearly died laughing. What a dickhead!"

A beautiful woman who used to be a dancer in the army owned a small boutique. She and her husband had changed professions to come to Shenzhen in search of new opportunities. Two years later, her husband became the "boy toy" of a woman manager at his work place. After their divorce, she was constantly being harassed at job interviews. Disheartened, she ended up becoming the mistress of a small Hong Kong businessman. Short, fat and ugly, he came from an average family.

"Ugly men from ordinary families are simpler," she said. "They don't have three or four mistresses hovering around them to complicate your life."

The man bought her an apartment, and she opened a small boutique with his financial support. When she talked about him, she kept saying: "My husband this, my husband that." However, three years later, she found out that he was cheating on her. She organised a "family reunion" made up of ex-mistresses who had been jilted by their lovers. They would meet up every week to sing and pray together. They asked God to inflict punishment on these "bastards."

For several years, you were spoilt for choice at the "general headquarters of the prostitutes' association," as the ex-mistresses called their reunions. There was a broad range of women of all genres: stylish and well-bred; hot chicks; the young and fresh; the shy and virtuous; the devoted wife; the nanny-type; the university student; the housemaid-type; those you have a weekend fling with; those who are hot in bed but otherwise frosty and hung up; the secretary-type... You name it. After the stock market crash in 1997, I heard that groups of prostitutes of "premium quality" had left Shenzhen on several charter flights to seek their fortunes in far-off horizons.

SIXTY-ONE

Diary
Thursday, 11th March 2004 11:23 am

The "depression season" is back again, I am in such bad shape. I catch cold easily and have aches and pains all over: sore throat, headaches, dizziness and feelings of suffocation. Can't concentrate, nor ease a kind of feverish restlessness in me. Had a nightmare a few nights ago.

It was bucketing down, and I was walking on the streets. Road workers were repairing the gutter and drainage channels. They were surrounded by a group of bystanders who were watching them work. The dead bodies of two workers were lying on the ground next to the gutter. A third worker with a heavy build fell from the sky and landed on the storm drain. He was dead on impact. The bystanders cheered: "Yes! Another one bites the dust!" Scared and not knowing what to do, I kept my distance. Suddenly, sewage water was gushing down the streets, rising up to my chest. The bystanders were wading clumsily across the streets. Can't remember the rest of the dream.

No matter what happens, I mustn't let myself relapse into depression during the months of March and April. I make an effort to take Lele out for a walk in the morning and afternoon.

According to David K. Reynolds, the author of *Constructive Living*,[1] those who suffer from mild depression can practise Morita Therapy and Naikan Therapy to reinforce the effects of medication.

I must accept the state of my current health as a whole and not just focus on the symptoms. Then I won't be hemmed into a vicious circle of my own making. I should accept my situation and do whatever is necessary to recover my health. Stay active. Positive actions lead to positive thinking. The more active you are, the more likely you are to adopt a positive mindset.

I've been forcing myself to be active these last two days. When I am not too tired, I have the strength to resist the pressures that others exert on me.

Notes

Lately, I've been thinking a lot about a painting entitled *The Toilette of Esther*.[2] It was part of a life-size calendar with world-famous nude paintings that a friend gave me in January 1999. Flicking through it, I realised that I was familiar with most of the paintings except for the one representing the month of June: *The Toilette of Esther*. Neither did I know who Esther was. In June or

July of the same year, through the inspiration of the Holy Spirit, I came across the Dongshan Church, where I bought a copy of the Bible. I spent three months reading it, and it was only then that I realised who Esther was. But I was yet to know what *The Toilette of Esther* was going to mean to me, for I hadn't yet grasped the significance of the story of Esther. It's only now that I'm beginning to understand.

Esther was a Jewess who lived in Persia. She was an orphan and was brought up by her cousin Mordecai. One year, the Persian king Xerxes was looking for a new wife. Esther and many other beautiful women were taken to the harem in the palace to be chosen. According to the custom, they should spend one year preparing their bodies with beauty treatments: six months with oil of myrrh and six with fragrant perfumes. When the preparation was over, the women would wait their turn to be received by the king, one by one. Days went by slowly.

The selection process commenced three years after the beginning of the reign of King Xerxes. It was not until the tenth month of the seventh year of his reign that Esther was received by the king. Following the palace protocol, when a woman left the harem to go to the king's palace, she was given anything she wanted. Esther was not avaricious: "[...] She asked for nothing other than what Hegai, the king's eunuch who was in charge of the harem, suggested. And Esther won the favour of everyone who saw her."[3] "Now the king was attracted to Esther more than to any of the other women, and she won his favour [...]. So he set a royal crown on her head and made her queen [...]."[4]

The story was just beginning. On the first month of the twelfth year of his reign, King Xerxes, under the influence of his evil minister Haman, gave the order for all the Jews in the kingdom to be killed on the thirteenth day of the twelfth month. Mordecai went to see Esther to ask her to beg the king to spare her people. According to the palace rule, anyone who approaches the king without being summoned must be put to death. Through a messenger, Mordecai said this to Esther: "If you remain silent at this time, relief and deliverance for the Jews will arise from another place, but you and your father's family will perish. And who knows but that you have come to your royal position for such a time as this?"[5] Esther was deeply moved. She approached the king without being summoned, risking her life, and uncovered Haman's conspiracy, thus saving the lives of all the Jews in the kingdom.

The story is compelling, the plot well-constructed and filled with suspense. I read it in one go. About the Book of Esther, I will quote from *What the Bible is All About*: "If God puts you in a hostile environment, it is part of his intentions."[6]

I listened to a sermon given by a pastor at the Dongshan Church about "Esther's situation." The key points are: Through the grace of God, He puts us in a given situation not at random, but through His will. He teaches us through warnings, trials, sicknesses and disasters, so that we may serve Him. Thus, we learn what obedience, prayer and sacrifice are.

Every one of us has our own destiny to fulfill. We can all be like Esther. At each stage of our lives, we strive to learn, to bide our time, to purify and better ourselves. Then when the right moment comes, we take on the task that has been given to us.

I like being alone at home.

When I am sick, I need to go into "hibernation." I unplug the phone, switch off the light, the television and my mobile phone and turn off the music. I don't see anyone; I don't talk; I lie down, unmoving, like a corpse. From time to time, I get up and potter around the apartment with all the lights switched off. At moments like these, I feel relaxed and at ease.

For many years, it was impossible for me to live with my family for longer than a month. Every month, I had to spend at least a few days at my place in Shenzhen, otherwise I would be edgy, anxious and restless. I would be ill at ease and my mind would become foggy, as if I weren't living my own life, but someone else's. I didn't belong to myself anymore. I had lost myself. It was only by spending three or four days alone in Shenzhen that I could find myself again. I got used to being alone as a child. Solitude became a way of life for me. During my adolescence, I was accustomed to staying alone in hospitals with no one to visit me. No one called me to ask how I was, and I had no one to exchange correspondence with. The lively and noisy districts in Shenzhen made me uncomfortable. It was only by being alone at home that I could find Li Lanni again. But after a couple of weeks, a kind of terror would set in. Negative emotions would gnaw at me: profound dismay; feelings of being abandoned and no longer existing; being totally at sea, adrift and aimless; no sense of self-worth. All these toxic emotions would end up driving me out of my own home. I needed to eat out in restaurants; listen to gossip; see people moving and walking; drink and smoke with them; throw myself into different kinds of distractions, so as to diminish my sense of self.

I was torn between two states of mind: the need to be alone and the need to be surrounded by life.

23rd June 2007

Correlations

Excerpts from *"My Budgies"*

Bao Erye was bursting with Yang energy. He was shrieking, and his eyes were bright and sharp. His green and yellow feathers were more striking and splendid than a tiger's coat. He liked to hop around in his cage. Sometimes he would groom Miss Bao with his beak, and sometimes he would gently nudge Miss Lin with his head. As for these two "Misses," one would stand facing east while the other faced west. Bao Erye, not wanting to neglect either of them, was busy attending to them both.

Miss Lin was beautiful, gentle and elegant. Her soft fluffy feathers were of a blue so pale and tender that it existed only in dreams. Dainty and fragile, she had a small head and body. There was something human in the look of melancholy in her eyes. Miss Bao was round and chubby. Her feathers, white like the snow, lent her an air of nobility. She was fond of her food and ate enough for two. Once she had her fill, she would peck at the metal cage. Was it a quirk of hers or did she want to peck open the cage to fly away? She liked to spread her wings and shriek, as if to say: "It's me, the mistress of the house."

[...] I decided to train my budgies. Every day, I would teach them to say: "Good morning," "Are you home?" "Let's eat," "Smile," and "Bye-bye." Incapable of understanding that it was for their own good, they ignored me completely. Perched on his ring, Bao Erye was swinging happily; Miss Bao was pecking away at the cage; and Miss Lin, eyes half closed, was thinking: "What a bunch of half-wits!" I wanted to train them for my own amusement. Once, they pecked and scratched me on my hand. I yelled out in pain. Then I heard screeching and, suddenly, flashes of white, blue and golden light were whirling around me, as if the sitting-room had been turned into a battle field. I managed to catch the budgies and put them back into the cage. I switched on the light and saw the scratch marks on my hand. The sofa and sideboard were splattered with bird droppings, and grains of corn were scattered all over the floor. The birds had given me a dose of my own medicine [...].

From that moment on, hearing their cries would grate on my nerves. To punish them, I put the cage on the balcony, exposing them to the sun and rain. I began to neglect them, giving them a big cup of seeds once every few days. I didn't clean their cage anymore, leaving it to the housekeeper, who came for half a day once a week. She was sloppy and always left it to the end. She would spray the cage and birds with a water hose. Poor Bao Erye and the poor Misses would hop around inside the cage, distraught, their feathers all ruffled. I confess I was slightly upset seeing them in such a state but did nothing to stop the housekeeper.

One day, I had to leave for an assignment and would be away for five or six days. I put a cup brimful of seeds and a big cup of water in the cage. I left Shenzhen in high spirits. But there was a setback and I ended up being absent for two weeks. During that time, I thought about the budgies twice. The first time was on the eighth day. As I was having breakfast, it suddenly struck me: Were there enough seeds for two weeks? The second time was when I was watching television. The weather forecast announced that there would be thunder storms and heavy rain in the next few days in Shenzhen. I thought: "The birds will suffer on the balcony. I'm a bit worried... You're thinking about them, but are they thinking of you? There's no point in losing sleep over it. If they die in the rain, there's nothing much I can do." I tried to reassure myself, but it was weighing on my conscience.

As soon as I walked through the door, I rushed to the balcony. The cage was a mess and gave off a foul stench. The cups were empty. Miss Bao had melted away. Eyes closed and shivering, she looked wretched and forlorn. Bao Erye's feathers were dull and splattered with excrement. Still alert, he was uttering sad and melancholic cries. Following his sad gaze, I saw an inert pile of blue ruffled feathers at the bottom of the cage. It was Miss Lin. I put my hand inside the cage to touch her. She was dead. It looked like she had been dead for a while, because she was no more than a frail and dried-up mummy. Did she die of thirst or from sickness? Had she been drowned in the rain or struck by lightning? There was no way of knowing. And as for Bao Erye and Miss Bao, how had they survived these last few days beside Miss Lin's dead body?

Overwhelmed with grief, I cried: "I'm sorry. I'm so sorry. What did I do? I'm so sorry..." I looked hurriedly for an unused white envelope and carefully put Miss Lin inside. Miss Bao opened wide her haggard eyes and looked at me with indifference. I quickly filled the cups with seeds and water, cleaned the cage and took it into the sitting-room.

Bao Erye drank some water, and with his hoarse voice squawked at me twice, as if to say: "You're cruel. You killed Miss Lin." At the same moment, Miss Bao glared at me with her big eyes filled with hatred. I felt a wave of panic. I was scared that they would suddenly start speaking human language to say goodness knows what to me. I ran into the study to look for a piece of red string to tie the white envelope with.

I said: "Pure, she came into this world, and with purity in her soul, she leaves this world."

As I was rummaging through the drawer, I suddenly heard a plaintive cry. Filled with a sense of deep unease, I ran into the sitting-room. Miss Bao was lying next to Bao Erye. She was dead. What did she die of? Devastated, I looked at Bao Erye.

He looked at me with the eyes of someone with a broken heart. There was no anger, nor bitterness, only an immense pain and profound sorrow. Tears filled my eyes, and I was afraid to look at Bao Erye.

I put Miss Bao in a white envelope and, with trembling hands and a heavy heart, I tied the two envelopes up with red string. I couldn't help but recite a Buddhist prayer, so that the souls of these two Misses would go to heaven. I went out, holding the two envelopes, and buried them at the foot of a redbud tree that was growing on the lawn in front of my building.

Inside the apartment, a hushed silence hung in the air. There was an atmosphere of death and loss. My knees gave way and I slowly sank to the floor. There was no need to go and see Bao Erye. For he, too, was no more.

Summer of 1994

Complementary Notes

I didn't want to reread this story. For it forces me to remember. As I was writing the story, I was filled with shame. These last two or three years, whenever the memories of my budgies came back, I would immediately shut them out of my mind.

An immense guilt has been gnawing away at me. I didn't know what had caused their deaths until I read an article saying that, for birds, water was even more important than food. I was so stupid and ignorant.

What was appalling wasn't so much my stupidity as my indifference towards another living thing. If I had had an ounce of respect for life, I would have tried to understand something as essential as that before taking on the birds. I should have been better informed and, to look after them properly, should have assessed their vital needs using mine as a touchstone. But I didn't.

I kept the budgies, not because I loved or appreciated them, but because I felt bored and lonely.

These last few years, when I look into my own conscience, I realise that I, Li Lanni, had in my subconscious mind the intention to do harm. You could say it was negligence, forgetfulness, ignorance, or even "manslaughter." But I know the real reason that had pushed me to behave as I did. The budgies gave me a channel to externalise my hatred. It could be that, unconsciously, I hated them and wanted them dead.

We have all experienced moments when we feel blind rage rushing up in us. As part of society, we are often subject to humiliations, hurts and contempt, which trigger in us the constant struggle between good and evil. When evil, this ugly and heinous thing, has the upper hand, it allows hatred to grow in us and transform us into diabolical beings.

According to psychiatrists, depression can lead to anger and aggressiveness directed towards the outer environment. It manifests itself in different ways depending on the individual, but the principle is the same. Some take it out on innocent and defenceless animals, others on those who are weaker than themselves.

Sometimes I hear on the news stories of cruelty to cats and dogs. There was an incident where someone threw sulfuric acid on some bears at a zoo. Stories of animal cruelty are common. But I don't pay a lot of attention to them. Firstly, because I have a bad conscience and they remind me of the despicable and unforgivable things I have done. Secondly, I am so full of shame. And thirdly, stricken with remorse, I have no right to condemn others. Cruelty to animals is becoming increasingly common and shouldn't be taken lightly. It's a warning sign that a growing number of people are suffering from mental illness. I have, on several occasions, repented of my sins or asked for pardon through prayers of repentance at church. But it is not enough. For I cannot offer forgiveness to myself. Never. Never.

SIXTY-TWO

Diary
Thursday, 1st April 2004 11 am

On 1st April last year, I was in the waiting room of the psychiatric department situated on the ninth floor of the Third Sun Yat-Sen Hospital. I had an appointment with a psychiatric specialist. It was during the SARS epidemic, and this hospital was among the few that were treating SARS patients. But the waiting room was full of people who had come to consult a psychiatrist. Luckily, my friend, Rui Lin, had called the head physician, Dr Zhang, beforehand to make an appointment for me.

The doctor received me at five past midday. I was the second to last on the list and the consultation lasted for 10 minutes. I called Rui Lin immediately afterwards to tell her that I wasn't suffering from depression. In the afternoon, rumours were circulating that the Hong Kong singer, Zhang Guorong, had committed suicide by jumping from a window. I refused to believe it, thinking it was a sick April Fool's joke concocted by spiteful journalists. At dinner time, a Hong Kong television program announced that Zhang Guorong's suicide was due to depression. It chilled me to the bone. I kept telling myself how fortunate it was that the doctor had ruled out the possibility of depression and that I had no suicidal thoughts. Otherwise I couldn't imagine how I would have taken Zhang Guorong's suicide. I couldn't bring myself to watch the television coverage, look at his face, see his eyes, nor listen to his songs.

Yesterday evening, a Hong Kong television channel announced the unveiling of a wax statue of Zhang Guorong. It wasn't until then, one year after his death, that I had the courage to look at images of him. Today, during my morning prayers and daily reading of the Bible, I prayed that his soul may rest in peace.

There's a thunderstorm, and Lele is frightened. The day before yesterday, in the afternoon, he was discharged from the veterinary clinic.

On 31st March, I had lunch at Shunfeng Village with President Dong and the two vice presidents, Yang and Xie, of the Guangzhou Cultural Federation. They were in Guangzhou for a meeting. I am immensely grateful to them for the interest they show in my work.

Notes

Have stomach pains and a high fever. I suspect it's mild heatstroke. The sun is pouring into the study and the heat is stifling. I drew the curtains and turned on the air conditioner, but the heat is still unbearable. In the afternoon, sitting in front of the computer, I still had nagging stomach pains, so took several capsules of *huoxiang zhenqi*.[1] I'm in bad shape: heaviness in the chest, sore throat, tension headache, nausea. I stopped my bloodletting sessions yesterday. Don't feel like it anymore all of a sudden. I was alone at home and took out a syringe but lost all incentive. It's beyond me.

Still can't get down to work. Writing these last two chapters, I have had to face up to the dark side of Li Lanni. It's torturous. I wanted to explore the darker nature of the people in Shenzhen, but to my dismay, I found nothing vile or tenebrous in them, only what is caliginous in my memories.

I am in the middle of reading *Chinese Characteristics*.[2] According to Arthur Smith, the Chinese are defined by the following characteristics: we dislike losing face; lack the notion of time; give little importance to comfort or the practical aspects of life; practise filial piety, etc. Smith was a perceptive and astute observer. If his grandchildren were to visit China today, they would discover a country in full economic development, as well as the emergence of a new type of Chinese who are capable of pushing certain notions to the limit. They are willing to do anything to make a profit and aren't afraid to lose face in the process. They don't care about losing face if it means they can move up in life. They are thrifty and cautious. For time is money. They can't afford to dilly-dally, because an hour spent doing nothing is money lost. As for filial piety, that's ancient history. As long as you have money, there will always be someone to show you filial piety. With no money, it is you who will have to show filial piety to someone else.

As for the other characteristics Smith talked about, they are taken to their extremes: an ability to deceive others; lack of civic sense; mutual suspicion and distrust; polytheism; pantheism and atheism.

On the news, in the newspapers, everywhere you turn, a tragic event is taking place: an accident in the caves in Shanxi, an incident with the mafia and the tanks in Tangshan, a young man killing his parents with an axe. Nowadays, we pray and make offerings to God in the hope that we will be rewarded with material wealth. We talk about so-and-so who is ill, or so-and-so who is broke, but how many of us ask: Are our minds sick? Are our souls unwell?

I worked as a journalist when I first arrived in Shenzhen. A year later, for better or for worse, I joined a newspaper's arts and literature team. In hindsight, if I had pursued my career in journalism, I would have had more confidence in myself. For I have failed as a writer.

There are no fairy tales, only fables. Trying to depict the realities of Shenzhen in a novel is an impossible task.

People have often encouraged me to write, saying that Shenzhen has many interesting topics and that I would do a good job of it. But I felt overwhelmed by the wealth of thematic ideas, as if I was buried in the mud after a landslide or submerged under a mountain of ashes from a volcanic eruption. I had the skills to write, but feeling burdened and smothered, I was fighting for my mental survival. I felt disorientated, insignificant, small and humbled.

I ran away. Very, very far away. As far away as possible from Shenzhen.

Before settling in this city, I used to write novels. For the first three or four years, I wrote novellas on the theme of youth entrepreneurship. And when Shenzhen seemed to me so alien and terrifying, instead of writing stories, I began to write essays. I described my impressions of living in a strange and unfamiliar city. When you are far away from home, you see yourself with surprising lucidity. However, I couldn't earn a living just by writing essays. A professional writer needs to produce longer works. The truth is, essays are poorly paid and difficult to write.

My maternal grandmother liked to remind us of this popular saying: "The heavens always watch over blind chicks." There is some truth to it. When I thought I had come to a dead end, someone flew in from Beijing to offer me a job as a film script writer with a competitive salary and generous benefits. My first script was an instant success. My life changed overnight. I was earning a decent living and had won an award. It was like in the folk tale, "The Horse that Sai Weng Lost." Sai Weng had lost his horse, which came back, bringing with it two foals. It was a blessing in disguise. But I am not wise like Sai Weng. He understood that the heavens always guide us out of an impasse, and that fortune and misfortune are interconnected. But I didn't understand. I thought that hard work would invariably lead to wealth, that three horses would automatically multiply into six the following year. I am not a greedy person. You don't steal the fruit of someone else's labour. There is a time for everything. A time to build, a time to destroy. A time to reap profits, a time to incur losses. Between 1996 and the end of 1999, I was writing film scripts in Beijing. In February 2000, I had a surgical intervention followed by chemotherapy. That year, I spent all the money I had earned the previous years. Can you call this fate?

I've just received an invitation from the liaison office of the Writers' Association. It's for a visit to the military barracks of the 2nd Field Regiment, 27th Division of the Armed Forces, 5th Division of the Air Force, and the National Navy of the northern sea. Two years ago, I visited the satellite launch centre with the Writers' Association. What moved me the most wasn't the control room, nor the accommodation where the astronauts stayed the day before their departure. Instead, it was the cemetery in Jiuquan, where soldiers who had died in service are buried. Hundreds of grey headstones stood in a desolate landscape. Be they of generals or foot soldiers, these headstones are, without exception, a testimony of endurance, simplicity and quietude. These military men and women lived in mud huts, suffered hunger in the desert and, cut off from the rest of the world, served their country with dedication, loyalty and intelligence. Their names are synonymous of devotion and sacrifice. They have given up their youth, children and grandchildren and, in turn, their children must sacrifice their parents. When the space shuttle was launched, the entire country celebrated. But few knew of Jiuquan cemetery, and even fewer of us remembered these soldiers, their parents and their children.

27th June 2007

Correlations

Excerpts from *"The Road to Spring"*

The friends who took me to the construction site of Binhai Boulevard in Shenzhen were all graduates of different professions from the Universities of Qinghua, Nanjing and Tongji. Some of them had already earned their Master's or Doctorate degrees. Our jeep drove through muddy paths saturated with rain. Then we climbed onto the concrete foundation that had just been put down. The first phase of land reclamation and the paving of the foundation were over, and you could see the initial outline of the boulevard that stretched 9.6 kilometres. The road took a sharp turn in the northern section. In the south, birds were flying in circles above a forest of red trees. In the north, I saw vaguely in the distance the Eiffel Tower of the Window of the World.[3] Culturally, Shenzhen is on a par with other international cities. It brings together nature, culture and urban vitality, integrating them into a whole from which a beautiful modern city can be developed in a methodical and scientific way.

During my visit to this construction site that would take us into the next century, I asked a boy of five-and-a-half years old: "Binhai Boulevard, how do you imagine it will be?" The little boy, the son of one of my fellow students, is gifted in drawing. Taking his coloured pencils from his bag, he drew a long road with flowers and fruit trees growing beside it. There was a patch of land where you could pick mushrooms and, by the sea, a beach with seashells.

July 1998

Complementary Notes

I would like to talk about my friend and fellow student, who is a PhD graduate, and about his five-and-a-half-year-old son, both of whom figure in the excerpt above.

One day in 2001, a colleague told me that this friend was under investigation. One week before that, he had talked about his plan to organise a reunion for his writer friends. When I learnt shortly afterwards that his wife was also under investigation, my first thoughts were of the little boy, whom I had met only once. At the time, when my friend gave interviews relating to the construction project for Binhai Boulevard, people were surprised to see a young child in the director's immaculate and austere office. Every project needed his authorisation before it could go ahead. Highly regarded for his competence and strong management skills, he was extremely demanding of himself and others. He commanded respect and had the dignified and distinguish air of a Doctor of Philosophy, which meant there was always a distance between him and other people. It was only through his son that he showed any hint of emotion. According to his subordinates, he was extremely lenient with his son, indulging in all his whims. But I think it is a bit of an exaggeration on the part of his subordinates, mainly due to the striking difference between his two extreme attitudes. I understand why he made a point of keeping a distance between himself and others. Life isn't easy for a man of his position. My experience living in Shenzhen all these years has taught me this: Opportunities lie behind each challenge, and behind each opportunity lies a trap. The greater the challenge, the more opportunities there are; the greater the opportunity, the deeper the pitfalls. In order to succeed in a challenge, one must know how to elude the snares. My friend understood this principle, but he fell into a trap nonetheless. He wasn't the first, nor will he be the last to make such an error. Someone else living in the same environment, where the elements are out of his or her control, would also be caught in a trap sooner or later.

I thought of the little boy who had drawn the colour picture of Binhai Boulevard. How did he live through the changes in his family? The people his parents socialised with must have been very different before and after their troubles began. Did these psychological changes leave any emotional scars on him? And as for children who are in similar cases, are their psychological wounds being treated? I said "similar cases", because in a city like Shenzhen, where people's fortunes are constantly being made and undone, a case such as this is far from uncommon.

Since my arrival in Shenzhen in 1983, society has undergone dramatic changes. Celebrities and prominent entrepreneurs change once every 10 years. I spent the greater part of 1999 away from Shenzhen, because I was on assignment elsewhere writing film scripts. When I came back, it was through my discussions with friends that I learnt that some of the trendsetters and industry pioneers of the 1990s had lost their place in society. Some had moved abroad and were never heard from again, while others were caught with their hands in the cookie jar and were convicted. Then there were others who were so riddled with debt that they were unable to repay their creditors. These stories have become so commonplace that they don't surprise me anymore. But they can affect the subconscious mind of those who suffer from depression or have depressive tendencies. They will shut themselves up in their distrust of others, which can have a detrimental effect on their psyche.

Before writing this book, I had already carried out preliminary work on myself on a psychological level: I warned myself against paying too much attention to these kinds of stories, for they could only have a demoralising effect on me. They have become so widespread in a society such as Shenzhen, where challenges, opportunities and pitfalls go hand in hand. Hell and paradise, fortune and misfortune. They are interchangeable.

SIXTY-THREE

Diary
Monday, 5th April 2004 10:40 am

Finally, a sunny day. It's been rainy and humid for the last two weeks. It's muggy and feels unhealthy, especially at home. The clothes stink of rotting marinated vegetables. The air conditioner can't dehumidify the air. According to the newspapers, the number of patients in hospital has gone up. And I know the number of depression sufferers has also increased. I try to eat properly and not tire myself out. Every day I pray, give thanks to God and put my hopes in Him. "But if he remains silent, who can condemn him?"[1] If you believe you'll succeed, then you will. On this beautiful sunny day, I've come to realise how much there is still to learn: patience, devotion, humility, faith, hope and forbearance.

Had a dream the night before last. I was walking on a road made of the kind of yellow earth that you'd find in the mountains on the island of Hainan. Suddenly, a military jeep with its roof pulled back stopped behind me. My fellow students Zhu Sujin, Jiang Xiaoqin and Deng Hainan were inside. They greeted me, and we were happy to come across each other so unexpectedly. They asked me to jump in and take a ride with them. We left the mountainous region and arrived at a village beside the sea. After grabbing a bite to eat, we reserved two sampans from the local fishermen. However, when we arrived at the beach, there were seven or eight people taking the sampans too. They were already on board and had taken the best places at the gunwale. I said to Deng Hainan: "Quick, tell the other two to hurry up. For our own safety, we have to get on the same boat." Deng Hainan called out to them, but it was very noisy, and they couldn't hear us. We beckoned them to come over and they waved back, saying they had gotten the message. But it was too late, because another group of people came running over and scrambled onto the boats. We signalled to each other not to get on the boats. Then more people came running. Grabbing the boats by the gunwale, they pushed them into the water and jumped aboard. For a few seconds, I was caught in the stampede. I tripped forward a couple of steps and almost fell. When I regained my balance, the boats, filled with people cheering and yelling, were already far away. I was alone on the beach and didn't know what to do. It was no good crying. The boats were sailing further and further into the distance. I was staring at them, hoping that my friends would realise that I wasn't on board and stop the boats. But the boats showed no signs of slowing down. I told myself that in the confusion, my friends must not have noticed that I wasn't with them. Looking at the strange village and empty beach, I asked myself: "What am I going to do?"

Notes

I am lucky. Fellow students that I met in my creative writing courses at the Lu Xun Literary Institute and Nanjing University have often been kind and helpful. Before my chemotherapy in 2000, I was self-reliant and independent, asking for help only as a last resort. Because it's not fair or honest not to give back what you have received. With no money, no social standing, I had no means to return any favours. It made me feel ashamed, anxious and uneasy. I often refused help and pushed away the friendships that others offered me. After my surgical procedure, several friends said to me: "We talked on the phone before your operation, why didn't you tell us?" It never occurred to me to ask them for help. Some of them had the financial means to help, others had social connections, but I was too embarrassed to ask for their assistance. Modern society, founded on mutual benefits and interests, has become highly commercialised. Even between parents and children, husbands and wives, it is money that matters above all else, not feelings. People like me, who lack material resources, are afraid to ask for help.

That year, I was suffering from hypothyroidism and myxoedema and had to be hospitalised in Guangzhou. Accompanied by my mother, I went through the administrative formalities while waiting to be admitted: consultations, medical tests, waiting lists for a bed. We stayed in a hostel, where a bed cost five yuan per night. My mother, who was retired, received only 30 yuan a month in pensions. We waited in Guangzhou for almost 10 days before a bed was allotted to me. To save money, my mother and I shared a bed.

"It would have been nice if someone could have put us up for a few days," she said.

I stayed in a hostel during my third year in Shenzhen. Once, I had acute gastroenteritis at 2 o'clock in the morning. I had diarrhoea and was vomiting. Not wanting to bother anyone, I didn't ask for help. I left for the hospital, my hands pressed against my stomach. Taxis were few and far between at that time of night, but the hospital wasn't far. I walked a few steps, fell down on my knees in agony, my forehead, back and chest covered in cold sweat. After throwing up, I carried on walking, almost bent double. The lampposts and buildings were swaying around me. I was afraid of fainting and being left for dead. I spent most of the night under perfusion at the hospital. Then, back at the hostel, I stayed in bed for two days without eating. I didn't leave my room until someone, thinking that something was wrong, knocked on my door.

After my operation in 2002, I received a phone call from a few of my fellow students: Zhu Sujin, Jiang Xiaoqin and Deng Hainan. They invited me to visit them in Nanjing, but not wanting to impose, I declined.

"You must come. We'll send you the money for the trip," Zhu Sujin insisted.

"Come. We mean it. Don't be embarrassed, we're friends, right?" said Jiang Xiaoqin.

"Medical expenses cost an arm and a leg, we want to help out," said Deng Hainan.

I was most touched by their gesture. I assured them that if I ever needed help, I would ask. The four of us visited the Jiangnan region. But we had an accident on the motorway; the collision triggered the airbag. It opened in Deng Hainan's face, which swelled up. Other than that, he came away unscathed. His family, who held a dinner to celebrate Deng's good fortune, joked: "He escaped death by the skin of his teeth!" After my trip to Jiangnan, the word "trust" and the expression "thank your good fortune" took on a new meaning.

20th July 2007

Correlations

Biopsy Report

Name: Li Lanni

Lymph nodes on the right side of the neck: thyroid cancer metastasis: mainly follicular carcinoma and, to a lesser degree, papillary carcinoma.

Dated 18th December 1998

Complementary Notes

In the summer of 1998, the Writers' Association of China organised a creative writing workshop for 21 people. The participants came from all over China and every one of them was in the midst of writing a novel. Today, looking at the group photo taken at the end of the course, I realise I was as thin as a rake but in good shape. Standing in the middle of the second row, I had a big smile on my face. What I didn't know was that three or four months later, I was to undergo two surgical procedures in the space of six months for metastatic cancer. I didn't pay much attention to my fellow students and never thought that one day they would offer me their help and support. For, later on, about 10 of them would write a letter to the oncologists at the hospital, who, in the end, agreed to postpone two operations that had been planned for me in 2001.

When I was in primary and secondary school, my family moved from place to place, and I changed schools often. I learnt never to look back each time.

Greatly weakened by my illnesses these last few years, I've become hypersensitive to temperature changes. But I count my blessings.

Regarding the biopsy report I cited in "Correlations," I only found out about it much later, just before the Chinese New Year in 2000. Even though lymphatic cancer usually spreads quickly, a lymph node dissection for cancer metastasis wasn't performed during my operation in 1998. In March 1999, I began to have a persistent low-grade fever and chronic cough. Was it pneumonia, a kind of "whooping cough," tuberculosis or emphysema? I imagined all sorts of possibilities, but it never occurred to me that it might be cancer. I was coughing for about six months. My chest, neck, abdomen and back were painful to the touch. I had the sensation that every single cell in my body was immersed in pain and that my epidermis had become a thin layer of membrane that was constantly sore and tender. I had lost so much weight that you could see the bones of my rib cage. My abdomen had shrunk and was no more than a hollow; my hip bones were jutting out. My parents felt guilty but still wouldn't tell me the truth. They tried to persuade me to have a chest examination. They were worried that the cancer had spread to the lungs, but pretended that it was to rule out the possibility of tuberculosis. In fact, my cancer hadn't spread to my lungs, but was active in the lymph nodes of my neck. What good would a chest examination have done?

Shortly before my operation in December 1998, I was extremely busy with my writing assignment in Beijing. I was immediately hospitalised upon my return to Guangzhou. My cancer had spread, and follicular carcinoma was more malignant than papillary carcinoma. I had an emergency operation, and as I felt perfectly normal afterwards, I went straight back to work and began writing a script for the film *Children of Macau*. The work was both physically and mentally demanding. Looking back, I realise that I was like a patient who, before being diagnosed with terminal cancer, went through a period of abnormal hyperactivity. In psychiatric language, it is called the "manic phase." There is a sudden overcharge of creative energy that is likened to burning firewood. Before dying out in the stove, its glowing embers rekindle and blaze up, sending flames dancing and leaping into the air.

You feel a surge of life from inside, intense and resplendent, but a moment later, it disintegrates into ashes, falling silently into a void.

SIXTY-FOUR

Diary
Monday, 12th April 2004 11 am

Leave this world. These words keep going round in my mind these last few days.

On 11th April last year, I began taking Seroxat, albeit with reluctance. I was going to pieces and felt there was no other choice but to take antidepressants. One year ago to the day, I was slumped on the sofa, completely wiped out by the severe side effects. Plagued by hallucinations and by my own obsessive-compulsive behaviour, I heard the voices of people who had committed suicide. They said: "Why don't you leave? Come. Quickly, come. There's nothing here for you." They explained to me why they had left this world and, thinking they had made the right decision, were telling me to do the same. In my head, I kept talking to them, saying how I understood. For three days, between 12th the 14th, I was a nervous wreck. Alone at home, I kept shouting: "I don't want to die. I don't want to die. Not like this. Help me, God. Help me!" But Satan hung on to me, pushing me to give way to temptation. He egged me on, whispering in my ear: "Go on. Jump. Just jump. You've suffered enough already. You're better off dead. What's the point of living like this?"

Even now, I'm afraid to recall the morbid state of mind I was in. Stop. Don't think about it anymore.

It was Easter Sunday yesterday. I attended a service at Dongshan Church and ate the Easter eggs the church gave out. I was in high spirits and in good form. It was a beautiful day. I felt the soft spring breeze on my face. Although I was enjoying the spring air, my mind was elsewhere. I kept asking myself: "Was it only last year that I was going through my physical and mental hell?" One year on, and I am much farther along the road to recovery. It's a miracle. Lord, I thank You with all my heart. Praise be to God. "We went through fire and water, but you brought us to a place of abundance."[1] Salvation is beautiful and mysterious. Those who believe in You know what happiness is. Amen.

Notes

The heat is stifling and it's humid. For the last 10 days, the temperature has been above 35 degrees in Guangzhou. Newspapers warn us about catching 'emotional heat stroke,' becoming restless and irritable because of the heat. The ultraviolet index is sky-high. They say people with depression suffer a lot in the summer. It's a risky period, in which they can inflict harm on themselves and others.

The sun is beating down, so I rarely go outside. I tried working on my computer several times but couldn't sit still in my chair. The sun is pouring into the study. Even with the air conditioner on, I can still feel the heat outside crushing against the windows, becoming thicker, heavier, more intense, forceful and ferocious. It penetrates through the windows, curtains and walls. It invades the house, scorching its way into my heart and brain. Heat creeps into every nook and cranny, oppressive and stifling.

The enemy is strong, but I am weak; the enemy is advancing, but I am retreating. You must stay calm, know how to wait with serenity and not fight blindly just to move forward. Those who have faith don't let themselves be eaten up by anxiety. It's a learning experience. Everyone understands this principle, but few can put it into practice.

I lack self-confidence. An inner dialogue with myself:

"Li Lanni, you're really lazy. You're doing nothing with your life. How can you live like this? Stop whinging. If you're suffering so much, then why don't you let yourself die? If you don't want to die, that means your suffering is just an excuse."

"I just want some peace. Leave me alone."

"But I worry about you. You so want to finish this book and tell others how you escaped from the valley of death, don't you? What a fool. You'll never finish it. Because you're going to have a cancer relapse and spiral back into depression. You're trapped, and there's no way out."

"No, no. I don't want to listen. You're mean and nasty."

"Li Lanni, how can you not listen to me? As long as you live and breathe, you'll never get away from me. I'll follow you to your grave. I know what you're thinking. If you don't want to say it, let me help you."

"Don't bother. I can do it myself. I am terrified that my cancer will spread to my brain and that I'm going to die ugly and disfigured."

"Li Lanni, even if you do, you'll be no more than a corpse. After death, there's only chaos and anarchy. Better to die sooner than later, and you'll be doing others a favour. Just imagine: Your brain will just be a mass of cancerous cells, your face all bloated and smeared with blood, putrid water dripping from the bed onto the floor. It's disgusting. You'll be a nightmare for your family. It's dying without dignity."

"Let me talk. I'm also terrified that my cancer will spread to my bones."

"Li Lanni, use your head. Do you really think there will still be bones left in your body? How can anyone cut them up? And which ones? A bit here, a bit there? Seriously. You're funny. A doctor should just cut off your head. Crack! How do you like that?"

"Go away! Scram!"

"Li Lanni, you can't accept me, can you? Because I am real. I am the real Li Lanni. I never lie. When you do your bloodletting, it's me who tells you to be careful, how to insert the needle, how to make sure the blood flows out properly. Hidden in your subconscious, I'm watching over you. But when you die, I'll live on."

"My head is splitting."

"Li Lanni, it's true what you said. If you want to write, you must grab this chance and get on with it. Who knows when you'll be hospitalised again? You go in through the main entrance, lie down, give up the ghost, and leave the mortuary through the back door, straight to the incinerator. In my opinion, you won't die from jumping off the top of a building. You say your prayers and take your antidepressants, but one day you're going to trip and fall off the roof. You'd never know. Here are some home truths: Don't bother writing. Your work is worthless. I really don't understand why I hate you so much. I wish you were dead. As long as you're alive, I'll never have any peace of mind. I'm going to talk, talk and talk… until you drop dead!"

I am going to pieces. I am… shaking…No, hang on…Don't lose your mind. I want to howl… want to rip out my face with my fingers, crack open my skull… Go on… Go… At the point of no return, a soft, peaceful and brilliant light fills my heart. The dark malevolent spirits are silenced. They fade away. I feel the Holy Spirit brushing against me, like a cool breeze. A radiant smile opens up in me, like a flower blossoming.

Relax. Stay calm. Stay centred. Focus your mind. Take a deep breath… Li Lanni, there's a soft warm light hidden in your memories. You must find it.

At the beginning of summer in 1999, I spent most of my time resting at home. I had a chronic cough and didn't have the strength to go to work. My coughing fits made it impossible to even talk on the phone. I was laid up on the sofa, spent my days leafing through books, but inside I was sick with worry. The cough wouldn't go away and stopped me from working, which made me even more anxious. I was a human wreck.

Sometimes, when I was alone at home, I would lie in bed on my stomach, my head dangling off the edge with a cushion beneath my chest. I stayed like this for hours on end, because it used up less of my physical energy when I coughed. Sometimes I coughed until my eyes started watering. Or I would lose control of my bladder and spend hours on the toilet in a daze. At other times, the coughing fits almost stopped me from breathing and I was afraid I might suffocate. Feeling helpless and vulnerable, I would recite any Buddhist sutra that came into my head. I asked God to watch over me. What should I do? I was in great pain. Who could I turn to? I just wanted the coughing to stop.

One day, I was flicking through *Streams in the Desert* by Lettie Cowman. I had bought it a couple of years earlier, but when I got home and started reading, the words refused to sink in. That day, as I was leafing through the pages, I came across a verse from the Bible: "Be still [...],"[2] which, trivial as it may sound, struck a chord in me and brought me some comfort.

There are passages in the Bible that teach us how to seek rest. Fate had put this book in my hands. Lettie Cowman says: "We endure sufferings in order to understand the need in others to find comfort. For example, one must live through the sufferings of being sick before understanding the pain of those who are sick. One must live through the hurts [...]. When you are in deep pain and despair, seek rest and do not fight against it. Know that God is by your side and is guiding you through trials and hardships."[3]

This passage spoke to my heart. When I am overwhelmed with feelings of helplessness and despair, the education I received as a child urges me to never stop fighting. But no one ever taught me how I could come through if I didn't have the strength to fight, nor the will to live.

Seek rest. Know how to wait, hope and trust in God.

I've learnt that life can be made up of moments of wisdom and illumination. So wonderful. Be serene and you will receive the strength, support and comfort that holy water brings. Just reading Lettie Cowman wasn't enough. I had an urge to read the Bible, but the bookshop was out of stock and I didn't know where I could get hold of a copy. One month later, my cough began to subside. I was still coughing when I talked or at bed time, but other than that my coughing fits became less frequent. This verse, which brought me peace and comfort, was always on my mind: "Be still [...]."

In the early hours of a perfectly ordinary Monday morning, I felt a voice saying to me: "Go out and buy a Bible." The call of God is wonderful. He is watching over me, so that I'll learn the right lessons at the right time. Six months later, I had an operation to remove a cancerous tumour, followed by chemotherapy and a relapse into depression. But I knew how to pray and believed that I would be saved.

3rd August 2007

Correlations

Excerpts from my interview notes

From 15th to 21st December 1999

In the Shenzhen office of the Young Communists Committee. Volunteer Association's general situation. High-level exchanges in the exhibition hall.

I gave people directions. Got lost the first day. Extremely crowded. People gathered together, like a human wall. Not enough volunteers. A young woman working as a guide. Absolute chaos.

Seeing a volunteer with a badge, everyone rushed over to ask: "Can we buy the tickets now? How do we get there?" Twenty years old. Very mature for her age.

But being selfless isn't necessarily a good thing. Must do things for the mutual benefit of both parties.

She wants to volunteer as a teacher to gain experience. Because she plans to give private tutorial lessons later to earn a living.

Young boy, well-behaved and hard-working. In two months, obtained high scores: 90 percent.

Told the young woman the good news straight away. Father sells shoes at the market. Has a handicap and likes gambling.

Mother called the young woman. Hopes her son will go to university.

Young woman hesitates. Sense of responsibility. Goes to see the mother after phone call.

Complementary Notes

The interview notes are fragmented and somewhat disjointed.

At the time, I was collaborating with the director He Qun on a film about young people. The main thread of the story was volunteer work in Shenzhen. After finishing the first draft, I was constantly plagued with dizziness and nausea. Too weak to continue, I had no other choice but to give up the project.

I didn't know that the cancer cells were active and multiplying in my body.

I quoted from my interview notes because I want to talk about another story. One day, I was attending a forum on volunteer work in Shenzhen. All the speakers and participants were busy.

Since I wasn't participating and was feeling unwell, I went outside for some fresh air.

There I met a middle-aged man in a tracksuit. I asked him if he was a volunteer. He said he was working on the emotional support hotline. He was quite talkative and said he used to be a bureau director of a certain committee in Shenzhen.

He told me this: "I became an assistant director in my thirties and quickly climbed the ranks in the 1980s. I had already read Hegel and Karl Marx's *Das Kapital* before I turned twenty. When I left the public service, I enjoyed more perks and benefits than most of my ex-colleagues and my business was flourishing. It was the good life: alcohol, prostitutes, gambling...You know what I mean? I often had over a million yuan in cash stashed away in my car. Amazing, right? And I wasn't the courier. If I wanted to set up a project, I only needed to bribe the other party and it'd be done. It was really exciting at first, but with time the voracious greed of these people disgusted me. I despised them, but I was young and ambitious."

"To tell you the truth, I have an ulterior motive in coming here to work on the hotline. It's like someone hiding behind his tiles in a mahjong game. I was tired of my life. I'm hiding here, and these people will never find me. And also I gain some experience at the same time. There're two sides to me: the good and the bad. People going through tough times call for help and I give them support. In helping others, I also help myself."

"Doing good deeds is gratifying. Look at me, my morale is high. Who would have thought I was that kind of person in my previous life?"

His face was beaming.

SIXTY-FIVE

Diary
Tuesday, 13th April 2004 10:35 am

Lele is seven months old. I wonder how old a seven-month-old puppy is in human age. Probably the equivalent of a child in his last year of kindergarten.

It was his birthday yesterday. He played with Bobbie in the afternoon. Bobbie is a three-year-old Papillon that belongs to Yan Zi and her husband. He is in his prime: proud, well-educated and fit as a flea. Lele loves playing with him. Yesterday, they were running around on the municipal lawn chasing after each other and had a whale of a time. Passers-by couldn't help smiling at them. Lele was prancing around with joy. With his mouth opened, lips slightly pulled back, smiling eyes, his fur ruffled by the breeze and the tip of his tongue sticking out, he looked like a little angel from fairyland.

Lele has character. He is extremely proud and likes to put on a show, but can be fearful at times. He has a habit of nestling in the gap between the cupboard and wall in the sitting-room. When he's in there, it's impossible to get him out. I wonder what he thinks about, snuggled up in his corner.

He also likes to lie on the windowsill in my study, watching the pupils play and attend classes in the primary and secondary schools opposite. He understands human nature so well that it leaves me puzzled at times. It alarms me even, for I am not sure how to deal with him.

I think God loves little children. One must have the purity and innocence of a child to go to heaven. Lele is a gift from God. I should learn from him. Learn how to live in happiness, love, trust and hope. Be innocent and carefree. And with forgiveness

Notes

Six months ago, I bumped into Bobbie's mistress's mother. She told me that Bobbie had run away, and that his owners were separated.

In 2004, I often saw them on my walks with Lele, and the three of them looked like a happy family. Bobbie is the first dog Lele became friends with. Bobbie's mistress is in her 20s, attractive and friendly. She and her husband made a lovely couple together. They advised me to take a bottle of water on my walks, because the dogs were often thirsty. Usually it was Bobbie's mistress who would be holding the bottle of water, and his master a rolled-up newspaper. They were always well-equipped to train and look after their dog.

Soon after that, Bobbie and his owners left the university campus and moved into an apartment. From time to time, his master would drive to the campus and let him play there. One year later, they stopped coming, because Bobbie had disappeared.

Could his disappearance have had anything to do with his owners' separation? He was probably so devastated that he could have left with any stranger.

The fact that Bobbie had once had a happy family life makes it even sadder. Dogs live for love, and they are happy because of love. Their loyalty comes from their love for us. But when they lose our love, they become depressed and unhappy for the rest of their lives, and die in sorrow and loneliness.

Westerners think that dog haters have a psychological flaw that is indicative of mental problems. In the film *As Good as It Gets*,[1] the main character suffers from obsessive-compulsive disorder. He mistreats dogs, but through psychotherapy, he changes himself and begins to love them.

A woman, who is a cobbler, told me she once found a stray dog. She kept it at home for several days, but the dog was doing its business all over the sitting-room. Unwilling to waste her time house training it, she abandoned it in a marketplace. Some labourers found it and had it for dinner.

"But that's so cruel. Why didn't you have it adopted by someone who likes dogs?" I asked.

"I could have let it live, but it would have become a burden for me eventually. So I let it go," she said.

Someone offered the little brother of a dog that lives in my building to an old lady. When the puppy was one year old, the old lady, thinking it was costing her too much money, had it put down.

The little dog knew what was going to happen and refused to go. When the final moment came, it was crying silently, its eyes filled with sorrow.

Such cases are common, and I become sad and depressed every time I hear stories like these. For they tell of the monstrous and loathsome nature of mankind.

25th July 2007

Complementary Notes

Before reading this article, I was thinking the same thing.

Animal haters have something dark and warped in them. Most of the time, they live in a subjective world, where they feel they are threatened by an outside enemy.

They have personal issues and feel exploited by others, believing that they always lose out in life. They have a pathological desire to control everything; want everything to be carried out exactly according to their will; and pick on the little things as a test to see if others love and respect them. But they themselves lack the ability to love in return.

I often come across people like this on my walks with Lele.

It's a habit of mine to always hold Lele's leash firmly in my hand. He carries a small light-yellow rucksack with cartoon characters on his back. Inside there is water for him and paper to pick up his poop. And I always take the quiet streets away from the hustle and bustle.

As soon as we leave home, Lele is all happy and bouncy. His little pink tongue is sticking out of his mouth and his little tail is perked up proudly on his behind. School children and even mature middle-aged teachers who walk past smile at him. Some of them come up to him, stroke his head and shower him with compliments: "You're a good boy!" or "Oh, he's so cute!"

Lele understands that he is being complimented. With a big grin on his face, his little flower-bud tail wags merrily. But there is an old woman I see who isn't as friendly. I always make sure that there are at least 10 metres between us and her. Sometimes I even cross the street, and both of us carry on walking as if we hadn't seen each other.

However, one day, this old woman started hurling insults at us. Pointing a finger at Lele, she cursed him: "Get away from me! Scram! You filthy mutt, I'm going to skin you alive!"

There is another old woman of the same ilk I sometimes see. She swears at us from a distance: "Bloody dog, I'm going to kill you! Go to hell! Don't let me see you again!"

Once, a couple in their 60s was walking past. Lele was being friendly; he looked at them, wagging his tail. But the woman screamed, and I nearly jumped out of my skin.

I was still in a state of stupefaction when the man walked forward a couple of steps and kicked Lele. He rolled over twice, yelping loudly. Usually mild and easy-going, I saw red and burst out:

"Why did you do that? He didn't bother you!"

"If I hadn't kicked him, he would have bitten me. What was I supposed to do?" the man said smugly.

"He's a pet. Look how small he is. You could have hurt him," I retorted.

They gave us a dirty look and left.

Then there is a boy, who must be in the first years of primary school. At the end of a school day, he would hang around with a bunch of rowdy and unruly kids. Seemingly the leader of the pack, he would taunt Lele and me: "Hairy little monster! Dirty mutt, I'm going to kill you."

Sometimes, not satisfied with just insulting us, he follows or runs after us, trying to kick Lele's behind. His friends, all fired up, yell and cheer him on.

It's sad to see incidents like these. I feel sorry, not so much for Lele, for it doesn't hurt him to be bullied a bit, but for the lack of humanity in these people.

It's troubling to see the lack of education in the schoolboy and in children like him. You can tell from his behaviour that his parents haven't taught him how to love nature, or at least how to respect life. His education is flawed and inadequate.

I also feel sorry for some old people, who, at their age, should know how to live at peace with themselves. But instead, they are bitter, petty and small-minded, lacking love and consideration towards others. With years of life experience behind them, they still don't know how to behave like human beings.

You can see the depth of a person's soul from his or her attitude towards others. But then, such extreme dog haters are quite rare in Shenzhen. People here are generally more generous, caring and open.

SIXTY-SIX

Diary
Monday, 19th April 2004 10:36 am

Had a dream in the early hours of the morning:

Yi Ling invited Ququ and me to spend the spring holidays in Beijing. Yi Ling asked me to write a short novel for children and gave me several elements to be included in the story. We agreed that it would be easy to achieve and signed the contract straightaway. Then the three of us visited the city, went boating and walked in the hills. But my mind was on the story that I was going to write. The more I thought about it, the more I felt incapable of integrating the required elements into the story in a natural and interesting way. It was bogging me down and I couldn't enjoy myself. I told Yi Ling that I wouldn't be able to finish the manuscript in time for the deadline. She told me not to worry and to enjoy my holiday. Then she asked Ququ to write a similar story for me. Ququ accepted and continued to enjoy herself without a care in the world. Soon afterwards, she announced that she had finished the story. I admired her, but at the same time, I felt ashamed of myself. I told them that not only was I incapable of producing such a work, but I was unable to take the pressure and didn't want to do it anymore. I offered to reimburse the publisher for the travelling and accommodation expenses. But Yi Ling and Ququ told me to wait, saying that since the first draft was finished, I could take my time and write at my own pace back in Guangzhou. But I felt uneasy and couldn't stop blaming myself for creating so much trouble for them. The kinder they were to me, the more useless and guilty I felt.

In my dream, I couldn't stop heaping reproaches on myself. I woke up with a splitting headache.

On Sunday, I listened to a pastor give a sermon at the Dongshan Church.

Psalm 42 of the Bible: "Why, my soul, are you downcast? Why so disturbed within me? Put your hope in God [...]."

There are seven reasons that can explain why modern man is plagued by depression and anxiety:

1. Anger
2. Fatigue
3. Distrust
4. Fear
5. Anxiety

6. Jealousy
7. Lack of will to live.

Faith helps us to overcome our worries.

It's already mid-April. I am confident in my ability to survive the "depression season." With all my heart and with the deepest sincerity, I celebrate, worship, thank and praise God. Every day, every hour, wherever I may happen to be.

Notes

1999 was a turbulent year for me. I published two books with Writers' Edition; attended the premiere of a television series in Beijing and Macau; and took part in the production of several programmes for the national television channel CCTV and for the Beijing television channel. I watched the shooting of a film for which I'd written the script, and was nominated for a high-level official post. I accepted CCTV's offer to write the commentaries for a documentary on Macau; did several interviews with the volunteers in Shenzhen; and finished the first draft of a script. I was also hospitalised several times for a cough and low-grade fever; was put under perfusion and had a battery of pathological tests. On top of all that, my mobile phone kept overheating, and the battery would be drained after a long-distance call to Beijing. I was so exhausted that I couldn't even lie down for a rest, because I would feel like all the limbs in my body were dislocated and broken and impossible to put together again. I was a machine running on full speed. The 365 days of the year went by in a flash and suddenly it was 31st December. But I wasn't happy; it was as if my life was devoid of meaning. I often asked myself: "Why aren't you happy? You should be, shouldn't you? What more do you want? What do you want from life?"

What I didn't know at the time was that my parents were more than busy. They were busy worrying themselves sick over the report of the operation I had in December 1998. They were asking themselves: "Has her cancer spread? If it has, how is she going to take it? Should we tell her the truth? What if she can't take it? Are we going to tell her she'll die in pain?" They couldn't agree on whether or not to tell me the truth about my cancer.

"We're both getting on," said my mother. "We can't protect her anymore. We must tell her. I can't take this anymore."

"It's out of the question," said my father. "It'll put her under too much pressure. If she doesn't die of cancer, she'll die of worry. We'll keep an eye on her. Just wait a little."

"I'm at the end of my tether. Maybe we're hurting her by not telling her the truth."

"What do you mean, hurting her? It won't hurt her at all."

They were fighting all the time and didn't see eye to eye about what they should do. My mother tried to find a middle-ground solution. She would go to the hospital with the biopsy report stating there was a cancer metastasis and observe the patients, and how the doctors treated them. From hanging around the hospital so often, the nurses at the reception came to know her. When she spotted a nurse who looked kind and friendly, she would wait until she had a free moment to show her my biopsy report. The nurses, as well as the matron, were unanimous that I should see a specialist without delay. Mother told Father what these medical professionals thought, and they began arguing again. Then she went back to the oncology department at the hospital, found a doctor that looked the most "specialised" and made an appointment with him. Obviously, my time hadn't come. For at the end of the year, my parents received instructions from the specialists that couldn't have been clearer: The patient herself must come to the hospital for an examination, because it was pointless to have the parents asking all of these questions. Instead of worrying, they should act. It served no purpose torturing themselves and wondering if she was going to die. It was a matter of the utmost urgency that the patient should come to the hospital in person. The sooner the better.

Shortly before Chinese New Year in 2000, my parents finally decided to tell me the truth. First, they had a long discussion with Fanding before talking to Xiao Bing, our close family friend. Then Xiao Bing called me:

"Hello, your parents want to tell you something. They had kept it quiet until now. It's...er...Do you remember when you had your operation in 1988 and the doctor said the tumour was benign?"

I didn't pay too much attention to what he was saying at first, but seeing that he had stopped talking, I asked:

"Yes, I was under general anaesthesia. What about it?"

"Well, your parents say that in fact the tumour was malignant."

For two seconds, my mind was a complete blank. I couldn't react. It took me a few seconds before I could understand the implications of what he had just said and react in an appropriate way. That explains it, then. All the doubts I had about my state of health at the time suddenly evaporated. That was why I was put under general anaesthesia. That was why my friend's cousin hinted at the possibility of cancer; why my parents insisted on coming to live with me in Shenzhen for a while; and why every time I fell ill, they would be sick with worry and start imagining all sorts of things.

"What kind of cancer is it?" I asked. My heartbeat quickened before going back to normal.

"Thyroid cancer. But it's not aggressive and doesn't spread easily," Xiao Bing replied.

"Er... well... It's probably nothing then. It's been so many years now. No need to get worked up about it."

"You're right. It's probably nothing. But they should have told us the truth. They could at least have told Fanding and me."

"They're like that. They like to keep secrets."

"When are you coming back to Guangzhou? They'd like to talk to you."

"What is there to say? All this time, they hid the truth from me because they were afraid I wouldn't be able to take it. But I'm not scared. I could have died ages ago. It's probably nothing."

But I was uneasy. My parents had been lying to me right from the beginning. I felt so stupid.

Back in Guangzhou, I read the letter the surgeon had written to my father, but I felt nothing. I didn't give it much thought, either. Several friends told me that the hospital had wrongly diagnosed them with cancer and that their lives changed overnight. They spent sleepless nights worrying and were tormented by a sense of injustice. But I didn't think too much about it, as if I couldn't focus my mind on my cancer. With no conscious effort on my part, my brain had switched itself off as far as my cancer was concerned. I was, however, slightly alarmed by my indifference. Something was wrong. I should be upset. What was happening to me? My indifference was a bad sign.

Our instincts drive us to flee from danger. Before my operation in 2000, I was incredibly obtuse, and my indifference stemmed from an instinctive reaction. Even when my parents showed me the biopsy report from December 1998, I was incapable of rousing myself from my indifference. The thyroid cancer may have spread, why? Didn't they remove it? Normally, metastasis only happens 10 years later, right? My parents insisted that I should consult the oncologists at the hospital to rule out the possibility of a metastasis. But I couldn't be bothered. They pestered me until my life became impossible. To have peace of mind and to prove to myself that chance was on my side and that everything was alright, I consulted a specialist on the morning of 17th February. The doctor palpated my neck and said: "Don't go home. You must be admitted into hospital." I laughed. It was funny. He made a mistake, right? He found a small lump in my neck and said I had to be hospitalised. Incredible.

"Hospital? What, today? But I'm very busy..." I said.

"Take her to do the admission paperwork," the doctor said to a nurse.

"What if I can't stay?"

"There's at least a two-month waiting-list for a hospital bed. There's one available for you right now and you don't want it. How stupid can you be?" the doctor said sternly.

"But is it really necessary? We can do tests in the outpatient department."

"You're going to have pre-operative examinations. Your operation will be in two days."

Then the doctor wrote the word "metastasis" followed by a question mark in my medical file. All my attention was focused on the question mark. I couldn't believe my bad luck. I was operated on at the end of 1998, so how could there be metastasis just after the Chinese New Year in 2000? It didn't make sense.

"I don't have enough money on me to pay for the deposit," I said. "I have to go home first."

I thought to myself: "God gave me a poisoned gift. I'm going to be operated on in two days' time without resorting to contacting my social network or being on the waiting-list. I got lucky then! A small incision, three or four stiches and, who knows, I could be home the next day."

Pleased that I was admitted into an oncology hospital with minimum hassle, I followed the nurse into the admission office. The nurse there said:

"Where's the patient? Tell her to come in."

"I'm the patient," I said.

"You? You're going to have an operation?" she asked, surprised.

"Yes, me."

"Well, you don't look like it," she said, looking me up and down.

From time to time, people who don't know me try to give me advice: "Be optimistic and don't let your worries eat you up. Then you won't be depressed. Maybe it's because you're weak. Don't pick holes in everything. Take a step back and you'll feel better." In situations like these, I just smile politely. It would be useless to explain myself, for they would never understand. Some say: "There's no point in getting depressed. Cancer is quite common now. There's nothing to be scared of." Then there are others who say: "Don't be sad. Depression, you just have to hang on, that's all." I answer them all with a smile and let them criticise or make fun of those who suffer from depression. Sometimes, a wicked thought will cross my mind: What if, one day, the doctors make a wrong diagnosis and tell them they have cancer? Will they be able to take the shock? But afterwards, I have pangs of guilt. To be tolerant and have the ability to forgive oneself and others is a difficult thing. It's easy not to harm others, but almost impossible not to have unkind thoughts. For having spiteful thoughts is also a sin. Who amongst us can say that we have never sinned?

8th August 2007

Correlations

Excerpts from *Illness as Metaphor*[1]

Illness belongs to the dark side of life. It has a complex social identity [...] Sickness awakes in us an ancestral terror [...]. Because if we have cancer, it becomes a cause for shame. It can affect our sexual and professional lives, or even jeopardise our chances for promotion. Those who have cancer do not like to talk about it and are extremely discreet about it.

Death is difficult to face [...]. If the cause of an illness is unknown or if medicine is powerless against a serious illness, then this becomes fraught with meaning. Firstly, all that terrifies us to the core of our being is related to illness: physical and mental decline, process of decay, contamination, abnormalities and weakness. Illness thus becomes a metaphor.

Susan Sontag (United States)

Complementary Notes

In the introduction to *Illness as Metaphor*, the translator wrote that Susan Sontag, a scholar at the American Academy of Arts and Sciences, was hailed as the conscience of the American people. Browsing through this book at a bookstand, I came across a sentence that made me buy it without a second thought. Sontag said: "We can use a military metaphor to talk about the shame associated with an illness such as cancer [...]. When I was diagnosed with cancer, what made me angry the most was seeing how the bad reputation of cancer made the patients suffer even more." Knowing that Sontag also felt anger brought me some comfort. Even though our anger arises from different causes, I appreciate her choice of words. It touches the anger that resides in the deepest part of me, making me feel that I have an affinity with her. Using a military metaphor to talk about medical procedures to treat cancer hits the nail on the head. It expresses precisely the psychological wounds that are inflicted on the patients by aggressive and invasive medical procedures. In the majority of cases, we don't die from the cancerous cells that are eating us up, but from the psychological wounds of having our dignity destroyed, and of being treated with contempt.

Many publications on cancer also address this issue. Doctors and nurses should look at the patient as a human being, and not just see the tumour and think of ways to remove it. They should make it their priority to help others, focussing on the patient as a human being and how to improve the quality of their lives.

Once I read the notes of a foreign doctor. Young and talented, he prided himself on carrying out many difficult and complicated surgical procedures. But when he was diagnosed with cancer, he was treated in a military and inhumane way by his colleagues. Filled with shame and remorse, he thanked God for the lesson he had received and that, through cancer, he was able to examine his conscience and understand what it meant to be a good doctor. At the end of the book, he regrets that too few doctors understand this, and he hopes more doctors won't have to go through cancer to understand. At the end of the day, we come back to this same principle: Love thy neighbour as thyself. Without compassion, you can't even be a veterinary doctor. Just a butcher.

Once, I asked an oncologist:

"You perform a lot of operations every day, do you ever get tired?"

"Never," he said casually. "It's like a pupil doing his homework. It's easier than slaughtering a chicken. I perform operations every day, but I don't have the stomach to slaughter a chicken. I've never killed one."

"Really?"

"Yes, really."

"Why not?"

"Can't bring myself to do it."

SIXTY-SEVEN

Diary
Friday, 23rd April 2004 11:23 am

Only one more week and the month of April will be over. Peacefully. This time last year, I was a wreck. Every day, I was laid up on the sofa with nausea and stomach pains. Time crawled by at a snail's pace, and April seemed never-ending.

The words "leave this world" came to mind and I jotted them down immediately. Then I sat like a zombie in front of the computer, staring blankly at the screen until I managed to wrench my gaze away. Words to describe my feelings and sensations failed me. They were out of my grasp. In trying to force my mind onto my writing, I had headaches, nausea and dizziness. Don't look back, don't let yourself feel anything and don't analyse your emotions. Instead, be joyful, like a flower slowly unfolding its petals.

A year ago, I began my nutritional therapy. I've taken to drinking green tea and oolong tea and am pleased with my progress. I should also make a habit of eating two or three fruits a day. But it's easier said than done. My head knows drinking tea and eating fruit helps me to fight cancer, but my digestive system isn't taking to it. Only now do I understand what "nutritional therapy" is.

I have fewer nightmares these days, and the quality of my sleep has improved drastically. I am feeling much more at peace. Slowly. It's literally the most difficult state of mind to achieve. Impossible without the help of the Holy Spirit. Nowadays, we are brought up from an early age to compete with others. Feelings of serenity have become a sin, something to be ashamed of. Those who are at peace with themselves are considered to be incompetent and should be eliminated by society and by our times. This is the reason why, tucked away in our collective unconscious, there is a fear of feeling at peace. We become blind from seeing too many colours; deaf from hearing too many sounds. Our sense of smell, taste and touch are blunted. In truth, many of us have become, without knowing it, "handicapped." It's the tragedy of an entire generation.

"In repentance and rest is your salvation, in quietness and trust is your strength [...]."[1] These are the words of God. Amen.

Notes

Shortly before and after my operation in 2000, I was numb and indifferent. I wasn't interested in my cancer, nor its metastasis, as if it had nothing to do with me. In a way, I was "alienated" from myself. I felt no worry, no fear, but was sometimes overwhelmed with anger, without understanding why. I would tame this anger with all my vital energy, burying it deep inside me. Psychiatrists say that even though there are similarities between acute anxiety and post-traumatic stress disorder, the latter presents specific symptoms, including dizziness and spatial disorientation. The patient often feels indifferent and alienated from the events around them.

I was admitted to hospital on 17th February, and the operation was scheduled for the 20th. During these three days, I wasn't worried about my cancer, nor did I bother to find out if there was metastasis. I was more preoccupied with the fact that I lacked the financial means to offer red packets[2] to the hospital staff. I wanted to thank them, because hospital work is physically and mentally demanding, especially for those working in an operating theatre. And there is a large discrepancy between their salary and the energy they invest in their work. To show my gratitude, I wanted to give the staff a little something. I would like the medical fees to be clearly established according to the skills of the specialist doctors and the level of difficulty of the surgical procedure. It made me uncomfortable to give money on the side before the operation. And I was filled with shame. I thought most doctors didn't accept red packets, as it undermines their integrity. Unfortunately, it has become common practice for patients and their families to insist, even though the doctors refuse. Nonetheless, I tried to quietly find out more about it from the three other patients I shared my room with.

The first patient:
"Are you going to do it?"
"Of course!"
"What's the best way to go about it?"
"It depends. We did it through a cousin who works at the hospital."
The second patient:
"Did you do it?"
"Yes, we did. Just to have peace of mind."
"But if the doctor refuses, it'd be embarrassing."
"A relative did it for us. He knows a fellow student here."
The third patient:
"And you?"
"You shouldn't insist too much. It might get the doctor into trouble."
"Yes, you're right. Mustn't get anyone into trouble. But how do you do it then?"
"The thing is, you mustn't do it in front of others. You mainly give to the surgeon and anaesthetist."
"What about the nurses?"
"It depends. Do you have friends or relatives who can help you?"

"No."

"How did you get admitted into this hospital then?"

"I went through out-patient consultation."

"You mean you weren't on the waiting-list? You're lucky. A bed here costs three hundred yuan a day. You saved some money then. If you want to give something, do it quickly when you're alone with the doctor in his office. Without saying anything."

"Thanks. Thanks very much."

I was hospitalised in the afternoon of the 17th and talked to the three patients on the morning of the 18th. The operation was scheduled in the early morning of the 20th, leaving very little time to offer my "gift." My father had hypertension and couldn't set foot in an oncology department. For every time he heard or saw the word "tumour," his blood pressure would shoot up. So I couldn't count on him to do it. My brother, usually fit as a fiddle and never sick, was, by coincidence, down with a fever of 40 degrees. He was under perfusion and under observation in another hospital. My mother thought giving the doctor a red packet shouldn't be taken lightly, and that it could potentially put the doctor in an awkward position. My husband thought it had to be done in such a way as to not embarrass the doctor or expose him to being criticised by his colleagues. Otherwise it would have the opposite effect of the one intended. I suggested offering a gift voucher and a bottle of red wine, as it was more discreet. We had a lengthy discussion about it. Many people have no problem doing it, but it was a headache for my mother, my husband and me. Being the patient, I couldn't offer the gift myself. As my mother is clumsy and tactless, the task fell upon my husband.

On the afternoon of the 18th, and during the whole day on the 19th, in all the years I've known him, I've never seen my husband so embarrassed and ill at ease. We hadn't talked about how to go about it. Fit and healthy, he has little contact with doctors. He has always prided himself on his talent as a basketball player and on how easily he could score a goal. He boasted of his agility and visual acuity, and how he was both an excellent defender and attacker. But every time he came back into the room after hanging around in front of the doctor's office, without him saying a word I knew that he hadn't "scored a goal," so to speak. We were both embarrassed. We consoled ourselves half-heartedly, saying that it didn't matter and that we could catch him on his way out from work. Tomorrow would be another day. We'd make it.

It never once occurred to me that there would be complications with the operation. I never discussed with my family what to do if there was metastasis, nor about my post-operative diet. We only had one thing in mind: How to offer our gift to the doctor.

If only I had known what was about to happen, I would never have given my consent for a surgical procedure. This thought has been plaguing me ever since. I was angry. Whenever I felt anger welling up inside me, I would stifle it and return to my indifference. When it came to signing the consent form, the doctor explained the medical procedure to my husband and me. But I couldn't concentrate on what the doctor was saying. My attention was focused on the other two doctors in the office, hoping that they would go outside, either to the toilet, or to do the rounds in the rooms, or to make a phone call. But they seemed to be busy writing reports and showed no signs of leaving. Uneasy and fidgety, my husband and I glanced at each other, worried, and continued to play with time.

"The operation will proceed as follows," said the doctor. "There're two tumour nodules. We'll make an incision here in the upper part of the neck to take some tissues for biopsy. If the cells are benign, then we'll make a second incision in the lower part of the neck. This will leave a small scar. But if the results indicate that there is metastasis, then we'll do a second procedure, a lymph node dissection."

I said to myself that a second procedure wouldn't be necessary. Because there's never been a patient with metastatic cancer in such good health.

"What's a dissection?" I asked casually.

"We're going to cut open this part," the doctor replied and, with his hand, made a sweeping movement from the top of my neck to the bottom. "We'll remove all the lymph nodes on the right side, as well as the surrounding nerves and tissues, then we'll close up the blood vessels. The surgical incision will be quite big and the duration of the procedure relatively long."

Without thinking more of it, I told myself that I wouldn't be so out of luck.

"What are the risks involved?" my husband asked.

"Generally, there're no complications. But there's a possibility that one shoulder might be higher than the other."

"Will I be weird like this?" I asked jokingly. Then I lifted one shoulder while lowering the other. It made my neck lop-sided.

"Will it make my neck tilt to one side?" I asked playfully.

"Not quite like that," the doctor laughed. "But we can't totally rule out this possibility."

I gave the second procedure no further thought. My husband was paying more attention to the details than I was. He asked about the reason for not putting me under general anaesthesia and questioned the anaesthetist's competence. When he signed the consent form, I wasn't in the least bit apprehensive. I was more worried about not being able to offer a gift to the doctor before the operation. It was the weekend, and the doctor would be finishing work early. We could only give it to him after the operation.

"What do you want to eat after the operation?" my husband asked me.

"Get a packet of soda crackers," I said.

At 7:30 the next morning, I followed the nurse into the operating theatre.

It was divided into two sections, so that several procedures could be performed simultaneously. In front of the door was a woman who was scheduled to be in the operating theatre at the same time as me. The nurse said the doctors thought she had early stage breast cancer. She looked sad and bitter and was surrounded by a bunch of people who didn't want to leave her, as if she had been sentenced to death. One by one, they went up to kiss her, whisper in her ear, encourage her and wish her good luck. Several women with tears in their eyes wouldn't let go of her hand. I was in a hospital gown, waiting for a nurse to bring me a pair of sterilised slippers. The woman's farewell ceremony was going on forever, and the crowd was obstructing the passageway in front of the door, preventing the nurses and patients from going in and out.

"You shouldn't get a patient all worked up like that, right?" I asked a nurse quietly.

"The woman's husband is a director," said the nurse. "There's always a load of people around her bed."

"It's not necessarily a good thing to have so many people around you," I said.

But then, wasn't I just jealous that she was the centre of so much love and attention?

13th August 2007

Correlations

Excerpt from *On the Sense of Anger: Incentive for Self-Assertion and Self-Development*

Our anger comes from having our dignity violated [...]. Our body stores up energy. How much of this energy do we use up just to keep our dignity intact? Maintaining our dignity is essential to our lives and how we function every day [...]. In other words, in our society, human beings are considered to be like inanimate objects, whereas objects, endowed with vital forces, play a pivotal role in people's destinies [...]. Today's culture pushes to the extreme the tendency to put the material aspect of life above the human aspect.

Verena Kast (Switzerland)

Complementary Notes

The day before my operation, a nurse took me to the therapy room to prepare for the following day. A curtain separated me from the man lying next to me.

He was crying, but in such a way that you didn't feel sorry him. His weeping was strangely stifled and roused not compassion nor sympathy, but a kind of irritation. Annoyed, I sat on my stool, frowning. The nurse explained to me that he had a urinary catheter. I heard another nurse scolding him for his lack of cooperation, for being squeamish and for wasting other people's time. Listening to him, you'd think he had been reduced to a human wreck. As the nurse continued scolding him, his crying gradually subsided, seeming to have found strength in his shame and to exert some self-control. But suddenly, his crying grew louder and louder until it broke into sobs. I told myself that I must absolutely make an effort to empty my bladder by myself after the operation to avoid this kind of humiliation.

The young nurse looked inexperienced and kept asking the old nurse for advice. With her hand, the old nurse drew a half circle on the right side of my head, singling out an area that was about a third of my skull. "Shave off all the hair here, as well as this part before disinfecting," she said to the young nurse, pointing to the right side of my face, ear and neck.

The young nurse listened attentively, holding a razor in one hand, and with the other, she indicated a spot on my head.

"Up to here?" she asked.

"More."

Alarmed, I covered my head with my arms. "But half of my head is going to be shaved Yin-Yang style," I protested. "I can't go out like this!"

The young nurse gave me a sympathetic glance, then looked at the old nurse, as if to ask her to spare me this torture. "Shave it all off," the old nurse said dryly, ignoring me. "Careful when you go around the eyebrows and ears."

Smiling awkwardly, I asked her quietly and earnestly: "Can you shave off a little bit less? When I'm discharged from hospital, I might have to go to Beijing for an assignment to write screenplays. Or attend meetings in Shenzhen where I have to do presentations. With my Yin-Yang head, I'm going to scare the living daylights out of people."

She looked at me, a light of pity in her eyes, and with her fingers drew a half circle on my head. I had the unmistakable sensation that the circle had shrunk. As the young nurse was shaving the fine hairs around my ear, she cut me in the area behind the bone. The wound was wide, and blood was trickling down my neck.

"Oh, I'm sorry. I cut you and you're bleeding," she said, pressing a sterile piece of cotton wool against the wound.

"Don't worry about it. I'm a bag of bones anyway," I joked. "There's not enough meat on me."

The young nurse and I burst out laughing. I was so glad about not having a Yin-Yang head that it didn't matter if I bled a little. The wound healed one month later.

SIXTY-EIGHT

Diary
Monday, 26th April 2004 10 pm

I rarely write the "Diary" section in the evening. But today I must, otherwise I'll forget my dream from the day before yesterday.

I was in a kind of concentration camp located in the centre of a city. It was night. A crowd of people, who were about to escape, was standing at the foot of the city wall. I also wanted to escape, but was afraid of the punishment awaiting me if I got caught. Would I be able to endure the cruel and barbaric punishment that would be inflicted on me? I was still undecided when the crowd began to disperse. People were escaping through holes that had been made at various places in the wall. Not knowing these people, I didn't know if I should follow them. Then my instinct pushed me to flee through the nearest hole. Many wooden huts stood beside the city gates. The enemy soldiers charged out of the city, chasing after the fugitives. I hid inside a dark, dilapidated hut. In one corner was a latrine big enough to hold a coffin, across which a plank of wood had been placed. I slipped into the latrine. I could feel the plank of wood against my back and hear the soldiers shouting and walking around outside. A number of fugitives were caught. I was petrified, but had nowhere else to hide and had no choice but to wait it out. My strength was ebbing away, and desperation was setting in. I heard the inhabitants say that there were over 10 fugitives still on the run and that the soldiers had taken all the necessary measures to hunt them down. Then as I was dodging between the huts, I remembered there was a person who took in fugitives like me. Worried and at my wit's end, I set out to look for that person. I arrived at his hut, and on seeing several other fugitives inside, breathed a sigh of relief. But one of them told me with a grave face that the person who sheltered fugitives had disappeared, and that we had to find a way to get as far away as possible from the city. It was every man for himself.

I left the hut. Physically and mentally exhausted, I had nowhere to go, but couldn't stop running. I felt wretched and distressed, and had a bitter taste in my mouth. Too weak to walk, I slumped against a pavilion column. I was alternating between catatonia and mental confusion. Then I passed out. When I woke up, I saw a young man dressed in white standing in front of me. I didn't know him, but he seemed to be aware of my situation. He said his mother could help me escape and told me to follow him. I felt grateful, but worried that I might put him in trouble. After a moment's hesitation, I politely refused his help. He understood my concerns and explained to me that his family had been granted immunity from prosecution. The enemy soldiers couldn't arrest people inside their home. I was overwhelmed with relief. We arrived at a European-style manor. A number of European-looking men and women were coming out of the manor. The young man in white said that they were spending their holidays here and that his mother was taking them swimming. Then he hurriedly went over to his mother, presumably to talk to her about my situation. I was overwhelmed with gratitude. It was another world here; one was paradise, the other hell. Suddenly, I panicked at the thought that the mother could refuse to help me. I felt inferior, as if I wasn't good enough for them, and I didn't deserve to have someone risk his or her life to save me. Distraught and confused, I lost the thread of my dream.

What's the meaning of this dream? Is the concentration camp a symbol of my depression? Is the young man in white an angel?

Notes

I am against hiding the truth from cancer patients concerning the status of their disease. You can't keep a secret forever. And what's more, when you weigh up the pros and cons, there are more disadvantages than advantages to not telling the truth. Because then you are caught in a situation where you have to constantly weave a web of lies.

Why aren't we able to face death? Why can't we arrange funeral services in peace and serenity? Why can't we spend our last hours in trust and faith? Why can't we die and accept our fate with dignity? To lie is to cheat. It's entering into a conflict with oneself and giving way to weakness. It's also a waste of time. Lies make those who are dying sink further into depression.

A few years ago, I shared a hospital room with a 13-year-old girl who had leukaemia. At the time, communication wasn't as developed as it is today, and our knowledge on diseases, such as cancer, was limited. But the young girl understood the nature of her illness. In this day and age, how can we possibly hide the truth about cancer?

Lying on operating table number 4, I was lucid and wide awake. Under local anaesthesia, I was aware of what was going on in the operating theatre: disinfection, injecting the anaesthesia, the first incision, feeling the surgical instruments prodding around inside the surgical wound. I heard the surgeon asking the nurses to pass him this or that instrument and to give him regular updates. February is the coldest month in Guangzhou, and the operating table was icy cold. The hospital gown was so flimsy that the metallic coldness of the table penetrated through my back and into the core of my being. My limbs were numb, but the numbness had the opposite effect on my mind, making my consciousness sharper and more sensitive. When I was given a sedative intravenously, I felt the coolness of the liquid flowing through the catheter, as if my blood vessels were drinking something cool and refreshing to lower the temperature of my body. The first incision went without a hitch. I was aware of every step of the operation. The doctors and nurses stopped working and were talking among themselves. When work is well-coordinated, it isn't tiring. We were waiting for the biopsy results, which were supposed to take half an hour. Frozen to the bone, I was impatient for the operation to be over as quickly as possible. I was also worried about the doctors and nurses. Working in the cold warms you up, but once you stop, you lose feeling in your fingers and toes. It never crossed my mind that we would have to do the second procedure: lymph node dissection. I just wanted the biopsy results to come through and get the operation over and done with. Boredom began to set in. I was listening closely to what the doctors and nurses were saying, as well as all the comings and goings in the other sections of the operating theatre. I heard a nurse informing the family of a patient that the operation was over. Then I heard a clear feminine voice call out, drawing on the words like in a song: "Bed... num...ber... *four*...me... ta... sta...sis... *di*...*section*..." My mind went blank. It took a few seconds to sink in. Bed number 4 was me. Were they going to do a dissection on me? Was I that unlucky? Calm down. Wait and see.

The doctors and nurses went straight back to work. Yes. Lymph node dissection on the right side of my neck. My first reaction was that of shame. I felt sorry that the doctors were going to finish work late because of me, because it was a complicated procedure. They explained it to us when we signed the consent form, didn't they? They were going to cut out the nerves, close up the blood vessels and remove the tissues around the lymph node. The procedure would be difficult and couldn't be hurried.

My second thought was for my mother, who was waiting outside the operating theatre. I wondered if my husband had informed her that we were doing the second procedure and sent her to wait in the room. Hanging around the operation theatre would only add to the stress. She would have nothing to drink, nowhere to sit down and would probably have a backache.

My third thought was for myself. My body was frozen stiff because of the metallic operating table. It would be midday soon, and I was wondering if it was sunny outside. Why was it so cold inside? I wasn't even thinking of my cancer metastasis, but of how I was going to make it through the operation. There was nothing I could do, except to pray over and over again. As the anesthesia was wearing off and my body was warming up, I began to feel pain in the surgical area. Clenching my teeth didn't make the pain subside. It was still hurting, and my teeth felt as if they were going to break. Biting on my lips didn't help either; they had become rubbery from me chewing on them. Several times, I begged the nurses: "Please, give me some anesthetics! Please, more! Some more, please!" They gave me one dose, but it wore off after a while. I asked for another, and in total, they gave me five. When I was back in my room, it was already 1 o'clock in the afternoon. I didn't even have the strength to talk. The other patients were full of sympathy.

"Oh...you look terrible. Poor thing..."

13th August 2007

Correlations

Excerpts from *The Noonday Demon*

My mother was diagnosed with ovarian cancer in August 1989. After one week in hospital, she told us that she wanted to end her life [...]. But when she began chemotherapy, which was painful and humiliating, the subject was put aside temporarily. Ten months later, she underwent a surgical procedure to evaluate the effects of the chemotherapy [...]. Very quickly, she lost her beauty due to the secondary effects of the treatment [...]. She felt the pain of seeing her body deteriorate under the effects of chemotherapy: she lost her hair; her skin became allergic to cosmetics; her eyes were dull and lifeless; and she lost a lot of weight.

When she obtained the medication necessary for her suicide, she came to accept all that was unbearable to her [...]. Her decision to end her life gradually became a reality that we accepted with serenity [...]. My mother decided to end her life on 19th June at the age of 58 years old. She could no longer wait. She was becoming weaker by the day and a certain level of energy is needed to carry out the act in a private space outside the hospital [...]. My mother had control over her own death [...]. I can say, with certainty, that death had made her life more satisfying. But I never thought that it would be a catalyst for my own suicidal thoughts.

Andrew Solomon (United States)

Complementary Notes

As a depression sufferer, I understand what Andrew Solomon went through. As a cancer patient, I am filled with admiration for his mother. In the past, I've been reluctant to talk about the inner pain caused by my surgical interventions and chemotherapy. Not only would it have been detrimental to my therapy, but no one, my family included, would have understood. Mr Solomon describes with so much insight and sensitivity the death of his mother, as well as her feelings during her chemotherapy: pain, humiliation, anger and fear. He also talked about the destructive effects that chemotherapy has on your morale, body and face. In reading his book, I felt there was an intimate connection between his mother and I. Yes, that's right. Perhaps I shouldn't use the word "intimate," but it's the only word that expresses the close connection between fellow sufferers.

The feelings that Mr Solomon went through, I have felt them too. But I kept them buried and hidden inside me. Because I didn't want to talk about them, nor did I know how.

I admire Andrew Solomon's mother and the way she expressed herself. She had the support and understanding of her friends and family and wasn't alone. She also had the unconditional love and support of her husband and two sons. Andrew Solomon quoted from a poem by Rilke: "In love, one must learn to let the other go. Keeping the other is easy, one does not need to learn." The father and sons helped the mother leave this world. They watched over her with love, making her life more fulfilled.

After the assisted suicide of his mother, Andrew Solomon fell into a depression. He wrote: "If, following my mother's suicide, there were major advances in the treatment of ovarian cancer, it would have been horrendous." No, Mr Solomon, I can say with certainty that you are wrong to think that. Having lived through the pain and humiliation of chemotherapy and the despair of depression to the point of contemplating suicide, I can tell you this: Your mother was happy. Your love and support made her life more fulfilling. I can also say that many cancer patients are filled with respect and admiration for your mother. You have our support. We know that quality of life is far superior to its duration. One year lived in dignity and freedom prevails over 15 years of suffering and humiliation. Even if there had been significant progress in the fight against ovarian cancer following your mother's death, it would not have been horrific, as you have said. Your mother would not have regretted her decision. Because she left this world in the warmth and plenitude of love that you brought her.

SIXTY-NINE

Diary
Wednesday, 28th April 2004 11:20 am

I really don't understand. Why is it that I almost never feel happiness in a spontaneous way? It's as if being happy isn't part of my life. A happiness that gushes from the inside, brimming over with plenitude, drowning me. Where I can lose myself, be at one with the universe, in communion with nature.

As a child, I must have lived a kind of untainted happiness, but I have no memories before the age of four. My first memories are of my trip to Beijing with my parents. I was so tired after having played all day that I wet my bed. Frightened and upset, I was fretting over how to hide the huge pee stain. We were on our way to the Li family's native village. It was the first time I accompanied my parents to visit my father's family. The village of Yuquan is located in the Xindian district of the department of Bing in the Heilongjiang Province. I still have recollections of this trip: the delicious taste of water chestnuts, round like young girls' lanterns; the sweet, refreshing cucumbers that we picked from their foliage; the familiar smell of corn roasting in the oven. My mother said Grandmother didn't like me, because I was a girl. But I never had that impression, and I don't even remember what she looked like. I think I was happy then. No, wait. I got it wrong. These memories are from my second trip to the northeast. So what are my first memories of happiness? I don't know. When did I lose the untainted, spontaneous happiness of a child? There are only a few childhood photographs of me smiling. Earlier on, I talked about the photograph taken of me on my 10th birthday. The expression on my face was not that of purity and innocence. I wasn't the rising sun, or the precious little flower of my fatherland.

I make an effort to be happy and keep reminding myself: "Li Lanni, you should be happy." But I chide myself at the same time: "Why do I always have to remind myself that I'm happy? What you're feeling can't be happiness." Stop brooding. Think of happy and cheerful things.

Notes

I dread the moment when I have to sit down in front of the computer to work on this book, *A Crowded Silence*. I always need a strong cup of tea mixed with coffee beforehand. I don't feel like doing bloodletting these days. And as I am afraid of stirring up painful memories, my writing has come to a standstill.

My stomach hurts; my belly is hard and bloated; there is a dull pain around my navel. Sometimes, it hurts so much that I have to switch off the computer to take a rest. I've stopped my medications, which weren't doing much good anyway. I lie on the sofa, legs against the wall, my head hanging on the edge of the sofa to facilitate the blood flow to my brain. Unable to do much else, I wait with feverish impatience for the pain to subside. I often have headaches and an urge to throw up, even if there is nothing in my stomach. It's an instinctive reaction to stress. Sometimes, I can feel my primitive soul standing to the right of my forehead, at a hand's distance away. It's looking at my body, coldly and silently. What is this separation between body and soul? It's when my soul manifests itself in the form of light that flashes by in front of me in a series of ellipses-like dots, and then fades away into the air. My body, like a mud statue drenched with rain, melts and disintegrates into a lump of mud to become just a watery puddle... I no longer exist. I am a repulsive glass paper octopus dangling in the air.

I admire Andrew Solomon. In spite of going through three episodes of major depression and being on the brink of a nervous breakdown, he was able to write *The Noonday Demon* in such a creative and methodical way. I couldn't do that.

When I use the *pinyin* input method on the computer, I hear a muffled sobbing sound. Maybe there is a spirit in my throat that wants to cry but can't, as if it's being stifled by a malevolent force. Where did this spirit come from? Who is it? Sometimes, I am frozen in front of the computer, my hands hovering over the keyboard. Even when I start to have cramp in my hands, I still can't move. Is it fear, or am I in the grip of an evil force? You can become incapacitated by fear. Paralysed and rooted to the spot; like a rock, you can't react.

My Depression[1] by Elizabeth Swados is translated into Chinese by Wang Anyi. I bought it without even browsing through it, simply because I liked the title. I was wondering if Wang Anyi had the required level of English to translate such a specialised book. It was only when I got home and opened the book that I realised how intelligent the author was. It's, in fact, an illustrated text and an excellent form of expression, for drawings can touch the readers much more directly than words. It's a shame that I am so lousy at drawing. I would like to have been a dancer and express my emotions through my body. But do dancers suffer from depression?

14th August 2007

Correlations

**Taken from the invoice issued by the oncology hospital
(from 17th to 24th February 2000)**

Multichannel electrocardiogram (premium quality) 1
Evaluation of abdominal lymph nodes by ultrasound (premium quality) 1
Ultrasound of the liver, gall bladder and spleen (premium quality) 1
Pelvic ultrasound 1
Surgical sutures (foreign import) 15
Mammography (premium quality) 1
Chest X-ray (premium quality) 1
Class II treatment (premium quality) 5
Class I treatment (premium quality) 3
Local anaesthesia (premium quality) 5
Strong anaesthesia (premium quality) 5
Lymph node dissection of the neck (premium quality) 1
Atropine 1
Diazepam 2
Phenobarbital 1
Pethidine 1
Batroxobin 6
Lidocaine 2
Moxiclav 13
Use of monitoring machine of the brand Bainuodai 1
Use of digital blood pressure monitor 19
Use of monitoring machine 19
Use of electric bistoury (foreign import) 1
Use of pneumometer 19
To monitor fresh blood oxygen saturation 1
Negative pressure suction (premium quality) 3
Preoperative disinfection of the skin (whole body) (premium quality) 1

Complementary Notes

I have the hospital's invoice right in front of me, but I won't list out every single item. I want to stop writing. Have stomach pains, nausea, chest tightness and inner agitation. Feel distraught and angry, not because of the pain caused by the surgical procedure, but from being treated like an object. Can't even express the anger simmering inside. What would it achieve anyway? As a cancer patient, I was just bed number 21, and then bed number 4 in the operating theatre. I was no longer a human being, but some sort of waste product that had to be disposed of, a burden to be removed, a living corpse that was cut up and its pieces sewn back together. Every time I read: "Local anaesthesia: 5 times," and "Strong anaesthesia: 5 times," I feel faint and queasy. I hear myself again, begging the nurses: "It hurts... really hurts. I can't take it anymore. Give me some more anaesthesia!"

I had a full-body bone scan on 29th May 2000. Can't understand the technical jargon in the report: medical radioisotopes, radioactive tracers, etc. I suppose it's all part of nuclear medicine. A bone scintigraphy involves injecting radioactive tracers into the body and is more complicated than a CT-scan. I felt a lot of discomfort. Maybe it's not such a positive thing. I was overcome with dismay on seeing all the bones in my body in one sweeping glance: big, small, thin, thick. It made me think of a decomposing corpse inside a coffin. I was wondering if I would see my skeleton covered from head to toe in cancerous cells the next time I had a bone scan. If there were a metastasis, I would refuse to be operated on. I wouldn't let myself be butchered, have one bone here chopped off, another one there sawed in two, until there's nothing left of me.

I needed respite from all the worries that were gnawing at my insides and sapping all my energy. The surgical wound was painful. But not wanting to impose on my family, I stayed alone in my apartment in Shenzhen. I would get up in the middle of the night to take pain-killers; pace up and down in my apartment until I was exhausted, and then lie down on the sofa. I bothered no one and my conscience was clear.

After seeing my medical file and biological results at the hospital, my husband brought home the photocopies. Three out of the four lymph nodes that were removed during the dissection had metastatic cancer. Upset and shaken, I asked Quan Wei for advice. Conscientious and prudent, he told me to do further tests. On 12th May, I had a CT-scan of the brain, lungs and neck. I passed out on the table and had to be transferred to the resuscitation room. Some of my friends said that I was too sensitive: Others don't faint, even after several CT-scans. According to them, it's my weakness and lack of willpower that have led me into a state of depression.

It's not just the doctors and nurses who lack compassion. Patients also suffer misunderstanding and contempt from family and friends. It's a problem in society that reflects an individual's level of education. As Susan Sontag said in *Illness as Metaphor*: "The word 'cancer' gives us the impression that it is an illness that degrades us, destroying our lives and our reputations. Some diseases are considered to be an evil that cannot be vanquished. And subsequently, they are not treated like any other diseases. When diagnosed with cancer, many patients feel that they are morally inferior to other people."[2]

For two days, I hesitated before adding the list of items from the hospital invoice to this chapter, because I thought no one would understand, that I would be criticised even for being petty over something so trivial. But it's my duty to do it. Susan Sontag says: "I am angry;"[3] "It hurts me to see that [...];"[4] "I am writing this book to alleviate unnecessary suffering."[5] She continues: "In order to liberate people and bring them comfort, we must remove all connotations and metaphors associated with an illness. However, to be rid of these metaphors, it is not enough to hide them. They must be exposed, criticised, analysed and dispelled."[6]

The results of the CT-scan of my neck came as a blow. It showed the presence of cancerous lymph nodes on both the right and left sides of my neck. This in spite of the fact that I'd had a lymph node dissection on the right in February. The surgical intervention didn't remove everything, leaving a malignant tumour of one centimetre.

"What's this supposed to mean?" I asked Quan Wei. "Is it cancer metastasis or is it because the dissection didn't remove everything?"

"Both are possible."

After that, I began chemotherapy, which, like a military invasion, savagely destroyed everything during five long courses. It decimated the good as well as the bad. A course lasted 21 days, during which I was on daily medication. It was followed by a pause of seven days. Kill. Massacre. Slaughter. Everything.

SEVENTY

Diary
Thursday, 29th April 2004 11:50 am

On reading the Bible this morning, I came across Verses 1 to 8, Chapter 3 of Ecclesiastes, which they say was written by King Solomon. I keep reciting the verses in my head and copied them down:

> *A Time for Everything*
>
> *There is a time for everything,*
> *and a season for every activity under the heavens:*
>
> *a time to be born and a time to die,*
> *a time to plant and a time to uproot,*
> *a time to kill and a time to heal,*
> *a time to tear down and a time to build,*
> *a time to weep and a time to laugh,*
> *a time to mourn and a time to dance,*
> *a time to scatter stones and a time to gather them,*
> *a time to embrace and a time to refrain from embracing,*
> *a time to search and a time to give up,*
> *a time to keep and a time to throw away,*
> *a time to tear and a time to mend,*
> *a time to be silent and a time to speak,*
> *a time to love and a time to hate,*
> *a time for war and a time for peace.*
>
> *Truth. Memory. Forbearance. Acceptance.*
> *There is a time for everything. Amen.*

Notes

Before descending into depression in 2003, I was often plagued by this one thought: "Why is fate so cruel to me?" I had my fair share of problems and misfortunes after my operation. Two months later, I had a cancer relapse due to the fact that not everything had been removed during the dissection. I underwent chemotherapy and was faced with the prospect of another surgical procedure. There was no end to my hell. Was there no justice for the good, while the bad enjoy good health and a beautiful life?

I didn't get it. Was there no justice in this world?

A colleague of mine cried when she heard that I had cancer. Three years later, she said to me: "I'm so sorry that someone like you, who is so kind, has had to suffer from cancer. It was such a shock." Some people cried on the phone, not to comfort me, but to lament: "Why are the heavens so unfair?" There were others who said with brutal frankness: "Li Lanni, you have a good life. Work, family, recognition... It all came to you so easily. Then the heavens dealt you this nasty blow. Life is an equaliser." Then there were others who lashed out: "It'll teach you to spend all your time writing!" I would be naïve to think that everyone in this world is nice.

A person with cancer becomes inferior to him or herself, and also in other people's eyes. Even if you were a state president, people would think: "We'll see how long you can hang on." Those who hold you in disdain or hurt you don't necessarily mean to. This is how society is. You can't escape from reality. When you're down with a serious illness, more than at any other time in life, human nature reveals itself in all its starkness. People show their real faces so naturally, like the sun that shines or the rain that falls. When all is well in your life, there will always be people hovering around. They smile and say pleasing things. But when you're going through hardships, few come to your aid, and you realise that people aren't what they pretend to be. Some avoid you on the street, while others disappear altogether from your life. Those who usually say pleasant things become less friendly. Those who always had a smile for you smile awkwardly and without sincerity. But these are good people. Some treat you with contempt and look down on you, as if their heads have grown taller. As you no longer have any use for them, they don't need to put on an act. In truth, it's a normal reaction from normal people. Cancer brings out human nature in all its cruelty and kindness.

I have a friend who works as a cashier and comes from a humble background. She asked her friends to see how she could help me. Moved by her sincerity, her friends, in turn, asked their own friends. Drawn together by compassion, these people, whom I don't know well, tried to help and share my problems.

I usually have little contact with government officials. However, I received a basket of flowers from them after my operation. It was a gift the Communications Department in Shenzhen had sent to my home in Guangzhou. After my surgical intervention, several friends in Shenzhen raised money to help me out financially. Some donated 10,000 yuan, others 5,000. Even though I didn't accept, I was extremely grateful to them.

For two years, a fellow student in Hong Kong regularly gave me a medicine that strengthens the immune system, which cost a fortune. When he was unable to come to Shenzhen, he would ask his secretary to send it.

Around the same period, a woman called Xiao Wang did the housework at my home in Shenzhen. I had only known her for six months. Knowing that I would be in Shenzhen during my convalescence, she offered to clean my apartment for nothing. My friends were going to pay her 50 yuan for me, but she firmly refused, saying: "I can't help Ms Li any other way. She needs a lot of money to pay for her medical expenses. I can work for free."

My friends knew that Xiao Wang's family was poor. She had a young child, and her husband was unemployed and worked as a street vendor. Xiao Wang was the main breadwinner. She worked several jobs, doing cleaning even at night, and to save money, she ate only marinated vegetable buns.

After Xiao Wang had finished cleaning my home, my friends were so touched that they immediately called to tell me. I asked them to thank Xiao Wang and to give her 50 yuan, saying that if she refused, I wouldn't have the peace of mind to fully recover my health. This woman of modest means made me believe in human kindness again. She restored my faith in society.

Correlations

Excerpts from *"The Book of Life"* [1]

Life is extraordinary!
Do not be glad to possess material things and do not wallow in self-pity. When life calls upon you to resist, rise to the challenge.

It is like the sea on a beautiful day: the surface is calm, but undercurrents are flowing in the depths. True strength is thus. Do not be taken in by the calmness of the sea, nor be swept away by its undercurrents. This is life. [...].

I came to know her late in life, after learning that she was ill [...]. Li Lanni's life force is a story in itself. She is bold and strong, like a rock. As I came to know her, I discovered that she is gentle and attentive.

Those who have a fragile and sensitive nature tend to be weak and vulnerable. But Li Lanni is able to unite strength and sensitivity in herself. How can her slender, graceful body hold such an astounding heart?

She has changed my notion of what strength is. A rock cannot feel thunder nor lightning. It remains still and unmoving in a storm. But this is not strength. A person with a sensitive heart feels, more than other people, the hardships, suffering and pain. She fights against all odds. This is strength in the true sense of the word.

Cheng Wenchao

Complementary Notes

At the beginning of the summer of 2001, an art and literature newspaper published an issue on the professional writers of Shenzhen and had asked Cheng Wenchao to write an article of about 1000 words. He was very excited about it, but several passages were cut out from the published version. Chang Wenchao said: "They deleted everything that was essential in the article. What I wanted to talk about was the notion of strength."

Strength lives, not in me, but in Cheng Wenchao. He underwent several operations for cancer. We were brother and sister in our misfortunes. Between 2002 and 2003, we were often on the phone, discussing chemotherapy and other cancer therapies. After his death, many of his friends wrote articles praising his strength. But they hadn't known the fragile and sensitive side of him. I had witnessed his pain and despair.

There is no strength without fragility.

I remember an embarrassing incident that happened to me towards the end of the 1990s. My home in Shenzhen was burgled twice. Several of my close friends had either been burgled or robbed. I would even go as far as saying that those who have never been burgled or robbed don't know the people of Shenzhen at all.

However, the second burglary was highly distressing. The burglars were competent, efficient and, in all appearance, highly skilled. The front door, made of solid wood, and its high-security lock were left intact. They had removed the metallic gate and front door from their hinges.

When my upstairs neighbours saw this and called the police, the burglars had already fled. My apartment had been completely ransacked. All the renminbi and Hong Kong dollars in the drawer were gone. They had taken the video player, CDs, Oscar-winning films on DVD, name-brand suitcases, bed sheets and everything else of value. They went through my wardrobe and took my European-style leather coats, leaving all the 'Made in Hong Kong' clothes.

I was shocked to find my bed stripped of its sheets and covered with photographs. The burglars had taken the photographs out of the albums, which were in the drawer, and had spread them on the bed to study them closely. It made my flesh crawl.

There was a void where the doors had been. I was too shaken and upset to sleep that night. So I sat alone in the apartment with all the lights turned on, waiting for daybreak.

I had goose pimples every time I thought of my bed covered with my photographs. I felt that I was standing in the light, and the burglars were lurking in the shadows. They knew who I was, but I had no idea who they were. It made my hair stand on end.

At 2 o'clock in the morning, I heard the kitchen door creak. I darted out onto the landing, screaming. I was blabbering but can't for the life of me remember what I said.

I must have scared the living daylights out of my neighbours, for they came running from upstairs and downstairs in their pyjamas, looking terrified. They called the police, but said it was better to let the burglars get away, in case they came back to make trouble for everyone in the building later on. After inspecting the premises, the police said it was the wind that had made the door creak. It hadn't been shut properly.

SEVENTY-ONE

Diary
Saturday, 1st May 2004 5 pm

The "depression season" is over. Finally. April has been a lousy month. May will be much brighter.

This time last year, I was still struggling with my health problems. On 4th May, I plucked up my courage and went out for the first time since my operation. I attended a religious service at the Dongshan Church. Initially thinking I wouldn't have the strength to stay until the end, I nonetheless managed to stay with the help of the Holy Spirit. When I left, I was feeling so inspired and uplifted. It had been a long time since I'd felt such positive emotions. I called Fanding to say that I had prayed for the birth of his daughter, Li Jiean, hoping it would go smoothly. At the time, we were at the height of the SARS epidemic and all the religious services in Beijing and Shanghai had been cancelled. We received Holy Communion that day and every member of the congregation was given a pair of disposable transparent plastic gloves. My illness stabilised towards mid-May. I become emotional when I think of all the problems I went through last year.

I won't be going on holiday during the seven-day break. Too tired. People have a hard time imagining how a sick person spends his or her holidays. They ask me: "What do you do at home? Don't you get bored?" I say nothing, because the only answer I have is: "I do my best to stay alive." All my energy is channelled into just staying alive. I don't have the energy to get bored. Boredom is a luxury. It's harder to live than to die. Those who have never experienced a major illness can't imagine what it's like. Listening to me, people would think I am patronising.

So, shut up, then. Or smile.

Notes

Upon reading *The Noonday Demon*, what impresses me most about Andrew Solomon is the support and understanding his family and friends show towards sick people. Whether it was his mother's cancer or his own depression, his father and brother did their utmost to understand and help them with love, intelligence and unwavering support.

In a sense, you can say that Andrew Solomon is lucky. Relatively speaking, of course. His father works in the medical and pharmaceutical sector. Andrew

Solomon, a graduate of Yale University and Jesus College of Cambridge University, comes from an educated background, where people are well-informed and knowledgeable about the different types of illnesses. And he had the psychological and financial support of his family and relatives. Following his son's depression, Andrew Solomon's father started research projects on antidepressants in his company. Through his love, patience, intelligence and mental strength, he gave his son understanding and emotional support during the six years of his illness.

In China, the situation is disastrous for those who are sick. Many living in poverty don't even know what illness is killing them. Even when they do know they are suffering from cancer or depression, they don't have access to the most basic psychological support or financial aid. I can't afford to be sick, let alone other people. As my parents' income is sufficient for them to live on, I don't need to help them out financially. But my mother lives in constant fear of not being able to pay for her medical expenses, if ever she falls ill. She is paranoid about having kidney damage or some other disease. Or that she might fall and break something, requiring a foreign-imported prosthesis. Or that she'll be paralysed following a stroke. Scared that anything could happen, she lives frugally, scrimping and saving, putting money aside to prepare for any eventuality.

Luckily, I am an employee with a fixed income and no children. But since I have been unable to write for several years due to my illness, I have no additional revenue. A second operation has been scheduled, and the possibility of a metastasis is real. Goodness knows how much it will cost. I am scared of going under the scalpel again or having an injection of thymosin imported from abroad, bumping up the medical bill. If a hierarchical superior takes a disliking to me and decides to make trouble, using my illness as an excuse to fire me, I won't have an additional income to make up for my loss in revenue. I made up my mind long ago that if I can't afford the medical expenses, then I'll refuse to be treated. I don't care. I've had enough. But most of the sick must continue to live. Crippled with worry, how do they cope? They don't all have caring and devoted children at their bedsides. A burden for their family, they can't even rouse compassion in others. Many living below the poverty line wait for help to come. But human, material and emotional resources are lacking. Sometimes, relatives, neighbours and colleagues even feel sorry for the sick person's family.

"What a burden!" they say. "Isn't he dead yet? The whole family has to suffer because of him. What bad luck!"

As people like to say: "A sick person is someone who is dogged by bad luck. Stay as far away as possible from him. Why is it him who has been struck by illness and not others? Fate has turned against him. It's divine punishment."

17th August 2007

Correlations

Excerpts from *The Noonday Demon*

Depression has made us suffer even longer than war, cancer and AIDS put together. At the root of many problems, illnesses, alcoholism and drug addiction, we find the hidden face of depression [...]. Practising a religion is one way amongst others to free ourselves from depression. It helps us face up to disappointment, go through depression, giving us a reason to live [...] and, when we are alone and without help, it gives us dignity and a direction [...]. Recently, an editor of *The New Yorker* said that I didn't suffer from depression at all. I retorted, saying that it was impossible to pretend, but he didn't believe me.

"It's better not to see each other so often," he said. "This depression thing, it's nonsense."

After I recovered, I tried to erase all my unhappy memories, although I don't think there is a connection between my past and my depression relapses. I don't hide the fact that I take antidepressants on a permanent basis, which creates suspicion and distrust in others. Having a tarnished personal reputation is one of the peculiar consequences of depression.

"Depression, I'll never fall for it," the editor said, as if I had invented a fictional character just to make the whole world feel sorry for me. I know several other people who are just as intolerant as he is. Even today, I still feel hurt.

Andrew Solomon (United States)

Complementary Notes

Andrew Solomon knows "several other people" who are intolerant. As for me, I know quite a few of them. Their tone and choice of words are similar to those of the editor of *The New Yorker*. The difference is that their suspicion and distrust are even more blatant. Once, a person looked at me questioningly, studying my eyes and face.

"There's no such thing as depression," he said. "You're talking rubbish. I don't believe it all. It's a figment of your imagination. You made it up so other people will feel sorry for you. Or maybe it's because you're stupid and gullible. You got fooled by your doctor."

Some said: "It's hogwash. I don't feel sorry for you."

Then there are others who said: "You're not depressed. If you're not sick, you mustn't say you are. What's the point? What good does it do you?"

Not only do I find the expression on these people's faces and their way of talking upsetting, they also disappoint me. Uncharitable, callous and compassionless, they are the centre of their own universe. If they were a doctor or worked in the National Health Insurance or worked as an assistant director, director or director general of a rescue service, they could endanger the lives of many people, who might end up dying in anger and bitterness. Of course, I don't only know cold-hearted and small-minded people. Some have limited medical knowledge and, lacking time or the intellectual motivation to learn, they repeat trivialities, making an effort to appear sincere. As the maxim goes: "Smile, it saves you from thinking."

"The Book of Life" by Cheng Wenchao was published for the first time in the *Southern Daily*. My parents, who were in the province at the time, bought the newspaper. They called me.

"Why did he write an article like that?" they asked.

"Why not?" I snapped.

"Now everybody is asking us what kind of illness our daughter has and if it's serious," my mother complained. "Your father is livid. He doesn't even know these people. You can't tell people you've got cancer."

"The article didn't say I had cancer."

"But people know."

"So?"

"Shit doesn't smell, it only stinks when you stir it."

What could I say to that? My mother used a saying popular in the village of Ping in the Jiangsu region. Cancer is shit. I, who have cancer, am a pile of shit. Shit that smells.

Should I have answered back or flown into a rage?

I am depressed. Shit.

SEVENTY-TWO

Diary
Wednesday, 12th May 2004 11:15 am

It's Fanding's birthday today. I called to wish him many happy returns. He said that the family had gotten together to celebrate Li Jiaen's first birthday on the 7th and that they wouldn't be doing anything for his. Since he became a father, he's no longer living for himself, and he's happy. The *zhuazhou*[1] ritual took place in the afternoon of 7th May, Li Jiaen's birthday. In the family photo, she's holding a pen in one hand and a 100 yuan note in the other. She already knows that to succeed in life, you must have "both fists clenched."[2] She's got a promising future ahead of her.

While reading Chapter 9 of Ecclesiastes this morning, I came across two passages that spoke to my heart:

"Go, eat your food with gladness, and drink your wine with a joyful heart, for God has already approved what you do."[3]

"The race is not to the swift or the battle to the strong, [...] but time and chance happen to them all."[4]

Notes

Children today are extremely sensitive.

When Jiaen was three years and eight months old, her mother went away to study in the United States for six months. Jiaen attended the best kindergarten in Guangzhou and came home to sleep three nights a week. Her grandparents stayed at my brother's place to give him a helping hand. There was also a part-time nanny. My brother spent most of his time at home playing with Jiaen; he put her to bed at night and accompanied the nanny to fetch her from school. But I felt that her mother's absence was affecting her. Once, we were watching the documentary *Winged Migration* at my place.

"Auntie, why is the mummy bird not taking the baby bird with her?" she asked.

"Because baby bird has grown up and is flying next to his mummy."

"But why is the mummy bird not taking the baby bird with her?" she asked again, not believing a word I said.

"Yes, she is. She is taking him with her."

"Why is the mummy bird not taking the baby bird with her?"

This idea was stuck in her head and nothing could make her change her mind. She was expressing her unhappiness through her question. I stopped talking, but she carried on asking me the same question until I switched off the DVD player.

The family tried their best to distract her. Once, my mother called me.

"Last night, Fanding came home after a business meeting," she said. "He had a bit too much to drink and fell asleep on the bed. Jiean wouldn't leave him alone and tried to wake him up. I told her she must let Daddy sleep, otherwise he would be too tired and he would die. And Grandma and Grandpa would die too. What would happen to Jiean? This child, she understood right away. She nodded, and with tears in her eyes, she stopped being naughty, and hugging her blanket against her, she went to sleep in my bed."

"Mother, stop frightening her. When I was little, you really scared me with your nonsense. Don't do that with Jiean. It leaves psychological scars."

When my sister-in-law came back from abroad, Jiean was happy again. And I felt relieved to see positive changes in her. It reminded me of my lonely childhood and those long and never-ending days after my parents had left, without giving any explanation nor news of where they had gone. I cried, afraid to even call out their names. Many people of my generation have lived through similar experiences. We can't blame our parents. But we must undo the psychological knots and free ourselves from this mental burden. Better late than never. Thus, we can lighten the psychological load for the next generation.

My parents stayed with me for 10 days in August. I asked them to stay until the end of the month, but they insisted on going back home to Junya Residence, because they saw that I could barely take care of myself.

I admit, I just couldn't cope with them around.

I had difficulty concentrating on my writing. It's demanding work, and I need quiet and a certain state of mind to deal with the negative aspects of my memories. But I have to put on a happy face in front of my parents. Normally, I work from 10 o'clock in the morning to 1 in the afternoon. I then play with Lele for a while before having lunch. I take a nap around 2 o'clock and work from 4 to half past 6. Exhausted, I lie on the couch for half an hour. As my negative memories continue to circle around in my mind, I take a stroll outside with Lele for about an hour to clear my head. Dinner is at half-past 8. To unwind after a day of intense writing, I potter around the apartment, watch the evening news, changing channels with the remote control depending on my mood, looking for funny programs that make me laugh and calm my nerves. With all sorts of thoughts still racing around my head, I don't go to bed until around midnight or 1 o'clock in the morning. I take alprazolam half an hour before bedtime, and if it doesn't work and I wake up in the middle of the night, I switch on the light and flick through the newspaper or a magazine on domestic pets until I feel sleepy. I generally wake up around 6:30 am. In my half-sleep, I try to make out the time on the clock. Then at 7:30 am, still drowsy, I switch on the television to watch the news. At 8:30, I get up.

My father gets up at 6 every morning. A 6:30 am, he takes a stroll outside and buys sugar-free prepared meals for diabetics, such as chicken glutinous rice, vermicelli or fried noodles, etc. My mother gets up at 7 o'clock. My parents each make their own breakfast. My mother has eggs or savoury porridge with tomatoes or sweet milk porridge. I am easy. I wait until they finish and then I have a bread bun, half a sweet potato (Lele has the other half), strong tea and coffee. When my parents are at their home, they usually have lunch around midday, dinner at 6 o'clock and are in bed by 10. But when they were staying with me, Mother couldn't take the air conditioning, complaining that it was too cold in the sitting and dining rooms. The temperature outside had been 36 degrees for several days in a row, and the heat was stifling. As I couldn't bear the heat, I either turned the air conditioner up to 29 or 30 degrees, or I would have the fan at full blast in the sitting and dining room. My parents were thoughtful and tried their best to adjust to my habits. They had lunch a little later than they would normally, around half past midday or 1 o'clock, and dinner would be at 7. With their daily routine up in the air, they felt uncomfortable living with me. Mother complained of flu-like symptoms and said she couldn't take the air conditioning nor the fan. When I switched them off, she said the symptoms were gone. From then on, I was more considerate towards her.

Filial piety is a difficult ideal to attain. I could have been rushed to hospital, even before my mother had a slightest hint of her flu-like symptoms. But I'm being dramatic and facetious here. So saying, my parents were considerate and thoughtful. Realising that they couldn't help me and that I was absorbed by the writing of my book, they decided to go home. They've been extremely understanding towards me these last couple of years. "Blind" filial piety isn't such the positive thing. Those who suffer from a serious illness should talk to their parents, allowing them to have a better understanding of what their children are going through. It encourages mutual support between parents and children. When I was writing the "Diary" section in 2003, I had lost my bearings and was crippled by anxiety. My parents didn't know I was in mental pain, nor about the possibility of a cancer relapse, nor the fact that another surgical intervention was in the cards. They had no idea that I had fallen into a severe depression and was engulfed in such despair that I wanted to end my life.

It is a Chinese tradition to give only the good news to your parents to save them from worrying, and to keep the bad news to yourself. But if we were to keep everything to ourselves, they would fret even more. For they're far from stupid, and, sensing that you aren't quite yourself, would begin to imagine all sorts of things, often leading to misunderstandings. But if you manage to hide the truth so well that they don't sense anything unusual, you can end up doing countless errands for them. Like the time when my mother was spitting blood a couple of years ago. My father insisted that I should find a doctor to prescribe tests and accompany her to her medical examinations. At the time, I was going through therapy for my depression; coping with the secondary effects of my medication; and coming to terms of the prospect of another operation. Too tired to take care of my mother, I decided to tell my parents the truth. But gently.

First, I suggested that they should read *Us Three* by Yang Feng. I was hoping that, in their old age, they would learn from Mr Yang Feng and have the same attitude towards life and death. For the chances were, their daughter would die before them. Whenever there was an untimely death of a public figure, I would make a point of talking about it with them. Also, a few of my friends and acquaintances had preceded their parents to the grave. The cause of death was cancer, or acute myocarditis, or brain haemorrhage. Most of them had died of cancer.

That was how I told the truth about my illness to my parents. I talked about the subjective experience of my operations, chemotherapy and depression. While revealing the truth about myself, I was careful not to talk too much about my pain, allowing them to gradually accept reality and to know the truth, at least partially. I tried to be as honest as I could with myself: "Am I being selfish? Am I neglecting my filial duties by not protecting them from the truth?" Every time I reprimanded myself, Li Lanni reassured me: "You must do it. Because you'll probably die before them. Youth is on your side, and as parents, they have a right to know."

The number of people who die in mid-life is increasing. This is especially true among intellectuals. Compared to the older population, the number of young people suffering from depression is higher. It's impossible to close my eyes to this phenomenon.

18th August 2007

Correlations

Ultrasound Report from the Oncology Hospital

Date: 17 December 2001

Several flat-shaped NL < 1.0 cm are visible on both sides of the jaw and in the upper part of the neck.

Tissues of the left and right thyroid are homogenous with no detectable mass.

Conclusion: Several NL without suspicious tissue mass on both sides of the jaw and in the upper part of the neck.

Complementary Notes

The doctor who carried out the ultrasound scan wrote the report by hand. It's not clear whether he wrote Ca, or NL for "lymph node." The test took place in a well-known hospital in Beijing. The colour Doppler results confirmed the results of the CT-scan I had on 12th May 2000 in Guangzhou. These results were a warning signal. Was there metastasis or was there a problem of a different nature that called for a surgical intervention? Would I have to lie on the operating table again, waiting for the biopsy results to reveal the truth? It was wreaking havoc on my nerves.

I didn't know anyone at the oncology hospital in Beijing. We ended up contacting the mother of my husband's former student, who in turn called a neighbour she hardly knew. This neighbour worked in the hospital's laboratory. After I had bought my plane ticket to Beijing, my husband's former student called to say that his mother had fallen and broken a leg and wouldn't be able to accompany me to Beijing. He was kind and encouraged me to stick to my plans. The doctor who worked at the laboratory informed me that the most competent doctors worked on Tuesday mornings. I arrived early at the hospital on a Tuesday morning and went straight to the laboratory to look for the doctor. But a plump nurse there said he had been hospitalised the day before for a myocardial infarction. It left me rooted to the spot in front of the laboratory. If only I had known, I wouldn't have come all the way to Beijing, as the trip was paid for out of my own pocket.

I had consulted two doctors in Guangzhou. The first one suggested that I should wait until the tumour grows to three centimetres, because I had just finished chemotherapy and my body was too weak for another surgical intervention immediately afterwards. The second doctor, an oncologist from another hospital, advised me to undergo an operation as soon as possible to root out the source of the illness and eliminate any chances of the tumour growing any further. Both were famous doctors, so which one should I listen to? My only solution was to go to Beijing. I had a 50/50 chance of being operated on again. Someone unlucky like me, looked down upon, broke, with no social connections, had to take this chance to find an answer. I made up my mind to go to Beijing, even if I were to come back empty-handed.

I stood in front of the hospital entrance, not knowing if I should stay or leave. Pray; when you're desperate, there's nothing else you can do. At the end of my prayers, an idea came to me: Stay and hang around outside the consultation rooms. Don't be sad. Don't feel sorry for yourself. And don't give up. After checking out all the consultation rooms, I noticed a magazine for cancer patients that was on sale. Following a voice inside me, I flicked through the pages and came across an article written by a doctor. It said that doctors should take the patient's state of mind into account, instead of only focusing on the illness. This article spoke to my heart. It was exactly the kind of doctor I was looking for. I went back to the consultation room area and found the name of this doctor listed in both the Chinese Traditional Medicine and Western medicine departments. It was a woman specialist. People were waiting outside her office. Poking my head through the door, I saw a woman who looked kind-hearted and caring. This was the impression I'd gotten from reading her article. Sitting opposite her was a student, who was helping her write out prescriptions. I plucked up my courage, walked into the office and explained to her that I had come especially from Guangzhou to be treated. I asked her to give me an appointment and that I was prepared to wait to be seen last. She looked up at me, studied me with impartiality, professionalism and without judgement. It made me feel like a human being. She gave me an appointment.

Two stories that have inspired me:

The first one: A man was travelling on a journey with an angel. On the first night, they stayed with a poor man, who welcomed them with everything he possessed and gave them a golden cup to drink from. It was a gift from a neighbour who had hated him for many years, and, as a sign of peace, offered him wine in a golden cup. When they left the next day, the angel stole the golden cup. The second night, they stayed with a rich but wicked and greedy man, who was cold and inhospitable. But when they left, the angel offered the man the golden cup. On the third night, they stayed with a poor family. The brothers, whose parents were dead, were good-natured and hard-working. They welcomed the two guests warmly. However, that night, the angel set fire to the hut, which was burnt to the ground. Then the angel left with his travelling companion, who, outraged by his friend's behaviour, scolded him:

"The brothers are devastated by their loss. I don't want to travel with you anymore, because you can't tell the difference between good and evil. You punished the wrong people!"

The angel said:

"The golden cup the neighbour gave to the poor man was smeared with poison. That's why I gave it to the rich and wicked man. As for the brothers, there is gold buried beneath their hut. When they dig to rebuild their house, they will be filled with joy in finding the treasure."

Second story: Two angels came down to earth and arrived at a rich family's home. The master of the house received the two guests coldly and asked them to sleep in a dark and chilly basement. As they were lying on the hard and icy floor, the older angel noticed a hole in the wall, which he plugged up immediately. The next day, the two angels arrived at a poor family's home. The farmer and his wife were kind and hospitable. They shared all the food they had with the guests and let them sleep in the only bed they had in the house. The angels slept soundly. However, at dawn, they found the farmer and his wife in tears. Their cow, which was their only source of income, had died in the night. Furious, the younger angel asked the older one:

"Why did you let such a thing happen to these people? The farmer is poor but he shared everything he had with us. And you let their cow die!"

"Things are not what they seem," the older angel said. "On the first night, when we were staying in that opulent house, I discovered there was gold hidden in the hole in the wall. As the master of the house is a greedy man, I plugged the hole to stop him from finding it. Last night, when I was asleep in the farmer's bed, the angel of death came. He was going to take away the farmer's wife. But I let him take the cow instead."

When a colleague learnt that I had cancer, he said to me:

"We're no longer rewarded by the good deeds we do. Those times are over. These days, even malevolent spirits are afraid of the wicked. Otherwise, how can you explain what happened to you?"

When a friend heard that I was shutting myself away at home because of my depression, she said to someone else:

"I don't understand why she isn't in God's good graces. I just don't get it at all."

In the past, I never knew how to explain my situation to other people. But today, I can say this to my friends and colleagues: Things are not what they seem.

SEVENTY-THREE

Diary
Thursday, 13th May 2004 11 am

Lele is eight months old today. They say that a six-month-old puppy is equivalent to 10 years old in human age, and that one year in a dog corresponds to five years in a child. I wonder if Lele is like me when I was 12 or 13.

I envy Lele sometimes. He is happy, healthy and has known love from the day he was born. His breeder loves and takes good care of dogs. Since he came to live with me at one month old, he has been showered with love and affection.

I made the decision not to have children because I know I can't make them happy, nor bring them up in a healthy and balanced family environment. It would have been irresponsible of me. But it's within my means to give Lele a good life. I don't force him to learn tricks to entertain people; I let him develop naturally at his own pace. People love and appreciate him. He receives compliments from strangers every day.

Sometimes, it seems that the life of a dog that is filled with love is better than that of a human being, or a king of the animals. I even think he's happier than I am. I wouldn't mind being him for a change.

He has more good qualities than a human does: loyalty, joyousness, innocence, kindness, empathy, compassion, candidness, selflessness, etc.

Lele is an angel. I should learn from him.

Notes

It's because of Lele that I began to have more contact with other people on the university campus. The mischief he got up to helped me widen the scope of my experience.

When he was two months old, I often took him to play in the park. Everyone loved this little puppy. He's used to people complimenting, cuddling and playing with him. He loves people, sniffing at their feet, wagging his little tail, hoping they would play with him.

As Lele is my first dog, I have no experience whatsoever in canine education. I can't correct the bad habit he has of always going up to people. As the owner of this mischievous little dog, I often find myself caught up in disputes.

The first time: My housekeeper was in the lift with Lele. A little girl entered the lift, accompanied by an adult. The girl was frightened of him, but Lele, thinking she wanted to play, jumped on her and scratched her on the legs. The girl's parents and relatives complained to the building's management and hurled insults at me, saying the dog must be put down before he causes any more psychological trauma in children. They were literally hysterical. I accompanied them to a clinic for an anti-rabies vaccination and paid for the medical expenses. The little girl needed to go back to the clinic for a second shot. I wanted to pay for the taxi, but the family refused. I paid them a visit some time after the incident and offered them a gift. That was the end of the story.

The second time: My housekeeper was taking Lele for a walk. A man in shorts and T-shirt was doing his exercises. As they went past, Lele put his paws on him. The man, my housekeeper and two teachers who were present checked and saw that the man didn't have any wounds. Nonetheless, my housekeeper gave him my telephone number. But she had barely walked through the door when I received a call from the man saying that he had a slight wound. I said: "You must have an anti-rabies shot. I'll pay for the medical expenses and taxi fare." He agreed but didn't want me to go with him. But he got ripped off by the clinic, where they convinced him to do several tests and have two vaccinations. My housekeeper said to me: "Ms Li, you get taken in by people too easily. That day, I saw with my own eyes that he wasn't hurt. There were even two witnesses." I said: "My conscience is clear. I don't think he had any intention to deceive me."

The third time: I was in the lift with Lele when a little school boy came in. Lele's mouth brushed against the boy's leg. After dropping Lele off in my apartment, I went to see the boy, who was at home with his father. I said: "I wanted to check to see if your son is alright and make sure he isn't hurt. As a parent, you must be worried." The three of us made sure the boy didn't have any scratches on him, and I left them my telephone number. Then I took the train back to Shenzhen. But somewhere between Guangzhou and Shenzhen, the mother called me, swearing at me and throwing a hissy fit.

"Don't panic," I said. "Go home and you'll see for yourself that your son isn't hurt."

"If he's not hurt, then why did you come over?" she shouted.

"Because I was worried. I was being kind, but you call to scream insults down the phone at me."

"My son was wounded in the knee once and he has a scar. He must be vaccinated straight away."

"Alright. When I come back from Shenzhen, I'll reimburse the medical expenses and taxi fares."

The mother chose a foreign imported anti-rabies vaccination, which cost me 850 yuan. I apologised to the family several times, but the mother, who'd been scornful since the start of the incident, wouldn't even deign to look at me.

The fourth time: My husband was outside with Lele. He was chatting with a lecturer whose wife was French, and they had two beautiful biracial boys. Lele had scratched his leg and, without telling us, the man went to a clinic for a vaccination. When I heard about it the next day, I went over to their place to apologise and reimburse him for the medical expenses and taxi fares. But he adamantly refused. So I went to the bookshop, Learning & Excellence, and bought a collection of classic fairy tales for his sons. The price of the book corresponded to the medical fees I would have paid. Seeing that I was sincere in my apologies, the lecturer and his wife told the boys to thank me.

The fifth time: Lele was playing with a little boy who lives in my building. Lele accidently scratched him. The mother came and asked me politely, without the slightest reproach in her voice, if Lele had been vaccinated. I quickly showed her the vaccination certificate and gave her some money for the medical expenses, which she accepted. But she refused to take money for the taxi, saying: "The clinic is just next door. I don't need a taxi."

The sixth time: This time, a housekeeper, who only stayed for one and a half months, was the cause of my troubles. She took Lele to play with her husband. Lele left a red scratch mark on his wrist. I gave the housekeeper 400 yuan for an anti-rabies vaccination. After she took the money, she said that she also had dogs at home and that her husband wouldn't be needing a vaccine. Two days later, she offered to give me back my money, but I said: "Keep it. If Lele scratches you again and I'm not here, go and get yourself vaccinated."

The seventh time: This was the incident with White Sneakers. Even though I've already paid her 4,600 yuan for medical expenses and compensation for any psychological trauma, I never know when she's going to turn up on my doorstep asking for more.

Above are seven stories, seven characters, seven types of behaviour and seven ways of solving a problem. These human reactions reflect the different aspects of these people's lives: their moral values, family environments, upbringings and the social behaviour within a family.

Of the seven different reactions, six of them were normal. I feel grateful to two out of the seven people. I was lucky. Our lives are made up of small insignificant incidents, but which trigger an array of human reactions: fear, anxiety, disdain, comfort, tolerance, reconciliation and embarrassment. Remember this: Never be vanquished by evil; conquer evil with good.

21st August 2007

Correlations

Words That Spoke to My Soul from Mother Teresa

We need to grow up surrounded by love. This is why we never stop loving and giving to the point of feeling pain. Love is not only about giving assistance or money, it is holding out your hand – a hand filled with warmth. Do not aim high and aspire to do noble things. For love begins with oneself.

Complementary Notes

Recently, I read a biography of Mother Teresa, who won a Nobel Peace Prize.

Mother Teresa founded a hospice in India that provides palliative care. The fact that she established a service for people at the end of life was controversial. Many thought it was a waste of resources, because many people in India don't have access to adequate medical treatment, and Mother Teresa was spending money on those who were dying. People questioned the value of her work. But Mother Teresa said that all life is precious, be it sick, disabled or dying.

China has some ruthlessly ambitious people, whose words are hollow and meaningless. They lack respect towards their colleagues and neighbours and would never dream of lending anyone a helping hand. And yet, they are sometimes suddenly overcome with feelings of generosity and donate millions and millions of yuan to the most backward places in the country. They do this in order to gain the gratitude of those who live in abject poverty. This flatters their ego and vanity, allowing them to call themselves philanthropists. Sometimes, the money they give to the poverty-stricken people in the countryside isn't even enough to cover the expenses of hosting and entertaining them. These are highly-educated people, and I know several of them in my entourage. They utter pious words and give 500 yuan to those living in the remote countryside. But at home they mistreat their domestic helpers; are rude to the dustmen; swear at passers-by who accidently brush against them on the street and rumple their clothes; feel glad when their colleagues suffer from misfortune; and are jealous of those who are better than them. They think that they trip over themselves to do favours for others and that the whole world owes them. They engage in philanthropic activities, but haven't an iota of compassion in them. They chase after prestige, wealth and social status. For them, philanthropy is just another form of self-advertising.

SEVENTY-FOUR

Diary
Monday, 17th May 2004 11:10 am

Reducing the dosage of my medication hasn't achieved the desired effects.

I was afraid of lowering the dosage too much. Two days ago, I decreased the alprazolam by half a tablet at bed time. That night, I woke up three or four times, and last night I dreamt about a bloody massacre.

I was in a strange town, where I was on a training program for skydiving. The course covered various skills: finance, calculus, current world topics and skydiving. I only knew two friends in this town: a woman and a man. The woman friend had long arms and legs and was graceful when she ran. The man friend was the leader of the trainees and had a weak character. At the end of the training program, the three of us were selected to be part of an action team. Brimming with self-confidence, I boasted to my man friend that I had jumped from a helicopter ladder and landed on the reefs. I was positive that I would succeed in my next challenge but was worried for my woman friend, for she was terribly thin and could have an accident when she parachutes from an aircraft. The man friend just laughed, saying she was quick and nimble, like a shooting star, and was stronger than me. The two of them went home, while I went walking around town.

The streets were dim. I arrived at a lively district and went into a tea house to rest. Suddenly, a man went on a rampage with a knife, killing several customers. Heads, arms, legs and blood were everywhere, and a strong stench of blood hung in the air. The killer lunged towards me, and I ran outside as quickly as my legs could carry me. To my relief, I found a safe place a few streets away. I wanted to go back to the dormitory. It was daytime. I arrived at the public toilets. It was spacious inside. Killers were butchering people with a knife in the ladies' room. Knives were flashing everywhere. I ran into the men's, hands covering my eyes, screaming: "Murderers! Catch them!" Men came rushing out of the toilets, but the killers continued their massacre. A little boy was severed in two. It was absolutely heart-breaking. The layout of the toilets was like the inside a labyrinth, and people were fighting in the corridors. Knives were flashing, and lumps of human flesh were flying everywhere. I felt fear, anger and despair.

Three of the killers were finally caught. Coming out of the toilets, I congratulated myself on having the presence of mind to call for help in the men's room, which saved my life. But I was ridden with guilt, because I was a coward and gave in to fear in the face of evil. Upset, I needed to talk to someone who could reassure me. I hurried back to the training centre. In the meeting room, I found my address book in a cupboard beside the platform. But it didn't have the names and telephone numbers of my two friends. I woke up in a state of distress and panic.

Notes

In December 2001, I attended a meeting held by the Writers' Association of China in Beijing. Making the most of my stay in there, I made two appointments at an oncology hospital. The first was with a woman specialist in Traditional Chinese Medicine. The medicine she had prescribed me last time turned out to be extremely efficacious. The second appointment was with an otolaryngologist. It was relatively easy to get an appointment in Beijing, unlike in Guangzhou, where the otolaryngology department is saturated due to the high rate of nasopharyngeal cancer.

The day of the appointments coincided with the election of the association's governing board. My colleagues were thoughtful and had reserved a car to take me to the hospital. Touched by their gesture, I said I'd be back in time for the meeting. I told the driver to return directly to the meeting after my hospital appointments. Things would be relatively simple, as I'd already had a colour Doppler at this same hospital. I only needed to show the results to the surgeon and discuss the possibility of an operation. It was a mere formality.

As luck would have it, the waiting-room was almost empty. The otolaryngologist looked at the colour Doppler closely and examined my scar, and we chatted in a friendly fashion. He knew I was in Beijing for a meeting, and I felt comfortable and grateful. It was my first consultation with this specialist. He was pleasant, didn't treat me like a sick person and took his time to answer my questions. Doctors like him are rare.

When he had finished, he said: "After your meeting, you must come back to the hospital for an operation." Then with his hand, he indicated how he was going to make a long incision on the left side of my neck and an incision in the shape of an S on the right, going back to the nape of the neck.

I was stunned.

"I have to discuss this with my family first," I said. "And also, I can't claim medical expenses that are incurred in Beijing. The last time, when I had an operation in Guangzhou, I couldn't get a refund."

"You must stay in Beijing for the operation. I can tell from examining your scar that the lymph node dissection wasn't a success."

"I only had the operation in February. A test I had in May showed there were still malignant cells."

A patient was standing outside the office. The doctor waved for him to come in. He showed me how this patient's scar was different from mine, even though he'd also had a lymph node dissection. His scar went from the top to the bottom of the neck before going back up to the nape.

I was speechless. My scar went from the top to the bottom of my neck without going to the back of my neck. Maybe this explains why the lymph node dissection hadn't removed everything. The patient studied my scar, relieved that it hadn't happened to him. The doctor went out to look for a pathologist, and together they examined my scar. Then two young doctors came in, followed by another patient. They had come to look at the results of a botched operation.

When the pathologist left, a young doctor came in with a camera. He gave it to the otolaryngologist, then stood, arms crossed in front of him, waiting for the specialist to speak. I knew that pose only too well. When I was at the endocrinology department in another hospital, I became a medical case study for doctors in western and Traditional Chinese Medicine. The students were listening to their teacher in the exact same pose, with their arms crossed in front. Some were holding a notebook.

The specialist was full of enthusiasm. He started taking photos of my scar: "Do you mind if I take some photos for reference?" he asked. The camera was clicking away, and I turned my head, so that my face wouldn't appear on the photos. My reason was telling me that this was my contribution to medical education. "No, no. Go ahead," I answered, trying to keep my face as far away as possible from the lens. I didn't want my tired and pale face to be in the photos.

I felt reassured that the look in these people's eyes was kind, without contempt or malice. The specialist was friendly, and he told me to come back to the hospital as soon as the meeting was over.

I left the hospital in a daze. My mind was a blank. The driver was waiting for me. It was the end of December, and the weather was cold. It cheered me up to see the driver outside with the car. On the way back, just to fill in the silence, I talked and thanked him. He was doing his job, but was polite and good-humoured, and never showed any signs of impatience. Sorry that I had made him wait for several hours, I chatted away in an effort to provide him with some distraction.

I attended the meeting as if nothing had happened. I talked to my colleagues and discussed various projects with them. But my heart was heavy. I had the impression that Li Lanni's soul was staring at me from the right side of my temple. I was like a human puppet.

Read the newspaper. The *Yangcheng Evening News* talks about how difficult it is to make an appointment with a doctor. The article talked about how at 4:30

am on 14th August 2007, there were 46 people waiting to consult a specialist in the lobby of the Guangzhou First Hospital, which belongs to the Faculty of Medicine and of Chinese Pharmacology. The first patients had arrived at 1 o'clock in the morning to wait for an appointment, since the specialists only see out-patients once or twice a week, and accept no more than 20 or 30 patients. There had been a sharp drop in temperature after several days of rain. Some of the patients were wearing thick winter clothes, while others had brought blankets with them. One couple, who'd brought a suitcase, was making instant noodles in the waiting room.

I was still trying to decide if I wanted to go through another operation when the otolaryngologist who'd advised me to continue with my chemotherapy referred me to a Traditional Chinese Medicine physician. He took me to see her and asked her to give me an appointment. When the specialist left to go back to his office, I saw that she didn't seem too pleased about it. I felt awkward and didn't know if I should stay or leave. I waited for a long time in front of her office door. Then she looked up, glanced at me poker-faced, and wrote out a ticket for an appointment. Relieved and grateful, I quickly took the ticket and waited outside her office. I would be last on the waiting-list.

When my turn finally came, the staff was finishing up for the day. The woman physician took my pulse and prescribed some medication. She looked pale and tired. I felt guilty and understood her expressionless face. There were too many patients, but not enough doctors, let alone specialists. Doctors had to cope with enormous stress and a heavy workload. The medication she prescribed me was efficacious, and she advised me to finish the whole course.

The second time I consulted this woman physician, I went at the same time of day, but all the appointments had been taken. At the reception desk, someone kindly informed me that I had to be there before 5 o'clock in the morning to make an appointment. Because, unlike the other doctors, she didn't make appointments over the phone.

Physically, it would be impossible for me to do that.

Normally, I went to bed at 1 or 2 o'clock in the morning. I would often wake up in the middle of the night and only go into a deep sleep in the early hours of the morning. If a cycle of treatment lasted for six months, I would have to get up at 4 in the morning, twice a week, to go to the hospital to make an appointment. It wouldn't work out in the long run. Taking the bull by the horns, I decided to spend the morning hanging outside the physician's office and managed to get an appointment. She said I couldn't do that every time. She had many patients to see, sometimes up to 50 or 60 in just one morning.

I understood that she wouldn't grant me this favour the next time. After buying my medicine, it was already 1 in the afternoon when I got home. If this happened every time, it would wreak havoc on my nerves and I would be appalled by my own brazenness for days afterwards. At the time, I didn't know I had depression. All I knew was that my life made no sense. It wasn't at all what I had wanted for myself, and it felt humiliating.

The film *Titanic* came to mind. The woman physician was like a lifeboat with limited capacity. What would be the point of fighting for a place on it?

I decided not to make any more appointments with her.

I wanted to live and die naturally.

Going back to the Writers' Association of China in December 2001:

If my memory serves me correctly, the closing ceremony of the meeting was on the following day of my consultations at the oncology hospital. There was, as usual, a breakfast buffet. I was sitting at the same table as Deng Yiguang and Zhang Hongsen. They were my fellow students from the creative writing course organised by the Writers' Association of China in 1998. Out of the 20 participants, 10 of them were present at the meeting. Since many of them had read Cheng Wenchao's article "The Book of Life" published in *Literature Magazine*, they were asking after my health.

Deng Yiguang asked me if the consultations went well. I explained to him that the doctor wanted me to go back to the hospital to undergo two surgical interventions. I said I was afraid to go under the knife again. Zhang Hongsen asked me what I was going to do. I answered: "I don't know yet. I'm going back to Guangzhou first." I talked to them briefly about my last operation and my feelings.

"Don't worry," Deng Yiguang said. "When you come back to Beijing for your operation, I'll come with our other colleagues to see you and give you moral support."

"Not knowing the doctors well isn't a problem," Zhang Hongsen said. "The other colleagues and I, we can send them books as gifts."

They decided not to wait, and set about putting their plan into action. Zhang Hongsen suggested that I should call Zhu Sujin, the other writers of the Literary Institute, and my classmates from the creative writing course at Nanjing University who hadn't attended the meeting to ask them to also send books to the doctors. Zhang Hongsen said: "Screenplays for the cinema and television are immensely popular. Tell the others to send these kinds of books." According to Deng Yiguang and Zhang Hongsen, they would bombard the doctors with books, in the hope that they would be touched by their gesture and take good care of me.

At the time, many of the writers from the class of 1998 had written screenplays that had been warmly received by the public: *Team Leader* by Zhang Hongsen, *Turning Point* by Zhang Ping, *Sky* by Lu Tianming, *The Way of Man* by Zhou Meisen, etc.

Before the closing ceremony, I briefly explained my situation to He Shen, Tan Ge and Guan Renshan. They agreed to send the books immediately after the meeting was over. I gave them the names of the otolaryngologist and the other specialists in western medicine and Traditional Chinese Medicine.

In truth, I was neither too enthusiastic nor optimistic about their plan. But Deng Yiguang's and Zhang Hongsen's survival instincts were stronger than mine. For without their encouragement or support, I wouldn't have had the courage to ask this favour of my colleagues. I didn't want to bother other people. I was moved by the positive attitudes of Deng Yiguang, Zhang Hongsen and the "Three Horse Chariots" of Hebei. They helped alleviate some of my anxiety. I decided that I would only approach them if the opportunity presented itself, and that there would be no point in asking them once I left Beijing.

When the meeting was over, I was able to approach Zhang Ping, Lu Tianming and Zhang Pinchang. They all agreed to help. Lu Lei said he would ask the others, and managed to persuade Deng Gang, Qiao Liang, and from the Lu Xun Literary Institute to help, as well as two lecturers, Zhang Xianliang and Feng Lingzhi.

I don't know how many people there were in the end, but there were a lot: writers from the creative writing class of 1998; writers from the Lu Xun Literary Institute and Nanjing University; many other colleagues and lecturers.

Two months later, the Chinese Medicine physician told me she had received many books, as well as several letters, in which my colleagues had written: "Li Lanni is an excellent writer and a good colleague and friend. Please do your best to help her and make her well again. We would be deeply grateful to you."

The physician is a well-known specialist in her field. Overloaded with work, she was nonetheless touched by my colleagues' gesture. She conducted consultations via telephone with me, sent me prescriptions and even came to see me when she was in Guangzhou for a medical conference.

My colleagues and writer friends had held out a warm helping hand in my time of need. They stood by me at a crucial point in my life. From then on, my surgical interventions became less frequent and the intervals between them longer.

23rd *August 2007*

Correlations

Excerpts from *Depression Explained*

For those who suffer from depression, the fact that they are conscious of the negative influence they have on the people around them could heighten their feelings of guilt. But they are unable to change their attitude [...]. Most people do not have the patience to help and support a sick person for an extended period of time, especially when the person with depression does not appear sick [...]. What people do not understand is that the time needed to heal and recover takes much longer than they think. They might even think that it is because you are lazy.

Gwendoline Smith (New Zealand)

Complementary Notes

I realise that one of the things that contributed to my major depression in 2003 was my fear of undergoing another operation. Feeling helpless and in a constant low mood for a long period of time, I was, as Gwendoline Smith wrote, "in a permanent state of unhappiness or in a situation which [I could not] control."

Depression should have hit me in the spring of 2002. But my colleagues Zhu, Deng and Jiang invited me to spend the holidays with them. Then there was the collective effort to send the books as gifts to the doctors. All this delayed the depression coming to the surface. My situation then can be likened to someone who has accidently fallen from a cliff. The trees and bushes below cushioned the fall, saving me from shattering all the bones in my body. The fact that my depression was pushed back until a year later is crucial. Because in 2002, people in China knew almost nothing about depression, and didn't care to, either. They only began to take notice and try to understand more about it when Zhang Guorong committed suicide, and also when Cui Yongyuan[1] courageously announced that he was suffering from depression.

I learnt one thing. When I was confronted with insurmountable difficulties, those who I thought could or should help me, couldn't or wouldn't.

When God closes one door, He opens another. The blessings He has bestowed upon me are way beyond what I had expected. I no longer had to bear the brunt of people's contempt. He allowed generous and kind-hearted people to reach out to me. He made me go through suffering so I could learn precious lessons from it.

SEVENTY-FIVE

Diary
Wednesday, 26th May 2004 10:40 am

Didn't have any nightmares these last few days but had a dream about travelling: I was standing on lush green grass; colourful clouds were floating by above me; spring breeze was brushing against my face; and I was breathing clean, fresh air. I felt exhilaration at the sight of this beautiful landscape and thought: "It's so beautiful!" Suddenly, my body melted away and my soul was fluttering in the air, like a butterfly.

Unfortunately, I can only remember this part of the dream. What came before and after is a blank.

I've noticed there's a pattern: I can clearly recall the sequence and details of my nightmares, but as for my beautiful dreams, what little that lingers in my mind dissipates quickly. And that is even before I open my eyes.

Why is it that memories of fear and distress stay in my consciousness, whereas those of happiness and joy just vanish? Is it like this for everyone? Or does it only happen to those who have depression?

In reading *The Neurotic Personality of Our Time*,[1] I realised that, although this book was published long ago, many of the author's observations still apply to our world today. It's a classic that has the potential to deeply influence any given society and era.

Notes

Why must I have another operation again? To stay alive.

But why stay alive, Li Lanni?

On 20th February 2000, the evening of my lymph node dissection, I was lying in hospital with all sorts of tubes coming out of me. I had two tubes inserted into an incision in my neck. One was to drain the blood from my surgical wound and had, at the end of it, a transparent plastic bottle that was slowly filling up with blood. My chest, arms and the tops of my feet were covered with tubes and wires that were connected to different machines.

I wasn't allowed to eat or drink during the 24 hours before the operation. The tops of my feet were linked, night and day, via a tube to a perfusion bottle. But I wasn't passing urine. The nurse said my bladder was full and that they were going to insert a urinary catheter. I remembered how the man was sobbing in the therapy room the other day. Apparently, having a urinary catheter is more painful for a man than for a woman. But I was afraid of the shame and embarrassment, as well as the scorn and criticisms that would be directed at me. So I begged the nurse to give me some more time, so I could be spared the humiliation.

I was under general anaesthesia for my first cancer surgery in 1988. I woke up in the middle of the night and had no problems passing urine. I was under local anaesthesia for this operation. The surgical wound was long and deep. The blood vessels had been closed, and the nerves and tendons removed, which could have affected my nervous system. Either the signals from my brain were blocked, or I was in a state of temporary paralysis. I concentrated hard but couldn't trigger the flow of urine. The nurse came over several times and warned me that the situation was becoming critical. It was winter, and I was sweating, although I never sweat, not even in the summer. The humiliation of having a urinary catheter made me redouble my efforts.

For all my previous operations, I had never once asked myself the existential questions of life and death, but there I was, in distress over something that at any other time would seem so insignificant. Finally, to my enormous relief, urine began to flow. It was an emotional moment. I realised only then that passing urine demanded a great deal of energy.

The day after my operation, the doctor came to do his hospital rounds. First he saw the patients nearest the door and, walking past me, went over to the patient by the window. Then he left. I hadn't eaten for 24 hours. I followed him with my eyes, hoping that he would come over. But he left without checking on me. The nurse reminded me to be careful of the tube that was inserted into the surgical wound to drain the blood. She told me to squeeze the plastic bottle every 20 minutes to make sure that the blood was flowing properly.

I didn't know if the doctor had forgotten about me or if he had another reason for not checking on me. When my husband came after work, we discussed what had happened. He said it would be pointless to guess why, and that he would go to see the doctor immediately to express our gratitude. The following day, the doctor came to check on me. I asked him if one of the tubes in my neck could be removed and he gave his authorisation. I'm not saying that doctors become suddenly kind and more humane when you offer them gifts. Within the social pact that is implicit in all human relationships, I tend to see myself as being inferior. I talk about moral values and all that, but I am incapable of taking the slightest offence to my person. Is it weakness, or the kind of hypocrisy that is characteristic of intellectuals? How I loathe myself!

Squeezing the plastic bottle made me nauseous. It was filled with dirty blood. The thyroid tissues and lymph nodes that the doctor removed: Were they lumps of flesh, dripping with blood? Was the surgical wound like a hole in the wall of a house, through which you can see the steel structure, reinforced concrete, electric wiring and internet cables? The liquid in the bottle was sewage water, and I was a pile of rubbish.

Not wanting to bother my family, I didn't let them stay with me the night following my operation. I put the bedpan on a chair beside my bed. I was capable of urinating without help. Around 3 o'clock in the morning, the bedpan was already half full. It was revolting, having it right next to me. The surgical wound was painful and was keeping me awake. With my head pressed against the headboard, I thought: "Why do I have all these tubes stuck into my body? Some of them are pulled out forty-eight hours later, others seventy-two, and some a few days later. Why does it have to be like this? You call this a life? They saved my life just to put me into this state? It's not worth it. I am the mistress of my life and destiny." Then I ripped out the tube on my chest that was linked to the monitor, as well as all the other ones, leaving only the drainage tube in my neck. I felt decidedly better.

I dislike reliving all the emotions I felt after my operations.

When I began writing the "Notes" section, my intention was to talk about my depression. At the time, the subtitle of this book was: 'The Notes and Diary of a Woman with Depression.' But as the writing progressed, I couldn't help but include my personal experience with cancer and surgical procedures. After some hesitation, I decided to keep it in the book only where it's directly related to my depression. Now that the writing is coming to an end, I must untie this emotional knot in me. It is a knot of fear, hopelessness and shame. These emotions are like a bloodstain that I've reduced to the size of a sesame seed. But no matter how small it becomes, it still has enough strength to sap my vital energy and will to live.

As I was writing the last paragraph, I tried to avoid the word "despair." I am a sensible and level-headed person. I understand that despair can come from a lack of self-confidence. It is a weakness that is shameful, and I deserve a slap on the face for it. Every time I am about to write the word "despair," I tell myself: "No, don't write it. Don't say it like that, find another word. Li Lanni, you've lived through many disappointments, but you've never lost hope."

For me, "despair" has moral and religious connotations. It is a taboo word.

When I came across a passage on despair by Spinoza, I realised then that hidden in a dark corner of my heart were feelings of anguish and despondency.

Be strong.

Stop complaining. Every sick person is in pain. Li Lanni, you're not the only one.

Talk about something else.

I was prepping myself psychologically for another operation. This time round, I'd take my time to come to a decision. I wanted it to be clear in my mind, why I was prepared to go through with it. Was that how I envisaged my life?

Chemotherapy brought radical changes to my daily life. I had countless physical ailments, and certain events that were out of my control led to negative repercussions in my life.

I couldn't read or write. Not wanting to cause any inconvenience to conference organisers, I reduced my professional engagements to a minimum. When a group of 20 people from my unit took a trip abroad, I was the only one who had to sign a liability waiver form. Even my husband had to sign one. Before, I was invited to take part in activities because I could make myself useful, but now I was invited because people felt sorry for me.

Chemotherapy left visible signs of damage on my skin, hair and face.

The woman specialist in Beijing asked me to fill in a medical follow-up form, on which there were questions about the changes caused by chemotherapy. When I came to a question about my skin, I stopped writing and asked her: "Do you think my skin was better before I started chemotherapy?" She studied me, reluctant to give an answer. It made me sad. Because since I was little, I've always been told that I had beautiful skin. Sensing my sadness, she reassured me: "It's fine."

Once, when I was having dinner with friends in Shenzhen, a woman socialite joined us. My friends introduced me: "This is Li Lanni." Taken aback, the woman said: "Oh, I didn't recognise you." I said to myself that I didn't know the woman. She said: "We met six months ago at an event. You were in top form then. How are you these days?"

I almost never buy new clothes, except for important occasions, because I much prefer wearing my old ones. And it's also a waste of money. New clothes soak up my energy and, in turn, I must 'feed' them with my vital forces, whereas old clothes are already saturated with my energy and don't sap my strength.

My days were a constant struggle with my illness. If I didn't have insomnia, I had nightmares. Whenever I heard people complaining about being tired because they hadn't slept for a few nights, I thought: "What about those who have insomnia or nightmares every day?"

I would wake up groggy and with a headache. My scar was painful for two years; my right ear was numb for an entire year; every day my throat was red and swollen; and every time I ate out, I would catch some respiratory infection.

An electrocardiogram showed that I had bradycardia, cardiac arrhythmia and a right axis deviation of 110 degrees. Normally my heart rate is a little over 60 beats per minute, but when I was lying down or if there were changes in the weather, it would go down to between 40 and 50 beats per minute. I often felt I was suffocating, even when I was breathing through my mouth. Unable to lie down for long, I had to force myself to stand up.

A gastroscopy showed traces of blood in the stomach, erosive gastritis and superficial gastritis.

I had chronic gastritis. The organic function of the stomach and intestines was reduced.

The specialist in Traditional Chinese Medicine wrote in my medical file: The pulse is short and sinking, Deficient Qi of the Heart, Kidney, Spleen and Stomach, Excessive Fire of the Heart and Liver, Humidity and Heat, unformed stools, micturition problems, bloated abdomen, flatulence, asthenia.

[...]

That's enough.

I don't want to live like this. It's not a life.

I was a sick person without a soul who had been banished to the fringes of society. An ordinary citizen, who was lost and had run out of luck. I was of no more use to anyone, just another bit-part player in this world. I had been stripped of everything: money, power, social status, usefulness, medical insurance. A burden for my family, relatives, friends, unit and society.

The thought that my situation could worsen, and even last indefinitely, plunged me into deeper despair.

If I chose to go through with another operation, I would lose control over my life. I was filled with shame and anger. The worst was still to come. I had lost my dignity, which had been trampled on. My life was unbearable.

Why live?

In preparing myself psychologically for another operation, I discovered that I had no reason to live.

Family, relatives, friends, respect for life, the revolution... None of these reasons were enough.

Why not ask my family, relatives, friends, comrades of the revolution and all those who respect me to let me go? I asked myself with the utmost honesty: "Why should I live for others?"

But what made me hesitate was my faith and moral values.

I was torn between the will to live and the desire to die.

25th August 2007

Correlations

Excerpts from *A Short Treatise on God, Man and His Well-Being*[2]

If, however, the thing is regarded by us as good, and, at the same time, as something that necessarily must come, then there comes into the soul that repose which we call confidence; which is a certain joy not mingled with sorrow, as hope is.

But when we think that the thing is bad, and that it necessarily must come, then despair enters into the soul; which is nothing else than a certain kind of sorrow. [...]

Shame is a certain kind of sorrow which arises in one when he happens to see that his conduct is despised by others, without regard to any other disadvantage or injury that they may have in view.

Spinoza (Holland)

Complementary Notes

I found this passage while going through my books yesterday evening.

Recently, after switching off my computer, I've taken to lying on the sofa-bed with my head and neck hanging over the edge. I face upwards until my head gets tired and then turn over to face downwards. The purpose of this is to direct the blood flow to nourish my brain. I stay like this until the dizziness, caused by my writing work, subsides.

Sometimes, boredom sets in. To stop my mind from being flooded with my inner dialogue, I resort to the method of 'neutralising the virus one by one' – that is, I feed my brain with words. I put a stack of books on the floor and, my head facing downwards, I browse randomly through the books. Maybe it's symptomatic of my obsessive-compulsive disorder. Keeping myself busy like this stops me from feeling guilty and accusing myself of being lazy.

It's rather a strange position to read in, and also quite tiring. My brain has trouble registering the words. If I force myself too hard, my brain acts as if it has a goal keeper that stops the words from coming in. But this goal keeper isn't always on his guard. Sometimes, at the end of one hour or after finishing a book, my brain manages to register one or two sentences. It takes the goal keeper and me by surprise. We're both stunned that my brain had "scored a goal."

That was how the passage from Spinoza entered my brain. Kneeling on the sofa, my mind in a fog, I read the passage twice, asking myself: "What does it mean?" I leaned against the wall and closed my eyes. Rereading the passage again, I realised that what Spinoza was saying corresponded almost point by point to what I was writing in "Notes."

Who was behind this coincidence?

I began having trouble sleeping again this month. I try to live with it. When I turn the computer off at midday, my memories continue to go round and round in my mind. Fragments of my past roam around inside my head, rambling, drifting, aimless and unrestrained. My abdomen is so bloated that I can't eat. I walk around in the apartment for half an hour, rubbing my belly and taking deep breaths. I force some lunch down and continue to pace up and down, like a beast in a cage. At the same time, I practise self-therapy. Finally exhausted, I take a nap on the sofa-bed. But as soon as I lie down, memories come gushing back, like a convocation of eagles swooping down and ripping me to shreds. Eyes closed, mind focused, I try to tame and drive away my memories before they gather strength and become distorted. I pray, reassure and comfort myself: "Hey, little one, don't be afraid. Sleep, sleep. Relax and go to sleep."

But I can't sleep.

So, I practise cognitive therapy. It's usually between 2 and 3 in the afternoon. Then the break is over.

At night, one tablet of alprazolam isn't enough to make me sleep.

Dreams. Dreams that exhaust me. I wake up, drained.

SEVENTY-SIX

Diary
Monday, 31ˢᵗ May 2004 11:05 am

Today is the last day of May. Since the beginning of my therapy for depression, I've acquired the habit of looking at the wall calendar every day. Time is crawling by.

Between 1996 and 1999, I was working in Beijing, Macau and Shenzhen. I was doing interviews, writing scripts on my computer and discussing various projects: novels, essays, television scripts and the different ways to write them. Time passed quickly.

According to some of the books I've read, I was suffering from bipolar depression at the time and was going through a manic episode, during which my creativity was at its height.

After my surgical intervention in February 2000, the pace of my life slowed down. And since the onset of my depression, my biological instruments to measure time have all gone haywire: sun dial, clock and stopwatch alike. It was particularly bad between the end of March and the beginning of April of last year. One minute was no longer one minute.

These last two weeks, the pace of my life has been more or less normal. I keep telling myself: "Appreciate what you eat. Savour the wine and enjoy it." Feel serene and light-hearted.

To celebrate Children's Day, I took Lele to a dog grooming parlour. The groomer shaved the fur on his body, leaving his head and tail untouched. Lele looks even cuter than before.

Dogs are therapeutic for people with depression. They also have a positive influence on autistic children. Dogs are angels from God. They bring us love, well-being, comfort, warmth and confidence.

Notes

According to the newspaper, today is World Suicide Prevention Day. One of the headlines in today's issue says that 80 percent of suicide victims suffer from depression.

At the beginning of 2007, I read a report that said there are 287,000 suicide victims each year in China. According to this report, the primary cause of death for those between 15 and 34 years old is suicide, and there are 2,000,000 failed suicides attempts. The newspaper talked about the director who presided over the first suicide prevention organisation in China. He and a colleague worked together on this project for nine years, helping many people, but he ended his own life on 7th September 1997. Since then, there has never been another professional suicide prevention organisation in Guangzhou.

For half a century after the Second World War ended, deep post-war trauma gradually led to an increase in the number of people with mental illnesses in Europe and the United States. Following this logic, there will be an explosion of mental illnesses in China in the 10 years' time. Are we taking any measures to deal with this phenomenon? China has a population of 1,300,000,000. Will there be enough qualified psychiatrists to cope with this eventuality? The number of people with mental illnesses, as well as those who defy stereotypical thinking, are on the rise. Hidden behind our ever-growing economic numbers is a bomb ready to explode. Concealed behind the accumulation of wealth is a mass of volcanic lava ready to erupt.

The concentration of power, wealth and education is held in the hands of what kind of people? What type of mentality is embedded in our collective unconscious mind? How will the coming two centuries modify our mental DNA? Five centuries from now, will our descendants thank us or curse us?

I've been working non-stop on my writing for the entire month. But I am in bad shape.

The pains in my chest are sharp at times and diffuse at others. In the past, my heart was like a rosebud ready to bloom and unfold its petals, but now it's faded and withered. Even strong coffee can't bring it back to life. To give me a boost so I can continue writing, I take the Chinese medication Xinbao and gingko biloba, but with no effects whatsoever.

For years now, my habit has been to work from 9 in the morning until 3 in the afternoon. But these days, I can't even get started at 10 in the morning, nor even at 4 in the afternoon. When I write, I get all hot and agitated. And it's getting worse by the day. The thought of sitting in front of the computer makes my scalp prickle. I have goose pimples all along my arms and legs, and the muscles in my inner arms and thighs ache. One night a few months ago, I was on the rooftop of my building on the 16th floor. I stood on the security rail, looking down into the void. I had cramps in my inner thighs. It was an instinctive reaction to being up in the heights and meant that I was unable to control my fear.

I am unhappy with Li Lanni. Because she is only capable of expressing one percent of her thoughts and one millionth of her subconscious mind. And even that is nothing much to write home about. Admit it, you're weak. You've triggered a mechanism to delete the memories of your past. That is why you have chest pains, cramps in your limbs and the sensation that ants are crawling all over your scalp. It's a defence mechanism of the Self. Don't worry about it.

My rational mind tells me I am not worried, but my gut feelings tell me otherwise.

I need to rest and be more charitable towards myself. Be kinder to Li Lanni. Let her rest for a few days. I feel sorry for her. She is lazy and doesn't want to dig into the deep and obscure layers of her memory. Better leave her alone.

Alright, let's continue.

There were things to sort out before my operation.

I gave away the pretty clothes that I had never worn, as well as the clothes and accessories that I had worn only once or twice. With the way things were going, I wouldn't be needing them. Keeping them would be a waste. Better to get rid of them now than bother my family later.

Things that I threw away or tore up: documents, contracts, letters and photographs that could give rise to misunderstandings, manuscripts, diskettes, magazines, illustrations, small objects, old address and phone books, make-up and any personal objects that I didn't need anymore. I also emptied my wardrobe, bedside table drawer and desk.

To prepare for any eventuality, I had to gradually cut my ties with people. First, I went to say goodbye to Grandmother in Pingxiang.

During the summer holidays of 2002, I paid Grandmother a visit with my husband, brother and sister-in-law. It was the first time the two families went to Pingxiang together. My brother and his wife had been married for less than a year, and Grandmother was hoping they wouldn't wait too long to have a child. My husband and sister-in-law are both university lecturers, and Grandmother, whose husband was a school teacher, felt an affinity with them. She had a radiant smile on her face. I thought: "This is the last time I am in Pingxiang. I'll always remember Grandmother's glowing smile."

Grandmother didn't know about my health problems. Mother was adamant that I shouldn't tell her about my operation.

"But she'll see the scar on my neck," I said. "What am I going to say?"

"In that case, just tell her that it's a benign tumour."

Grandmother was overjoyed to see us and didn't ask about my scar. She didn't notice that I looked rundown and frail and even chided me for not doing enough exercises, because she walked and climbed the stairs quicker than me.

We went to a photo studio for a family photo.

Like Andrew Solomon's mother, I was preparing myself for the eventuality of another metastasis. I needed time and space. Many cancer patients have similar intentions but few go through with them.

Now, sitting at my computer, it suddenly dawns on me that maybe Grandmother knew I had cancer. She was an intelligent woman and could have understood my situation without mentioning it. In Chinese tradition, keeping silent is one way of easing anxiety.

There was one more thing to sort out before my operation. I had to take care of the formalities to ensure that my apartment would go to my husband.

The social housing reform act was introduced in Shenzhen in 1989, enabling me to buy an apartment in 1991. But this meant that my husband wasn't allowed to acquire an apartment in Guangzhou.

In 1985, I moved into a 77-square-metre apartment. The construction of a batch of residential buildings in the Sun Yat-Sen University was finished in 2000. My husband made a down payment of over 10,000 yuan for an apartment and acquired the right to pay in monthly instalments. In 2001, we moved into an apartment for lecturers that was fitted with a lift. Having a lift was essential for me, because Cheng Wenchao was so weak during the last stage of his chemotherapy that he could barely walk up the seven floors to his apartment. In the end, the university provided him with temporary lodgings until his death.

So, I had to settle everything related to housing. I wanted to sell my apartment back to the government and rent one between 30 and 40 square metres in Shenzhen. My husband could then buy an apartment in Guangzhou, which would solve our housing problems.

One morning, I went to the Housing Department to enquire about the necessary administrative formalities. Seeing the scar on my neck, the clerk was understanding of my situation and said:

"Rent in Shenzhen is more expensive than in Guangzhou. You should give it more thought before making a decision."

"Can people in my situation benefit from any measures that have been put in place?" I asked.

"You'll have to ask my boss," she said, pointing to an office opposite. "He'll tell you all the measures that have been put in place this year. He'll advise you."

I tapped lightly on the door, which was slightly ajar. But there was no reply. I turned around to look at the clerk, who gestured to me to go in. I knocked again, slowly pushed open the door and stood in the doorway. The director was reading the newspaper. I walked over to his desk and politely asked him a couple of questions. Looking bored, he interrupted me:

"No measures have been put in place this year. Don't bother asking."

I had intended to settle as many things as possible before my operation, but didn't expect to come up against so many obstacles. It made me think again.

Finally, I decided not to do anything about it. It just wasn't possible to plan and sort out everything before dying.

Let yourself die in peace. The living will find a solution.

27th August 2007

Correlations

Excerpt from *Our Inner Conflicts*[1]

Our inner needs are the most important. We must keep an emotional distance between ourselves and others [...]. In a society permeated by hypocrisy, deceit, jealousy, cruelty and greed, the weak and vulnerable suffer because of their sincerity. The emotional distance allows us to preserve our intrinsic nature [...]. There is only one reaction in the face of danger – flee or hide [...]. It reveals the fear of having your personality being split up and which manifests itself in dreams or in the association of ideas.

Karen Horney (United States)

Complementary Notes

The last time I went to get my antidepressants at the psychiatric department of the Shenzhen North Hospital, Dr Li told me that 50 percent of cancer patients fall into depression.

Personally, I think that over 95 percent of cancer patients have depression, with 65 percent suffering from moderate to severe depression. Many of them die at the end of one year. But the families only see the biological aspects of the metastasis without understanding that depression plays a role in accelerating the growth and spread of the malignant cells.

In a society that lacks moral values and faith, and where hypocrisy, greed and indifference reign, sick people with cancer don't count. It's not cancer that is frightening. It's society's and individuals' attitudes towards cancer that are terrifying.

SEVENTY-SEVEN

Diary
Wednesday, 2nd June 2004 11:25 am

On International Children's Day, at dusk, I took a photo of Lele on the lawn in front of the physics department. It was fun. Maybe it's my way of making up for an emotional emptiness left over from my childhood.

I don't remember ever having celebrated International Children's Day, let alone spending it with my parents. Those of my generation lacked unconditional and nurturing love in their childhood, giving rise to personality disorders later in life.

I didn't learn anything new from reading *The Neurotic Personality of Our Time*. The author has an in-depth knowledge of the different types of personality disorders that have become normalised and accepted today. Having a behaviour contrary to society's standards is seen to be abnormal.

People of my generation are different from those of the previous generation, and the generation that came after us. As children, we lacked the attention and sense of security that parental love should have provided us. In Chinese culture, it's a taboo to criticise your parents. Harbouring resentment towards them is literally a crime.

In our dysfunctional society, our parents' ignorance and mistakes have harmful repercussions on the family and the mental health of its members. Children suffer from deep psychological wounds, which they are unable to express. They can't cry or ask for help. Repressed emotions are transformed into tumours that become malignant and degenerate into cancer. The cancerous cells spread, invade and destroy us.

Psychiatrists and psychologists all agree that childhood wounds are at the root of many personality disorders.

The fear and anxiety that has built up in us undergo changes. We live in a purgatory, where neither life nor death could bring us peace.

We aren't the only victims. Our parents and children also suffer. We must save our souls.

The first step towards healing is to face up to our wounds and go through 'chemotherapy' with our parents. Chemotherapy is dangerous and painful. The idea is to use poison to kill off another poison. There is no other way to cure cancer. There is no escape from it. After chemotherapy, you enter into a period of convalescence, during which Stagnant Energy and Congealed Blood are dispelled, stimulating the blood's circulation. The road to recovery is long and unsteady.

How many of us have suffered from this kind of cultural taboo?

Notes

The theatre play *Assassin* is in Shenzhen. I went to see it out of curiosity.

A poster at the entrance of the Shenzhen Opera House said: "A man of honour dies for the person who understands his heart. A woman makes herself beautiful for the person she loves."

It was not until the end of the play that the audience learned why the assassin, Yu Rang, wanted to kill Zhao Xiangzi. When Yu Rang was serving his first master, he was a painter-decorator; when he was serving his second master, he was a foreign honorary advisor. Zhao Xiangzi killed his second master. Yu Rang, greatly physically weakened, swore to avenge his master, but his attempts were fruitless. In his determination to succeed, Yu Rang disfigured his own face in order to approach his target. Several times he failed to kill Zhao, who asked him: "Your second master killed your first, but you felt nothing. I killed your second master, and you seek revenge for his death. Why?" Yu Rang replied: "I was only a painter-decorator for my first master, but my second master elevated me to the rank of a public official."

This is why the popular saying: "A man of honour dies for the person who understands him" was the theme of the play. When Yu Rang died, Zhao Xiangzi gave him a state funeral.

I walked home after the play. Thoughts were racing around in my mind. As if I were under the grip of an obsessive-compulsive episode, I kept thinking what "a man of honour" meant. A voice was shrieking in my head: "Where is a man of honour?" The voice, vulgar and domineering, was spinning, charging around inside my head, slapping me, hitting my brain, pulling on my nerves and screaming: "A man of honour can accept death, but not humiliation. A poor man of honour is noble and virtuous, and doesn't let himself be corrupted by wealth. Where is this man of honour? Where is he?"

I had pain in my ears, head and temples, and the *baihui*[1] was boiling hot. I was having hallucinations again. My brain fluid was like tofu simmering in a pot. I was walking, my hands pulling at my hair. The more it hurt, the better I felt. I had to tame and bring to heel the Li Lanni that was in my brain. Suddenly, a strange voice spoke. It was neither in my heart nor in my brain. It seemed to be coming from outside, somewhere in the air. It spoke from behind my neck: "The person who understands you, where is she? I'm asking you, where is she?"

According to one article I read, the suicide rate in Shenzhen is higher than the number of deaths due to road accidents. It said that in the last few years, there have been on average over 2,000 suicides a year. Most of the suicide victims come from a middle-class background. Last year, there were 910 cases of death by road accidents. There are over 250,000 deaths by suicide in China each year. The article said that China has one of the highest rates of suicide in the world. There are 20,000 suicides a year in Guangdong Province alone, and over 100,000 failed suicide attempts.

In the same article, it said that when the Permanent Committee of the People's Assembly of Shenzhen was studying public health development projects, a proposal related to mental health was put forward. As a Shenzhen citizen and a woman suffering from depression, I welcome this initiative, which gives me hope.

Psychiatric research shows that anxiety, depression and criminality are closely related. Our intuition tells us that depression and violence are two facets of the same thing. In other words, aggression can be directed inwards or outwards. Following the hypothesis put forward by psychiatrists in other countries, Shenzhen would be the city most affected by depression and violence in China, and China would be the developing country most affected by this phenomenon. Sometimes, I wonder how many sane people there are, if we exclude the following: elderly people over 80 years old; children under five; people with mental disorders, depression, cardiac and blood vessel diseases; the physically disabled and those who are paralysed; people with AIDS, uremia or autism; the mentally disabled; prisoners and criminals. We live in a dysfunctional society, where there are quarrels and misunderstandings between brothers and sisters, husbands and wives. Love is fragile and transient. Sometimes, we give love but receive hate in return.

8th September 2007

Correlations

Excerpts from *My Depression*

> When I think of suicide, I think of famous people and the methods they used to end their lives.
> Virginia Woolf drowned herself in a river with her pockets filled with stones.
> Kurt Cobain shot himself in the head.
> Sylvia Plath put her head in an oven.
> Mishima Yukio committed hara-kiri.
>
> I've made a list of other possible methods:

Hanging.
Drink wine laced with sleeping pills.
Get beaten to death by the police.
Throw yourself off a cliff in your car.
Slit your wrists.
Cut your throat.
Heroin overdose.
Take the wrong medication.
Go on a date with a pervert.
Put your head in a plastic bag.
Throw yourself off a roof or from a window.
Swim for hours in the sea.
Drown yourself in a swamp.
Try a Houdini disappearing act.
Ride your motorcycle at high speed on an oily road surface.
Etc...

Elizabeth Swados (United States)

Complementary Notes

I agree with Elizabeth Swados when she said we should "learn more about other people's depression."

Since spring of 2003, I've been making efforts to learn how other people cope with their depression. When I go into a bookshop, I head straight for the psychiatry, psychology and medicine sections to see if there are any new titles. I prefer works that have been written by people who have experienced depression themselves. Up until now, all the books I've read on this subject have been written by patients in other countries, who come from all walks of life: psychotherapists, television presenters, script writers, film directors and best-selling authors. In this book, *A Crowded Silence*, I mention books that I've read and quote the passages that seem relevant. Many people wander alone in the dark wilderness, seeking to understand more about themselves and their illness.

The Chinese edition of Ms Swados's book is prefaced by Cui Yongyuan.[2] The preface begins with: "I cannot count the number of times my editor has urged me to finish the manuscript in the shortest possible time. I felt embarrassed, and the editor even more so. The truth is, I had finished the preface a long time ago but had torn it up. It was written with so much honesty that it made even my scalp tingle."

Standing in front of the bookshelf at my home in Shenzhen, I spent a few minutes flicking through *My Depression*. The drawings over-stimulated my mind and made me feel queasy. I was afraid to look at the illustrations in too much detail. Images stimulate the imagination more than text, speeding up the function of the brain. I put the book beside my pillow, so I could read it again before going to sleep. Bad idea. The book's crazy drawings acted like a grinding, ear-piercing sound that was pushing the Li Lanni in my head to scream. Impossible to read it. After switching off the light, I could still feel the presence of the book. I sat up in bed, felt around in the dark, found the book and pushed it towards my feet. But it was still bothering me. So I slipped it in the gap between the bed and the head board. The next morning, I put it back on the bookshelf in the sitting-room.

I took the book with me to Guangzhou. That afternoon, I was leafing through the pages on the train between Guangzhou and Shenzhen. The sun was pouring in through the windows, so I closed the curtains, creating a safe and peaceful atmosphere to help control my thoughts. When I read Cui Yongyuan's sentence: "It was written with so much honesty that it made even my scalp tingle," I realised that others who reread what they have written on depression also feel a prickling sensation in their scalp!

Not so long ago, the thought of getting down to work in front my computer gave me goose pimples all over. I always ended up cutting short my writing just so I could breathe. I was besieged with self-doubt and scolded myself every day. Li Lanni was weak, always looking for excuses to run away. Among those who suffer from depression, was she the most neurotic and cowardly of them all? I came down so hard on myself that despondency began to set in.

Cui Yongyuan wrote: "It made my scalp tingle." Li Lanni, I'll let you off the hook.

I like how other patients in other countries can talk about their weaknesses. Maybe it's because I'm fighting against my own failings and inadequacies. "Learn more about other people's depression" is part of the therapy that helps us heal from our wounds.

Reading the list drawn up by Ms Swados, I realise western and Chinese points of views differ. A western celebrity once said that there are two criteria to understand a man: the kind of woman he chooses to be his wife, and how he chooses to die.

Peasants in China kill themselves by swallowing insecticides, whereas most white-collar workers take sleeping pills.

Apart from the 15 ways to die on Ms Swados's list, there are many more. Every person, who suffers from depression has, at one point or another, thought about the different possible methods. Here are the 12 ways I've often mulled over:

1. Drink alcoholic beverages containing more than 50% alcohol laced with sleeping pills. (But experience shows that it is generally not

efficacious, because of too many failed attempts. Nine out of ten victims remain unconscious for several days, damaging the brain and memory. Then we become a burden for our families for the rest of our lives.)
2. Hang yourself with a silk stocking. (Not a reliable method. To fail at it is humiliating. Even if you were saved in time, the brain can lack oxygen and we become mentally disabled and totally dependent on others.)
3. Slit your wrists in the water. (The blood can coagulate, making it into just a self-harm exercise.)
4. Throw yourself off a 15-storey building. (Must be done between 2 and 3 o'clock in the morning. The higher the building, the greater the chance of succeeding.)
5. Throw yourself off a boat deck. (A rather stupid method. For you can saved by the crew at any moment.)
6. Throw yourself in front of a train. (If this is badly executed, the train driver could be fired from his job.)
7. Get run over by a car. (If you don't die, you might become disabled for life.)
8. Cause an aircraft accident. (This method puts other people in danger. You wouldn't be the only one to die in a plane crash.)
9. Bring about your own death by speeding up the delivery rate of the perfusion. (The chances of success are low. The medical staff will find out and give you a slap on the wrist.)
10. Put yourself in the line of fire. (The chances of finding yourself in such a situation is extremely low.)
11. Gas yourself. (This can cause collateral damage for the family, neighbours and the cleaning lady.)
12. Get yourself electrocuted. (It is not as simple as it sounds. An electric shock could just cause numbness, or you could be thrown backwards and nothing more.)

In considering all these different methods of suicide, one basic principle must be kept in mind: Never cause harm to others. For example: Blow yourself up in a station; contaminate drinking water by jumping into a well; self-immolation; put rat poison in the soup, etc. It wouldn't just be suicide, it would be murder. And it is a crime.

Since the onset of my chronic depression, I pay a lot of attention to stories about suicide.

The other day, I read in the papers that someone tried to set himself on fire at customs in Hong Kong. He didn't die, but a customs officer did.

Someone threw himself into a river, or the sea. He survived, but the person who tried to save him drowned.

In her book *Ordinary Days*, Ms Li writes about how she survived four suicide attempts: taking sleeping pills; gassing herself; slitting her wrists; and swallowing poison. Having looked into these different methods of suicide, I have come to the conclusion that throwing yourself off the top of a building has the best chance of success.

I heard on the news that a fourth-year student attempted suicide on the Guangzhou University campus. He wasn't suffering from depression, but acted on impulse, because his business project had failed. He himself didn't die, but a brilliant 19-year-old girl student did.

It is impossible for those in a deep chronic depression not to think of suicide. No one can stop them from doing that. I can say two things from first-hand experience: One, no matter what happens, you are capable of coming through difficult times; and two, never cause harm to others.

SEVENTY-EIGHT

Diary
Sunday, 6th June 2004 10:10 am

It's been a year since I began the "Diary" section.

But I'm reluctant to reread my previous entries. For I haven't been able to express what matters to me most; that is, to write about my feelings before and after my operations and all my dark thoughts during my depression. Maybe it's because I don't want to think about it, because it would drive me insane. Pain that is unspeakable and untold.

I seem to be living in three different worlds: reality, dreams and imagination. They are so different from one another that it's ripping me apart and sapping my energy. It's like I'm living three separate but parallel lives.

Am I, in fact, three different people?

Which one is Li Lanni?

I don't like any of these Li Lannis.

I wish to see a Li Lanni who is happy, in good health and about to embark on a new life.

Is it worth my while to continue writing the "Diary" section?

I don't know.

When are you going to reread your diary? Answer me, Li Lanni.

Notes

"Little rabbit, little rabbit, be good. Open the door. Quick, quick, hurry up and let me in."

"No, no, no. I don't want to. Mummy isn't home. No one can come in."

In my memory, this is the first song I ever learnt. I don't remember who taught it to me. It could have been the kindergarten teacher or one of the women at the military barracks. This song taught me that the big bad wolf ate little children and that I couldn't trust anyone. Because everybody has it in them to be a big bad wolf. Why do I have such a clear memory of this song? Because I felt anxious and uneasy as a child. What if the big bad wolf disguised itself as my mother and knocked on the door? How would I know that it wasn't my mother? And if my mother ate me up?

I attended a school for military children. Every day, we stood in line in front of the classroom, and a classmate would always count: "The first one farted and chased the second one two *li*[1] away, the third one sharpened a knife and pierced the arsehole of the fourth, the fifth one was flying a plane, bombarded the sixth and made the seventh one sweat, the eighth one played the trumpet and the ninth got blasted in the face." The classmates who were fourth and ninth in line weren't happy and wanted to change places. After a lot of shuffling around, the counting began, and we would all want to change places again.

The teacher never told us fairy tales or myths. I don't even know who taught me nursery rhymes.

The children in town went to an activity centre, where they learnt to recite poems, play the flute and violin. They would listen to Andersen's tales, whereas my friends and I, we would recite lewd poems like: "We told the commander we had no trousers to wear. We went to the general headquarters and took two pieces of cloth. We put one on the left arse and one the right. But you could still see our arses."

Every day, squatting over the latrine, we would hear a classmate, either from the front or the back of the hut, shouting: "Who wants toilet paper... Ah... Red sanitary napkins... Red sanitary napkins...Red... All red. Quick, scram!"

When the boys had nothing better to do, they would imitate the sounds Japanese soldiers made in the film *Landmine Warfare*[2] when they invaded the villages: "Bang! Bang! Bang!" Sometimes, the girls would grab me by the arm and sing: "Little doll Ni, sit down and we'll give you a wash. Scrub, scrub scrub-a-tub-tub, until you become a lump of mud."

When I was at boarding school, the girl on the upper bunk of my bed told me a story about a sleepwalker who ate corpses: "Do you sleep walk? You know what? Someone told me that at the hospital morgue, someone went around eating human flesh at night, but no one knew who it was. On the third night, the doctor told the nurse to smear iodine solution on all the corpses. The next morning, the doctor said to the nurse: 'Let's check everyone to see who has purple teeth.' The nurse screamed: 'It's you!'" Suddenly, the girl pointed a finger at me and shrieked. I nearly jumped out of my skin. Cackling with laughter, she said: "It was the doctor!"

The boarders loved to play these kinds of tricks to scare themselves and others. Sometimes, we would get out of bed in the morning feeling spooked and wondering who had purple teeth. For we were all afraid of being a sleepwalker.

This was the environment I grew up in. How can I describe the backdrop of my memories? Bland? Sterile? Dirty? Rustic? I only knew how to make war and catch spies. Words like 'science' and 'writer' weren't part of my vocabulary. I had never been to an exhibition, but was familiar with watch towers, knives, rifles, ships, binoculars, trenches, tunnels, canons and grenades. My toys were red-tasselled spears, wooden guns, plastic bands, bamboo arrows, stones, sand bags and batons.

They say that our memory is at the height of its function during childhood. For many scientists, artists, literary specialists, politicians and entrepreneurs, it was during their childhood that their intelligence was stimulated and the foundation of their knowledge laid down. It is a pure and uncorrupted heart filled with beautiful memories that determines your character and abilities, and the direction your life will take. The kind of fertilisers you use play an essential role when it comes to growing trees, vegetables and flowers. The fertiliser's type, quality, quantity and chemical composition (calcium, potassium, phosphorus, azote, zinc) determine how quickly the plants grow, their ability to yield fruits and flowers, and to resist disease or pests.

Let's say I was a turnip seed, and loyalty and courage were my fertilisers. Even if I had been fed with a bit of calcium, this little turnip shoot would still have been frail with yellowing leaves, covered in insects. Adding more fertilisers just before the harvest wouldn't have changed anything. I would still have been a turnip that weighed only a few grams - bland, soggy and with a peculiar taste.

11th September 2007

Correlations

Excerpts from *Memories, Dreams, Reflections* [3]

The story of my life is an attempt to fully develop my subconscious.

I dreamt that [...] I was talking in Latin. A gentleman, wearing a curly-haired wig, was talking to me and asked me a difficult question. Upon wakening, my first thought was of the book I was writing at the time, *Psychology of the Unconscious*, as well as the question that I could not answer. It made me feel ashamed of myself [...] It was not until many years later that I understood my dream and my reaction in my dream. The man in the wig was the spirit of an ancestor [...] He asked me the question, hoping to know all that he was unable to while he was in this world [...] If consciousness exists after death, then I think it serves to perpetuate the consciousness of the human race. In every period of history, the ability to change our consciousness is limited.

Jung (Switzerland)

Complementary Notes

I don't know how to interpret dreams, but the subconscious is a subject that interests me enormously. Research books on this subject are few and far between in China, and I haven't read any that talk about it in a compelling way. Nowadays, medical specialists attach great importance to cutting-edge technology, and their publications are aimed at specialists. They are not interested in popularising science for the general public. Even the cultural community pays little attention to subjects on the subconscious. It is a shame that we put so much focus on the superficial aspects of society.

You can gain a clear perspective on what readers are looking for, and the subjects they're interested in, from the best-sellers that are on display in bookshops. In one sweeping glance, I see: urgency, restlessness, impatience and carnal desires. In this materialistic world, every minute must be used to the fullest.

Many years ago, bookshops used to be empty and deserted. At the time, I wished they would be more lively and vibrant. But today, I wish they would be quieter.

SEVENTY-NINE

Diary
Tuesday, 8th June 2004 10:30 am

Didn't expect to pick up the thread of the "Diary" section so soon. Thought I could do without cognitive therapy for a while. Health is stable. No more nightmares, which always wreak havoc on my mind and nerves.

But I had a dream in the early hours of the morning.

The beginning and the end are blurred. Only one part keeps coming back into my head:

I came across an old warehouse by chance. A woman who had hanged herself was dangling from the roof of a building. She was attractive, in her 40s, and reminded me of Song, a classmate of mine. Suddenly, the woman was standing in front of me, at a near distance. I could see her so clearly: puffy, purplish-blue face; heavy and swollen eyelids; stiff body. I don't know if her chin was naturally fatty or if it was because the rope was too tight, but her double chin was quite peculiar. The second chin was sagging so much that it looked as if it was going to fall off. Her torso and limbs were slightly bloated. But the expression on her face wasn't scary, as if she felt relief at having been freed from this world.

Suddenly, I felt a rush of fear and quickly left. I decided not to mention it to anyone, as if I hadn't seen anything. I vaguely knew that the woman had committed a crime, that she was under investigation but didn't deserve to die. Maybe she had cracked under pressure and decided to end her life.

The next part was blurry. Then, together with some other people, I paid a visit to the woman's family. Her parents welcomed us warmly, offered us tea and invited us to eat with them. While doing the cooking, they talked and laughed with us, as if they didn't know that their daughter was dead. I found this deeply disturbing. Maybe the woman wasn't their daughter; maybe they didn't know their daughter was in trouble. When the meal was ready, the mother went outside quietly. When she came back in, she looked tired. You could tell she had been crying, but was pretending that everything was alright. I thought: "Maybe she untied her daughter and put her somewhere safe, waiting for the night to come to bury her." I felt comforted for the dead woman. She may have committed a crime, but her parents still loved her. I felt upset for the parents, for their daughter had killed herself. Her body hadn't even been buried, and they had to entertain guests.

In my head, I saw the bloated corpse with the purplish-blue face and was overwhelmed with emotions: sadness, fear, pity, understanding, confusion.

I woke up with a splitting headache, heaviness in my chest, and my mind in a fog. I lazed around in bed for a while.

Putting this dream on paper helps me to forget it. There's no point in delving into its meaning. I don't have the energy and have no idea what this dream might symbolise. I only know that I have to continue taking my medication.

Notes

Had a dream. Woke up at 5:45 am. Went to the toilet at 3 am. Had this dream between 4 am and 5 am.

Can't remember the beginning... I was staying in a holiday club in Beijing. It was autumn and the weather was cool.

The holiday club was manged by a family and was made up of flat-roofed bungalows and a big courtyard. To go to the rooms, you had to cross a big lounge that was located in the centre of the club. The rooms and furniture were old, antique-styled, but in good condition. In the lounge, an old woman in her 70s was manging the staff, who all seemed to be family members. She was friendly and courteous; she wanted to know why I had come to Beijing and asked about my family. She told me to make myself at home, that I could stay as long as I liked and that she knew my family. I was taken aback, thinking she had made a mistake.

It was an exclusive members-only club but was far from luxurious. The staff didn't speak and pottered around as if they were at home. From time to time, a couple of guests came into the lounge, but they didn't speak either. It was calm and quiet.

Wang Yun arrived. I was wondering how she knew I was there but was glad to see a familiar face. She said: "We'll spend the day together in Beijing."

I followed her outside, but instead of finding myself in a lively part of the city, I was on a main road. Pedestrians and cars were passing by, and I felt at ease in an environment that I was familiar with. Wang Yun was the senior writer and editor when I was script-writing for the Centre of Television Production of China, and I trusted her. Pointing to a sign on the side of the road with 'Huizhou – Hong Kong' written on it, she suggested we go there. I said: "No, it's too far. We can go another time." She said: "We'll go by bike to an interesting place."

Wearing a windbreaker, I was riding on a mountain bike on the main road and arrived at a crossroad. On the side of the road was an island, where pedestrians and cyclists could wait for the lights to turn green before crossing.

There was also a red and white railing on the side of the road. Suddenly, I noticed that a group of Chinese and foreign professional cycling champions were following behind Wang Yun. The bicycle in front of me was stylish; the cyclist was tall and wearing a bicycle helmet. Leaning forward, he was ready to pedal. I copied him and leant forward, my eyes on the red light. But the lights wouldn't turn green. At that moment, three or four children on roller skates glided in front of me and began to play on the railing. I thought: "Who do these children belong to, hanging around on the streets like this? Where are their parents?" I looked around me to see if their parents were anywhere nearby. The cyclist I'd copied was already miles ahead of me. Wanting to catch up with him, I pedalled as hard as I could and arrived at another main road. All the cycling champions were gone, and Wang Yun was nowhere in sight. She must have thought I was behind her. I continued on that road but suddenly stopped dead in my tracks. Something was wrong. I couldn't see the end of the road. Tall buildings, like the skyscrapers you see in Manhattan in New York, stood on both sides of the road. Beautiful, impressive and elegant, they stretched out into the horizon.

My vision became blurred, and my eyes were irritated and watery. I tried wiping them but still couldn't see clearly. Annoyed, I thought to myself: "Wang Yun will be looking for me. I'll go back to the crossroad to wait for her." But after a while, she still hadn't appeared. I noticed that next to the island for pedestrians was another road. Could Wang Yun have taken this route? But I went down another road that was empty and abandoned. The sea was on one side and several old houses were on the other. I couldn't see the end of that road either. There must surely be another crossroad, where the two roads met.

I got down from my bicycle and carried on down this road. But I felt uneasy. Why was the road empty? What if thieves were hiding inside these houses? Feeling nervous, I returned to the intersection but didn't know the way back to the holiday club, nor where these two roads led. Then I found a wallet and a packet of tissues in the pockets of my windbreaker. Glad and relieved to have some money on me, I could now go to a coffee shop if I became tired. I wiped the tears from the corner of my eyes with the tissues and felt much better.

I strolled along the empty road that led to a beach. I thought it was odd that Beijing had such a wide open sea. The water was clean and of a light-green colour, but no one was on the beach. I walked along the coast and saw a reef made up of huge clusters of large, powerful, sturdy rocks. They were a dull, dark brown but didn't have a single seashell on them. Waves crashed against the rocks, breaking up into tiny droplets of greenish-white sea spray that flew into the air.

Suddenly, a rush of anxiety swelled up in me.

I remembered the tunnels the soldiers had dug on the island. I was nine years old. Alone at dusk, on my way to dinner at the home of a division head, I had to walk through a cave in the reefs. The cave was slightly taller than an adult and was large enough to hide several people inside. It was eerie and sinister. I could hear the thunder of the waves as they thrust themselves with all their power against the rocks. I was terrified that a sea monster hidden in the cave would eat me up; or that the cave would be submerged by the sea; or that I would be carried away by the waves. I hung around outside the cave, not wanting to go, but night was falling, and waves were pounding against the rocks. I was afraid to look. My head and face were moist with sea spray. I peeped through my squinted my eyes to see if the waves were going to come thundering towards me. This experience left its mark on me. Since then, I hated seeing violent waves breaking against rocks.

I wanted to run far away from the reefs. I didn't dare look. The horizon was hazy with mist. Waves of white foam were rolling across the sea but, suddenly, they swelled up, rearing high into the air and came roaring towards me. I didn't have time to run or close my eyes and saw the waves crash against the reefs and break up, like a flower unfolding its petals. The flower's stigma was white. A cascade of light green petals came showering down, like a dazzling, resplendent firework lighting up the sky. I shouted: "It's so beautiful!" Bursting with joy, I felt happy and free.

I woke up in a state of exhilaration.

And my head wasn't aching.

12th September 2007

Correlations

Excerpts from *Tao Te Ching*[1]

Colour's five hues from th' eyes their sight will take;
Music's five notes the ears as deaf can make;
The flavours five deprive the mouth of taste;
The chariot course, and the wild hunting waste
Make mad the mind; and objects rare and strange,
Sought for, men's conduct will to evil change.

Therefore the sage seeks to satisfy (the craving of) the belly, and
not the (insatiable longing of the) eyes. He puts from him the
latter, and prefers to seek the former.

———

Thus we may see,
Who cleaves to fame
Rejects what is more great;
Who loves large stores
Gives up the richer state.

Who is content
Needs fear no shame.
Who knows to stop
Incurs no blame.
From danger free
Long live shall he.

———

Misery! — happiness is to be found by its side! Happiness! — misery lurks beneath it! Who knows what either will come to in the end?

———

Therefore the place of what is firm and strong is below, and that of what is soft and weak is above.

———

It is the Way of Heaven to diminish superabundance, and to supplement deficiency. It is not so with the way of man. He takes away from those who have not enough to add to his own superabundance.

———

Sincere words are not fine; fine words are not sincere […]
Those who know (the Tao) are not extensively learned;
the extensively learned do not know it.

[…] The more that he expends for others, the more does he possess of his own; the more that he gives to others, the more does he have himself.

With all the sharpness of the Way of Heaven, it injures not; with all the doing in the way of the sage he does not strive.

Complementary Notes

For 10 years, between 1989 and 1999, I took a particular liking to the colour white. It became something of an obsession.

The more the streets of Shenzhen were noisy and chaotic, the more I needed to find comfort in white.

Almost every evening during these 10 years, I was out attending parties or some social event. While drinking, smoking and laughing with friends, a little voice in me said: "Colour's five hues from th' eyes their sight will take... Music's five notes the ears as deaf can make..." It was unnerving.

After my lymph node dissection, we entered into a new millennium. I went out much less in the evenings. Several friends, who worked as directors and were studying at the same time, told me about the book *Tao Te Ching*. I asked them if the phrase: "Music's five notes the ears as deaf can make" was from Laozi. Then a friend gave me the book as a present, saying it was, in his opinion, the best edition.

Less than a year later, someone filed a complaint against one of these friends, and he was subsequently transferred to another company. He said: "I hope the good guys won't always be casualties of office politics and backstabbing. It reassures me that my successor is honest and competent." However, a few months later, his successor also fell prey to office intrigues and was ousted from his post. He said to me: "My conscience is clear. I hope the truth will come to light one of these days."

I asked myself: "Why do good people always come up against so many setbacks? Does it make them lose faith in life?"

EIGHTY

Diary
Thursday, 10th June 2004 10:40 am

What's happening? Many years ago, I had a dream that made me so sad. I dreamt of it again.

For 10 years, between 1992 and 2002, my dreams often made me unhappy. In these dreams, I felt humiliated, disappointed, upset and sad. My sorrow was so overwhelming that it would wake me up with a start. I would go through all the details of the dream in my head. And like someone who had fallen into quicksand, the more I struggled, the deeper I sank.

These dreams had a particular flavour to them. When they became painful, the images would be blurred and give off a sweet and sour smell. It's difficult to describe. Sometimes during the day, the air I breathed would be saturated with it. I never tried to analyse this sensation, but my instincts told me that it was sorrow.

There are no words for this sorrow. I've never talked about, let alone put it down on paper. If it's possible to write about it, then it wouldn't be the sorrow that I felt. Only my soul can understand. It's a pity that I didn't know how to ask God for help a few years ago and had to face up to the hardships alone.

I haven't had this kind of dream for several years now. And I keep telling myself: "Forget the past and move forward into the future."

Don't be afraid. Don't be worried. Don't be sad.

Who has never been sad? What matters most is knowing how to ask God to heal us. "We went through fire and water, but you brought us to a place of abundance."[1]

Notes

For many years, I took a particular liking to the colour blue. The whole spectrum – from light blue to dark blue. Everything in cotton, silk, and velvet was in blue. Bedsheets, pillow cases, quilt covers and curtains were all in blue.

Someone wrote this on a piece of paper, but I've forgotten where I came across it: "Blue is the colour most suitable for healing wounds." My brain said to my heart: "Li Lanni, you're blessed. You need the colour blue, you need to heal your wounds."

The colours that you like are determined by your subconscious. It has nothing to do with fashion, nor whether the colour itself is pretty or not.

One of my earliest memories was of liking the colour green. During the Cultural Revolution, bright red and khaki green were extremely popular. My head told me to surround myself with these colours, but my subconscious made me keep my distance.

When I am in a lively and vibrant city, or when I'm going through periods of intense activity, my subconscious needs the colour white to tone down my stress. It's a gut reaction. When the organs in my body and my mental capacities begin to malfunction, I instinctively seek comfort in the colour blue.

When I'm recovering from depression, I like to wear red clothes: pale red, cherry red, burgundy, scarlet, carmine red. Even my alarm clock, cushions, travel tumbler and suitcases are red. Because this colour lifts my spirits and gives me courage.

Our subconscious sends us signals according to our needs. But life in society is noisy and chaotic. If we are restless and agitated, we can't hear these signals. As time passes, we fall prey to illness, traipsing from one doctor to the next. It's better to be still and listen to what your body tells you. Listen to the voice inside and let it guide you towards joy and serenity.

18th September 2007

Correlations

Excerpts from *A Gift for God: Mother Teresa of Calcutta*[2]

If we cannot love the people we see every day, then how can we love those we come across in life? [...] First, try to show that you care for your children, husband or wife with a few kind words or by helping those around you, at work or at school.

Being hungry does not always mean that you hunger for food. You can hunger for love. Being naked does not always mean you have no clothes to wear. It can mean you are stripped of your dignity. Being homeless does not always mean we do not have a roof over our heads. It can mean being abandoned.

[...] I do not know what the world would be like if there were no suffering. People live in pain, while preserving their love and dignity.

[...] Today, I have come to receive a prize in the name of the poor, the sick and the lonely in this world.

Mother Teresa

Complementary Notes

I bought *A Gift for God* several years ago. After leafing through it, I put it on my bookshelf, finding it uninspiring and not compelling enough. Even though I admired Mother Teresa, I only had a vague idea of what she was doing.

But illness makes us grow.

Going through the book again, these words flew in my face: "[...] in the name of the poor, the sick and the lonely of this world." I saw myself in these words. I was sick, poor and lonely. She had received the Nobel Prize in the name of all of us. She understands, respects and protects the outcasts of this society.

EIGHTY-ONE

Diary
Thursday, 17th June 2004 10 am

Had a stroll around Xiju Gardens yesterday at dusk. When I left home, clouds were gathering in the sky towards the south. As the popular saying goes: "Clouds in the east, the wind comes up; clouds in the south, the rain falls in torrents." But the clouds seemed more towards the west. Thunder was rumbling in the distance, and people were walking briskly. I was still strolling along with Lele, who was chewing on grass here and there.

The drops of rain were hard like hail stones. Suddenly, the sky darkened. Shafts of lightning flashed through the air, and thunder rolled above my head. Lele and I, we dashed under a pavilion. Rain was lashing down, and I opened my umbrella.

I sat down on the stone bench with Lele lying at my feet. The gardens were empty, except for a few frogs hopping around. Lightning ripped through the sky, and the thunder cracked with violence. But Lele wasn't afraid. Looking up, he watched the rain fall, barking from time to time. I felt reassured.

Since my early childhood, I've been terrified of storms. Holding Lele against me, I shouted at the top of my lungs: "We're not scared!" The warmth of Lele's body soothed me. I was beginning to appreciate a world seen through this sudden rain storm and recited out loud: "The Lord has done it this very day; let us rejoice today and be glad,"[1] and: "Thanks to God for my Redeemer, thanks for all Thou dost provide [...] Thanks for pain and thanks for pleasure, thanks for comfort in despair."[2] Then I sang: "Hallelujah, praise the Lord... Hallelujah, praise the Lord..."

Lulled by a sense of spiritual calm, I felt free and happy.

It was still pouring, and my umbrella was soaked. A thunderous boom reverberated in the sky. I closed the umbrella and put Lele on the stone bench so he could stretch out, allowing me to quietly take in all the sensations the thunderstorm brought me. I was un-anxious, for I knew the storm would pass, making way for a bright, clear freshness.

The downpour subsided into a soft, fine rain. The grass was an emerald green. Thunder growled in the distance, and the flashes of lightning were no longer as dazzling. Lele and I came out from under the pavilion and continued our walk in the gardens, which was more refreshing and uplifting than usual.

This is my life.

Notes

Lele is four years old. He celebrated his birthday last Wednesday. His present was a soft toy horse. It has baby pink and blue spots on its light-yellow fur. Its tail is like a small flower, and when you pull on it, music starts to play: do re fa so ti la mi la ti do fa.

I clapped my hands to the tune and sang: "Lele is so handsome, so very, very handsome." Puzzled, he stared at soft toy horse, tilting his head from left to right, thinking: "Why is this thing singing?" With his mouth, he took it by the neck, as if it were his prey, and shook his head vigorously. Then he raced around wildly in the apartment, still holding it in his mouth. Suddenly, he stopped and looked at me happily with his bright sparkling eyes. He wanted me to take his toy. I ran after him, shouting: "The toy is mine! Give it to me! I'm going to catch you!" Lele was beside himself with joy. His mischievous, smiling black eyes were gleaming with happiness. We played "catch the thieves" together, running from the sitting-room to the study and then from the study to the bedroom. He scurried under the bed, holding the soft toy in his mouth, and looked at me, waiting to see how I was going to grab his toy. It felt a bit silly that an adult like me couldn't catch that little rascal. I have no authority whatsoever. I lay on the floor, looked under the bed and tried to squeeze myself in to catch him. But he was too quick for me. He scampered out and stood outside the bed looking at me. I tapped on the floor, laughing and scolding him.

We were so happy together.

I was catching up on my lost childhood. And living moments of happiness that I never had.

Correlations

Excerpt from "Military Base"

I received an invitation to visit a military base but hesitated before accepting.

I lived on a military base for the field unit until the age of nine. During their childhood and youth, military daughters like me feel closer to the army than to their parents. The military base was my world. In the years when my mind was beginning to open up to the world around me, my parents were assigned to a maritime outpost located on an island. The army was preparing for war. I was separated from my parents and lived as a boarder in an ugly and austere school for military children. When our teachers were denounced and sent away, I, together with a handful of children, had nowhere to go. Days went by in a kind of hopelessness, in an environment deprived of culture and education.

Many years later, I became sick with cancer and underwent three operations and five courses of chemotherapy. I also suffered from severe depression. Writing *A Crowded Silence* awakened dormant memories in my subconscious. I relived the sadness, pain and loneliness of the military child that I was. My parents were stationed on an island outpost. They had lived the glory of war, but I never witnessed this mysterious glory with my own eyes. Only its ashes.

I was in the middle of writing the sixth part of *A Crowded Silence* when I received the invitation. I hesitated before accepting, because I didn't want to be disappointed. When I left the military base with my parents to live in the outside world, the military system was in the initial stages of reform. Later, I settled down in Shenzhen alone, without my family. Economic reforms were being put in place. At the time, the army was going through a difficult transformation period. I wanted to visit a modern military base, but was afraid of being confronted with the negative changes that I had heard about. Deep inside, I knew that I would always be a military daughter. I disliked hearing people telling untruths about the army. For I wanted to protect the magical place that the army holds in my heart.

It was with mixed emotions that I visited the military base with a delegation of writers.

I visited the missiles division, land forces, parachute division, air force, submarine division and naval division. The military men and women I met were strong, modern, loyal and skilful in the art of war. The principle of "have no fear of hardships, have no fear of death" was still very much alive. The overall level of competency of the modern army was much higher than in the past. The officers and soldiers talked of 'scientific development,' 'the principle of the primacy of man over machine,' and of 'computerisation and digitalisation.' There were psychotherapists on the military base and health magazines in the reading rooms. The military men and women were fit and healthy, and enjoyed a high quality of life. I felt moved, seeing the army's scientific progress, military capabilities and humane advancements.

I admired the vigour and iron discipline of the modern army. I loved the look of determination and rectitude in the eyes of the soldiers. On seeing their tanned faces, faintly tinged with pink, I felt their loyalty, strength and courage.

Every day, I try to heal the wounds of my soul. And every day, I am filled with pride for the soldiers of the people. To have a modern army that is loyal to the Party allows China to develop in peace and stability, and have a voice on the international stage.

There was a photograph in the military culture club: A group of soldiers, covered in mud and dust, on their way back to the base. A military child of about five or six years old was walking in front of them. Wearing an outfit with cartoon characters, he looked mischievous with a little smile playing at the corner of his lips. His face beaming, he was looking up at the soldiers, eyes filled with joy and admiration.

When the army went south, Mother was 16 years old. One night, the troops were marching in the rain on a slippery and muddy road. With a rucksack on her back, she looked like a mud figurine. Close to exhaustion, she could barely walk. An old, experienced soldier walking behind her suggested she should carry her rucksack in her arms. He was responsible for the artistic regiment's make-up and costumes. The girl soldier asked: "Does Chairman Mao know that we're marching?" The old soldier replied: "Of course he does." That night, with strengthened faith, the young soldier marched into a new era of China.

In 2004, I visited the Jiuquan Satellite Launch Centre. But it was the military cemetery that left an indelible mark on me. It was empty, except for the rows and rows of neatly aligned grey-white headstones. They say that before the cemetery existed, soldiers who died in combat were buried in the desert. Many years later, no traces of their bodies could be found. On seeing the names of generals and foot soldiers engraved on the headstones, I asked myself: "How many of us know about these men's selflessness and spirit of sacrifice?"

My visit to the military base gave me the answer I was looking for. In the corridor of the housing unit, a phrase was displayed on the wall. It said: "No words are needed, our fatherland knows of our existence."

I am forever grateful to the soldiers of my country.

15th July 2007

Complementary Notes

On my visit to the military base, I had a little too much to drink and was drunk for the first time in my life.

Even though I am not a heavy drinker, I have a high tolerance for strong alcohol. In 10 years, I've only had two minor incidents. The first: After drinking cold beer, I had strong, stabbing pains in my stomach. As I can't take cold drinks and don't like beer much, it taught me not to touch the stuff again. I went to the nearest clinic for an analgesic injection. The second incident was during my chemotherapy course. The doctor had ordered me not to drink alcohol, but completely oblivious to the danger, I took my medication after drinking a glass of red wine. Several minutes later, I had chest pains, was vomiting and shaking. My friends called an ambulance, and I was admitted into the emergency services at the Shenzhen Futian Hospital.

Sometimes, I envy my friends who can drink. It's amusing to see them get drunk. They start babbling, and their true nature comes out: candid and endearing.

Before my visit to the military base, I had never been drunk. Sometimes, I would drink a little too much and start talking a bit louder than usual. But the more I drink, the more my subconscious mind usually tells me to stop. I drank some white wine at the military base and was soused after a few glasses. I remember seeing Zhou Xiaofeng's face. She helped me lie down on the bed. I heard Ye Guangqin saying they should keep an eye on my red wallet. I smiled inside and passed out, not knowing that my friends from the writers' delegation were fussing over me. Standing at the door of my room, they were discussing amongst themselves: "Should we ask someone to check if she's alright? Does she need to take any medicine? Did she break something?" Worried that the pin on my badge might hurt me, they took it off and put it on the bedside table. I was sound asleep, oblivious to the joy of being the centre of so much attention.

It was the second time in my life that a group of friends had shown so much concern for me. When I had my operations and was going through chemotherapy and, subsequently, depression, I never asked for help from my friends. But my subconscious wanted to ask, and felt that they cared. God had filled my emotional void by sending angels in the form of my friends from the delegation, who soothed the pain in my soul.

It was the first time in years that I had fallen asleep without taking any sleeping pills. I slept until 3 o'clock in the morning, woke up feeling refreshed and without a headache. After a shower, I had coffee and soda crackers in bed, wondering all the while why I'd gotten drunk. I had forgotten to take my hormones in the afternoon, and when my body lacks hormones, I become tired and drained, like a mobile phone that has run out of battery. My biological system breaks down easily and starts to malfunction. During my visit to the military base, which lasted several days, I was both excited and fatigued. Before drinking wine that evening, I had spent the whole afternoon in a car. Worn out physically and mentally, I slipped easily into a state of inebriation.

My visit to the military base was like going home again. The army is my spiritual family. And I felt serene and comforted. When I left the military base many, many years ago, I felt lost, as if my soul had flown away. But today, returning to a modern military base that has entered the 21st century, my soul has come back to me. I am whole once again.

EIGHTY-TWO

Diary
Saturday, 7th August 2004 9:30 pm

To get away from Lele, I dithered around at the Learning & Excellence bookshop before dinner. I often go there to browse through books and look for new titles. So glad to have such a first-rate bookshop near me.

I bought a copy of *The Count of Monte Cristo*. It's a luxury edition published by Yilin Publishing House. I bought it because of a phrase on the last page of the book: "[...] until the day God will deign to reveal the future to man, all wisdom is summed up in these two words – '*Wait*' and '*hope*.'"[1]

I first read this novel at the end of 1987. At the time, I was staying at the First Zhongshan Hospital. I prefer the translation of the phrase in that edition: "[...] before the day God will deign to reveal His plans to man, all wisdom is summed up in these two words – '*Wait*' and '*hope*.'"

This phrase spoke to my heart, but had been relegated to the forgotten realms of my memory during all these years.

Today is 7th August 2004. The time is 10:10 am. In the "Diary" section, I hereby write down my wish: "[...] before the day God will deign to reveal His plans to man, all wisdom is contained in these two words – '*Wait*' and '*hope*.'"

To wait and to hope. Li Lanni.

Notes

In truth, I don't like the novel *The Count of Monte Cristo* much. I've only read it once, and seen the film once. But the words "wait" and "hope" are etched into my mind.

I asked myself: Did Xiaotao read this novel? Did she know these two words? Her husband was away studying at Qinghua University for several years. Did hope help make the waiting easier and the hardships more bearable?

I remember the last letter she wrote to us, in which she said: "Know how to be content with what you have in life."

I had pushed Xiaotao to the back of my mind.

I wrote this passage yesterday. Couldn't continue.

For a long time, I made a deliberate effort not to think about Grandmother. After her death, I prayed that I wouldn't dream about her. I was afraid of seeing her unhappy in the next world. It would have broken my heart. Once, I dreamt that my parents had received a letter from her. It was written on paper with vertical lines, the kind that was used in the olden days. It said: "I've just moved. Now I'm living in apartment number 1308 in such and such a building." I said to my parents: "I think Grandmother is dead. But the apartment is somewhere nearby." My mother, brother and I went looking for her in this building, which was built like a labyrinth. When we arrived on the 14th floor, the people there told us to go down one floor. As the building had no lift, we were forced to go up and down the stairs. Finally, we arrived, tired and out of breath. It was dark, and the floor was covered in mud. We had to go down one more floor to apartment 1308. We were beginning to feel dizzy. Lost in the maze, we had to ask several people for directions. We arrived at the apartment 08 to find it occupied by a large family. The man said: "This is apartment 1208. You've made a mistake, you have to go up one floor." I said: "But we just came from there. The apartment there is 1408. That's strange, why can't we find 1308?" Upon waking, I felt relieved that I didn't see Grandmother in my dream. Seeing her face would have made me sad for days afterwards.

In the early hours of the morning, I saw Grandmother in my dream.

The landscape in my dream was blurred, and I didn't know which town I was in. Several people I didn't know came up to me to say that Grandmother had been sentenced to death, and that she would die by firing squad. A wave of panic and anxiety swelled inside, and I asked: "What crime did she commit? Why has she been sentenced to death? She's been wrongly accused. Where is she? When will the execution be? I want to see her." The people replied: "She's in hospital. She's too old. The doctors refused to treat her, saying they don't treat people who've been condemned to death."

I was heartbroken and filled with bitterness.

I found the hospital. There were crowds of people, and I recognised smells that were so familiar to me: iodine solution, formaldehyde solution, alcohol. All the consultation rooms were full. Distraught and confused, I was searching everywhere in the hospital.

As if my eyes were suspended from the ceiling, I was looking down at myself weaving in and out of the crowd in the lobby.

Who was I looking for? Ah yes, the administrative director.

Upset and angry, I was arguing with people. I couldn't hear what I was saying but knew that I was fighting to save Grandmother's life. What time was the execution? Couldn't it be postponed to another day? Would it be possible to repeal? How could I let Grandmother suffer such an injustice? Would it be death by firing squad or lethal injection? No one could give me an answer. I asked everyone why Grandmother had been sentenced to death. But no one answered. Exhausted and in distress, I sat down on the stairs. First things first. Never mind who sentenced her to death or the crime she had committed, I had to find Grandmother first and insist that she be treated by the doctors, and then ask her to explain this strange business.

Suddenly, I saw my mother, brother, sister-in-law and husband. My family was here, which reassured me. My brother said: "Grandmother is receiving treatment right now. Your sister-in-law is in the consultation room with her." Surprised and happy, I thought: "This hospital is better than I thought. They've agreed to treat her."

"Why has Grandmother been sentenced to death?" I asked my family. "Do you know why?"

"No, we don't," Mother replied.

"Does Grandmother know?"

"Yes, she knows. She feels peaceful. The execution will probably be tomorrow."

I couldn't understand why Mother wasn't beside herself with worry like I was. I was heartbroken. My mouth tasted bitter. I wanted to cry but couldn't. My heart was dry and empty. I had no tears.

"She's going to die, just like that?" I burst out, all of a sudden. "No, no, no, I won't let her."

"Have you taken your medicine?" my husband asked, grabbing me by the arm. "Go on, take your medicine now. There's no point in getting yourself worked up like that. I'll take you to see Grandmother afterwards."

I was afraid of seeing her. I had to take my medication.

"Last time you told me Grandmother was so sick that she had become unrecognisable," I said to my brother. "How is she now?"

I wanted to see her, but I was afraid.

"She's better. She's not frightening to look at anymore."

My family and I were standing in front of a consultation room. A nurse said to us: "Your grandmother has just finished her intravenous infusion. She's in the toilet." We went out into the lobby to wait. I was nervous and edgy. Suddenly, all the patients started to walk backwards, with their backs facing me, except for one person, who was walking towards me. She stopped a few steps in front of me, and the people around her moved away. Grandmother was standing before me.

Her face was expressionless. She was thin, had sunken eyes and a prominent brow bone, like a mummy. She was smaller than before and was wearing an old blue and black outfit. I didn't have the courage to go up to her. She looked nothing like how I remembered her. She must have been through immense suffering. She pursed her lips, and there were long, deep furrows around her mouth. She looked dry and withered.

My heart was heavy with sorrow. I wanted to take her into my arms but couldn't move.

Grandmother blinked. A light came into her eyes. They were no longer dry but moist. I recognised that those were Grandmother's eyes.

The whole family came over and stood around her. We wanted to take her by the arm to help her remain steady on her feet. But she didn't need our help. She sat down on a chair, and there was a look of sadness and joy in her eyes.

She was looking at me. Kneeling at her feet, my hands on her knees, I looked at her, thinking: "Grandmother, we're all here."

I woke up. It was still night.

A vague lingering sadness.

Mournful and in sorrow, but unconfused.

Sitting in front of my computer, my throat is dry and sore. My mouth tastes bitter. So very bitter.

20th *August* 2007

Correlations

"Jonah"

One day, God sent the prophet Jonah to Nineveh to preach to the inhabitants of this city, whose sins had provoked the wrath of God. But Johan disobeyed, boarded a ship for Tarshish and hid inside.

During the journey, there was a raging storm and the ship nearly sank. To lighten the weight of the ship, the sailors threw the goods and merchandise into the sea. Then, they decided to cast lots to find out who was responsible for this misfortune. The lot fell on Jonah, who explained to the sailors that he had fled from the will of God. At that moment, an immense wave rose up, as if to engulf the ship. Jonah said: "Throw me into the sea and the storm will cease." The men refused and rowed to bring the ship to shore, but their efforts failed. They prayed to God that His will may be done and threw Jonah overboard. The storm ceased at once.

God caused a large fish to swallow Jonah, who stayed in the fish's belly for three days and three nights. He cried out to God for forgiveness, and the large fish spat him out onto the shore. Again, God commanded Jonah to go to Nineveh, and he obeyed.

Jonah walked through the city all day crying: "In forty days Nineveh shall be destroyed!" The people of Nineveh believed in the word of God, repented of their sins, fasted and turned away from their sinful ways.

God forgave them and did not destroy their city.

A story from the Bible

Complementary Notes

Jonah was a prophet, who had a calling to fulfill. Though gifted with an innate wisdom, he refused. With nowhere to flee, he finally accepted his fate.

We all have a calling to fulfill in life. It is part of our destiny, whether we are rich or poor, whether we hold a position of power or otherwise. This is regardless of our talents or abilities. As the popular saying goes: "Man may act, but their fate is determined by the heavens." This simple truth lies behind all human experience and is one of the myriad laws that govern our mysterious and unfathomable universe.

One day in May 2006, I arrived back in Shenzhen after a trip to Beijing. On the motorway, the taxi driver told me a story he had just heard on the radio: A demobilised soldier passing through Beijing had lost his wallet. When his taxi driver learnt that the soldier had been part of the rescue operation during the floods, he gave him 600 yuan to pay for his journey home. Many years later, the soldier, who had succeeded in life, returned to Beijing. To show his gratitude and repay his debt, he managed to track down the taxi driver through a radio program.

My taxi driver said: "He did the right thing. They're good people, these two. But me, when I do something good, I always get screwed and end up regretting it afterwards."

I asked him what had happened.

He said: "It was last year. The weather was stifling hot. A client had left his laptop case with his computer inside in the car. I immediately told the taxi station, so the client wouldn't have to pay 200 yuan to make an announcement on the radio or in the newspaper. It would have been money down the drain. Apparently, the client had already contacted the taxi station, so I called the client. The heat was sweltering. I told him not to bother going all the way to the taxi station and told him to meet me at the Kempinski Hotel at one o'clock in the afternoon. I went all the way there to give him back his computer. He took it, thanked me and was putting his hand in his jacket to take his wallet out when I said something he took offence to. Then the bastard just told me to go. It really pissed me off. I had driven an hour in the bloody heatwave to give him back his thing. I hadn't eaten. And he didn't even ask me if I wanted something to eat or drink. Who wants to do good things after that? I'll never do anything stupid like that again."

I felt bad for him, as well as for all the others, who had done good deeds but were not paid back in kind.

"Have you heard of Cong Fei?" I asked him.

The taxi driver turned around, gave me a blank look and shook his head.

"Cong Fei was a singer and a volunteer worker in Shenzhen," I said. "He financed the education of over a hundred children. But he had cancer. Even towards the end of his life, the children were still asking him for money."

People say that Cong Fei was suffering from depression and that he had tried to commit suicide in 2002.

I can believe that. Being in a situation like the one he was in, it would have been difficult not to fall into depression. Alone in Shenzhen, with no fixed income, he had to provide for his family. With the scant resources that were at his disposal, he financed the education of 168 children, who were living in poverty. You can imagine the kind of pressure he was under.

When he was first admitted into hospital in 2005, Cong Fei relied on the financial support of his friends, who were also volunteer workers. His wife was pregnant, and he was supporting a young daughter from a previous marriage. He was sick and could no longer sing for a living. What's more, he was castigated for no longer being able to finance the education of those children. Without the intervention of the media, government and many Shenzhen citizens, what would have become of him?

I think he would have fallen back into depression. If he hadn't died of cancer, depression would have pushed him into taking his own life. He was worried for the future of these children and didn't want to be a burden for his family and friends. When his friends asked the journalists of *News of The Special Economic Zone of Shenzhen* for help, Cong Fei was suffering from severe insomnia but refused to be hospitalised. Plunged into depression, lacking the financial means to undergo medical treatment, he could have died in poverty, and may never have known that he had cancer.

The Shenzhen of today would never have left Cong Fei to suffer and die in silence. In a way, it is Shenzhen that had made him into what he was – a compassionate person with a heart of gold. Cong Fei is the light and soul of this city.

Every one of us has a calling in life. God sent me to this city to forge me. This city needs angels. Its inhabitants need to live in dignity.

I have often wanted to escape from Shenzhen or to change professions. In theory, I have the skills to go into another line of work. I've thought of applying for a job with *Southern News* or *News of The Special Economic Zone of Shenzhen*; I've also toyed with the idea of doing university research or working in a literary research centre, which would allow me to have a calm and stable life. But every time I made plans to change my life, something happened to ruin my project. At the end of 1999, I applied for work in the art and literature section of a newspaper and had been given the job by the director. But at the beginning of 2000, I underwent a surgical procedure for cancer. Around 2002, my friends were on the lookout for career opportunities for me. But in 2003, I plummeted into depression. At the end of that year, I had a revelation while reading the story of Jonah: It told me to stay in Shenzhen. My calling in life was to portray the soul of this city in my writings. To be plagued with cancer and depression is part of my destiny. I need to go through the experience in order to put it into words. It is like that glaring scar on my neck. The otolaryngologist took a photo of it as an example of a botched operation to show to medical students. The purpose is to help others live in health and happiness.

Mother's birthday was on 2nd August. I invited my parents to spend a few days with me on the Sun Yat-Sen University campus. We didn't eat in a fancy restaurant that evening. There were no presents or birthday cake. Mother had a toothache and stomach ache. Since she had her gallbladder removed 10 years ago, she doesn't like eating out. I asked the housekeeper to cook Cantonese-style soya sauce chicken. The meat was tender, melting and juicy, but Mother only ate a few mouthfuls. I didn't know what presents to give her, as I usually buy her things she needs without waiting for her birthday to come around. Feeling a bit stingy nonetheless, I ended up buying a couple of music CDs. She prefers instrumental music to songs.

After dinner, my parents sat down and made themselves comfortable on the sofa. I closed the windows, drew the curtains, switched on the light, turned the air conditioner to 29 degrees and put on the music. Then I announced: "Let the birthday concert begin!" Pleasantly surprised, my parents smiled, amused by my theatrical staging. Many years ago, our family shared happy moments together during musical evenings of our own. My brother and I would set the staging, and my parents sang. It had been a long time since we'd had a family musical evening. Waving my arms to the rhythm of the music, like a conductor, I began to sing: "Deep blue skies, floating white clouds...horses running..." Mother joined in: "... Horses' manes in the wind... bird songs quiver..." I got the lyrics wrong and sang: "birds fly away," but Mother corrected me, saying it was: "bird songs quiver." Merry and in high spirits, Father also joined in: "If I am asked what place is this... proudly I say this is my homeland..."

The concert only had one audience member. Lying on the glass coffee table, Lele was watching us with his big black eyes. We were singing along: "Deep blue skies, floating white clouds... horses running..."

Suddenly, I became distracted. It struck me: "This is my moment of happiness."

In my mind's eye, I saw the beach on the island of Neilingding. It was night. Moonlight was shimmering on the waves of the sea. Mother was working at the radio station and was playing a song that was a favourite among the soldiers on the island: "Red flowers on the trees, reflected on the emerald-green sea... Flames rise from the water... Coral-red sweet viburnum...Spring is forever... Petals scattered in the wind...on the waves..."

Li Lanni was five years old. She was sitting on the beach, barefoot and smiling. The wild grass around her was thin and sparse. Holding a blade of grass between her teeth, her heart was listening to the song her mother was playing on the radio. She watched the slivers of moonbeam on the water, in the hope that flames would surge out of the sea and burst into clusters of red flowers. She waited patiently, afraid to even blink. She had faith that a beautiful red flower would rise out of the emerald sea.

First draft was finished on 21st September 2007 at 1 pm
Proofreading and editing completed on 3rd March 2008 at 12 pm

POSTSCRIPT ONE

The day I finished the first draft of the manuscript, I felt light and serene. But the next day saw the beginning of a slow descent into anxiety, followed by severe depression. I was faced with a dilemma. On the one hand, I felt that it was within my capabilities to produce a mature literary work; however, I was unsatisfied with the results. But on the other, I was reluctant to edit the texts, preferring to leave the spontaneity intact.

In the early hours of the morning of 8th November 2007, I had what seemed to be a premonitory dream.

I dreamt that I had arrived in a strange town and that I was staying in an old and shabby room. The landlady trusted me and had given me the key to the house. As the lock was at the bottom of the door near the floor, I had to kneel down to put the key inside. I didn't want to keep the key, because I was planning to go over to the other side of the snow-capped mountains and not come back. I climbed into a heavy canvas truck with a group of strangers. I was in high spirits and looking forward to seeing beautiful snowscapes on my journey.

But as we went higher and higher up into the mountains, I became colder and colder. Frozen numb, I tried to stick it out as long as I could. But the truck started to skid. I felt a rush of panic, terrified that the driver would suddenly brake and cause a fatal accident. It felt as if the truck was about to overturn, and thoughts were racing around in my head. Then it skidded off the road and started to fall apart. The passengers were flying into the air, screaming. I hung onto the gearstick, eyes closed, afraid to even look at the other passengers to see if they could make it. I thought I was going to be smashed to pieces, but that if I hung onto the gearstick long enough, I could perhaps slow the truck down. Then everything went blank.

The last part of the dream: Back in town, I was standing outside the front door of the house. I was dying to go inside to take a rest, but someone had thrown away my key. Night was falling. Then I found myself in an alleyway at the back of the house. People going home after work were walking through the alleyway. I felt guilty that I had lost the key and was wondering how I was going to explain it to the landlady. Exhausted and anxious, I was heaping reproaches on myself.

Today is Chinese New Year's Eve. I can't write this postscript anymore. Lately, the forces of life and death are caught in a ceaseless struggle. Endlessly. Every day.

On 15th January, I picked up my biological test results at Shenzhen Hospital.

I had a dream in the early hours of this morning. I can't remember the beginning, except that I was on a street in Shenzhen. Towering buildings stood on both sides of the street. One side was against the light, while the other side was facing the sun. In the middle was a narrow, quiet one-way street with no cars. Several men and women were standing on the side that was against the light. They gave me a rope and urged me to go to a building opposite, about 10 metres away. There I was to end my own life.

"Quick," they said. "With this rope, you won't fail."

They told me to hurry up, because they wanted to make sure that I was dead before making funeral arrangements. In a state of euphoria and holding the rope in my hand, I rushed over to the building, not wanting to make these well-intentioned people wait. They had my well-being in mind.

But as I was approaching the building, a voice in my head suddenly said: "Is this how you're going to leave this world? Think for a second. Why are you in a hurry?" I slowed down and stopped, undecided and at a loss as to what I should do.

Then I noticed there was something odd about the hemp rope I was holding. Why did such a large coil of rope weigh so little? I could hardly feel it in my hands. You couldn't possibly jump off the roof and hang yourself with that! Were these people stupid or what? It was just as well that I hadn't listened to them.

I woke up with a start. Opening my eyes, I realised that I was in the bedroom of my Shenzhen apartment. It was night outside, and, inside, a thick, heavy silence hung in the air.

I felt a rush of cold air at the back of my head. The forces of death were advancing. The invasion had begun.

I don't know when I'll be able to finish this postscript.

Today is 9th March 2008. The time is 5:05 pm.

I'm practising cognitive therapy.

Li Lanni, you've made good progress in your fight against depression. Every day, you take one tablet of Seroxat and three tablets of alprazolam and Euthyrox.

Good news: After reading the first draft of the manuscript, He Shaojun says my book has literary value.

This year, the literary review *Literature of Shanghai* will publish an excerpt from the first draft in each of its issues. Li Hongxiong has already sent me the first two issues.

Li Lanni, in your fight against depression, the support of your friends is crucial. The Writers' Association of China has invited Cui Daoyi and Zhang Shouren, two highly respected writers, to do reading sessions of your book. On 4th March, you were told of the editorial board's decision. Your book will be published shortly.

Such encouraging news can only have a positive effect on your health.

Not such good news: I still can't bring myself to reread my manuscript. It makes me want to bang my head against the wall and tear at my hair until it hurts. Pull yourself together and take a deep breath. Don't be afraid. Have faith. Li Lanni, you're doing well. You are still alive. You must live. Smile. Entrust the task of writing the postscript to your friends Li Mei and Tian Huiping. "[...] Seek and you will find; knock and the door will be opened to you."[1]

Li Mei and Tian Huiping, it is your turn now.

POSTSCRIPT TWO

Lanni, when we last saw each other in Shenzhen, we agreed that if *A Crowded Silence* wasn't published in your lifetime, I would do my utmost to see it published in mine. A few months ago, I heard that your book would be published by The People's Literature Publishing House. It is such wonderful news. I never doubted that it would be published in your lifetime. For your book is forceful, profound and inspiring. It gives me a sense of relief, not because it dissolves our agreement, but because you are able to see the birth of your book into the world.

Lanni, I was afraid of losing you. Afraid that after completing your book, you wouldn't have the strength to live through your suffering anymore. I thank you for finding the courage and strength, and for providing an example to many people, myself included, as well as to all those who know and don't know you, to everyone, and to yourself.

We had a long conversation after my first reading of *A Crowded Silence*. The next morning, a thought came to me upon wakening: Lanni, entrust me with the task of writing your obituary. After reading your book, I am no longer afraid to talk about death. I have already shared my thoughts with you: Lanni, if, one day, you want to leave this world, then go. Do it for yourself and for life, which is beautiful. Do it, so that life can open up in all its splendour. *A Crowded Silence* made me understand for the first time that I was wrong in thinking that to respect life, you must live. On the contrary, in the name of respect and love, we can choose to give up on life in peace and serenity. Through your book, I have learnt that it is our duty to respect the unique traits that are present in each and every one of us. So many people suffer from depression, but we know so little about this illness. The lack of understanding gives way to intolerance, which, in turn, gives rise to disdain and disrespect. How many people are struggling just to stay alive? So many around us have fallen prey to depression. A book such as *A Crowded Silence* brings a better understanding of this illness to Chinese society. Lanni, this is your contribution to Chinese culture and civilisation. Your pain and suffering are worth more than gold.

I will never again try to convince you that life is beautiful. But I will try to convince other people to respect life in all its many facets. I will never again utter trivialities, such as: "You must live to feel the beauty of life." But I will show you through my actions how we must never disregard life. Thank you, Lanni. I wish you all the happiness. Whatever you choose to do, I am certain that it will be the best choice possible. Like sisters, we have this in common: We thrive on all that is beautiful.

The publication of your book makes me both happy and sad. I am afraid of losing you. Don't forget our agreement: to write each other's obituaries. I understand how difficult it is for you to carry on living, but you must. For it is your duty to write my obituary.

I cannot write anymore. I have never been confident in my own writing. My thoughts are confused. I am crying but don't know why. I cannot write anymore, be it good or bad.

With all my affections,
Huiping

22nd April 2008

22nd April 2008

(Tian Huiping: Director of the Xing Xing Yu Educational Research Centre of Beijing, founder of Education of Autistic Children of China – clinical intervention based on Applied Behaviour Analysis)

POSTSCRIPT THREE

I arrived in Shenzhen in March 1984. At the time, I had never met Lanni and only knew her by name, because people often compared me to her, saying we looked alike. When we finally met, I saw that there was not the slightest resemblance between us. Later, we both lived in building number 100 in the Yuanling district. I was on the fifth floor and she was on the second. I lived in Shenzhen for over 10 years and, during this time, Lanni was my best friend. As long as I have known her, she has always had a thin, pale face and has been unwell. I couldn't understand how a body that young could be in such poor health. When I lived in Shenzhen, I fell ill only once a year from some minor ailment. I was incapable of understanding the physical suffering she was going through. Illness and pain were her daily lot. Sick and frail, she faced up to the world with a smile. Every time I experienced problems and challenges in my life, I would go to her. But in the face of her suffering, I could only watch helplessly, incapable of alleviating her pain. It upset me.

I knew she was struggling to finish her book *A Crowded Silence*. It was only after reading it that I realised that her suffering was beyond anything I could have imagined. But she said that what she was able to express in her book was only one-tenth of what she had gone through, and that she would try to write the remaining nine-tenths. I advised her against it. It would destroy her. Would the nine-tenths left unsaid change the intrinsic value of her work? Why push writing to its extreme at the risk of destroying yourself? What is the point? Limits must be set down. I believe in the goodness of human nature. Is it possible to save humanity if we only see life through the cruelty that it inflicts on us? Can we not accept the realities of life within the limits that our sufferings impose upon us?

Words cannot express pain that is deep and intense. It is unspeakable and unfathomable, a mystery that God has bestowed upon mankind. For thousands of years, mankind has strived to describe it in writing. Same with death. It is indescribable. And what we do manage to describe is not the true face of death. For we do not co-exist with death; we only see its cadaverous remains. But Lanni has opened up a pathway for us. She spoke of all that is in her heart. With open hands, she gave herself to the world. She may not have said all that she wanted to about her illness and pain, but she has spoken of her love. Love made her plunge into the dark side of life... Lanni, you gave all that you had. You have given the best of yourself. Enough.

When we fall into the bottomless pit of despair, there is only death. But Lanni will not die. Not because she has not reached the depths of her suffering, but because she has kept her promise to God. Without it, she would not be with us today, but freed from the pain, trials and tribulations of life.

Lanni has delved into the fathoms of her heart through the words she has written with pain, one by one. She has given her blood and cut her flesh into small pieces, but has survived through pain and self-harm. For Lanni, who doesn't know how to cry, it is a form of self-preservation. Even the strongest among us cannot live in a hermetically-sealed world. If she had not been able to express herself through words, she would not be alive today.

We must thank Lanni for sharing with us her experience as a cancer patient and a woman plagued with depression. With sincerity and candour, she has shown the world her weakness, confusion, and vanity, even. Through her writing, I have come to know not Lanni the writer, but a woman, sick and in pain, and also a friend who has finally opened her heart. All these years, I have lived in the hope that she would open up to me. But unlike many of us, she cannot express herself with ease. I never imagined that she would lay herself bare in such a way, to the point of tearing herself apart. I thank the Lord that her work is now completed. The sky is bright and clear.

In offering us her heart-rending testament, Lanni nearly lost herself.

In a way, I almost envy her. She has reached the depths of her suffering, so how can life allow her to live in pain anymore? She is free. She will no longer be a slave to her torments, sickness or inner reality. A path filled with peace, light and felicity unfolds before her. She has nothing more to fear.

I wish Lanni joy and happiness. She has taught me to be grateful for the blessings and infinite possibilities that life bestows upon us.

Li Mei

11th April 2008

(Li Mei: Chief Editor of the magazine *Modern Photography*, director of the review *Central Point* and a photographic art critic)

ENDNOTES

About Li Lanni

1. Zhang Guorong (1956 – 2003): Also known as Leslie Cheung. A Hong Kong actor and singer who committed suicide on 1st April 2003 after a long battle with depression (All the explanatory notes in this book are written by the translator)

One

1. Philippians 4:13
2. Isaiah 40:29
3. Susan Aldridge, Seeing Red and Feeling Blue: The New Understanding of Mood and Emotion, Random House UK, 2000
4. Ursula Nuber, Depression: Die verkannte Krankheit, Kreuz-Verlag, 2000
5. A poker variant that is popular in China

Two

1. In Traditional Chinese Medicine, Heat and Humidity are Pathological Influences which cause imbalances in the body
2. Matthew 5:14
3. Norman Vincent Peale, *The Power of Positive Thinking*. 1953. Reprint, Vermillion, 1998
4. SARS (Severe Acute Respiratory Syndrome): Avian influenza or bird flu. It is a viral respiratory disease caused by the SARS coronavirus. An outbreak occurred in Southern China between November 2002 and July 2003

Three

1. Susan Aldridge, *op. cit*

Four

1. Lymph node

Five

1. Psalm 118:24
2. Romans 8:31

Six

1. In Traditional Chinese Medicine, this indicates an internal imbalance of the digestive system
2. Isaiah 28:16

3. Isaiah 40:31
4. Genesis 50:20
5. There are three levels to this system of refund, which applies to public officials and those with a civil servant status: level one applies to heads of governmental departments; level two is for governors of provinces, war veterans and those who participated in the revolution; and level three is for vice-governors of provinces, teachers and professors
6. Gwendoline Smith, *Depression Explained*, GSA Limited, 2002
7. Ursula Nuber, *op. cit*
8. San Mao (1943-1991): Novelist and travel writer from Taiwan. She is also known as Echo Chan

Seven

1. Mark 9:23
2. Susan Aldridge, *op. cit*
3. Eastern sea means a sea that is far away
4. "Fish stuck in a rut" is an idiom meaning to find oneself in a difficult situation and in need of help, like a fish stranded in the groove of a wheel track, desperately in need of water

Eight

1. *Dream of the Red Chamber*, written by Cao Xueqin (? – 1763), is considered to be one of the four great classical novels in Chinese literature

Nine

1. Toothpaste tubes were made from aluminum
2. Toothbrush handles were made from buffalo horn

Ten

1. Verena Kast, *Vom Sinn des Ärgers: Anreiz zur Selbstbehauptung und Selbstentfaltung.* 1998. Reprint, Herder, 2014
2. Matthew 21:22
3. From the poem "Red Rivers • With Comrade Guo Moruo" by Mao Zedong

Eleven

1. Jiefang is a manufacturing brand in the 1950s and 1960s that produced motor vehicles, bicycles, shoes and everyday items

Twelve

1. Psalm 37:1-7
2. A jacket with mandarin collar and four pockets in front
3. It is also known as Tomb Sweeping Day. On this day, people visit grave sites to pay respect to their ancestors
4. "Decoction of the Four Noblemen": composition: *renshen* (root of *Panax Ginseng* C.A. Mey), *zhigancao* (root of *Glycyrrhiza uralensis* Fisch) grilled with honey, *fuling*, (*Poria coco* (Schw) Wolf), *baizhu* (rhizome of *Atractylodes macrocephala* Koidz). Indication: Deficient

Spleen Qi and Deficient Stomach Qi characterized by indigestion; diarrhea et weakness in limbs
5. "Decoction of Suanzaoren-Ziziphus": composition: *suanzaoren* (stone of *Ziziphus sativa spinosa* (Bge) Schneid), *gancao* (root of *Glycyrrhiza uralensis* Fisch), zhimu (rhizome of *Anemarrhena asphodeloides* Bge), *fuling* (*Poria coco* (Schw) Wolf), *chuanxiong* (rhizome of *Ligusticum wallichii* Franch). Indication: insomnia

Thirteen

1. Corinthians 12:9

Fourteen

1. Genesis 50:20
2. In Buddhist terms, the "pagoda of seven storeys" represent the good deeds we do in life. The more good deeds we do, the higher we climb in the pagoda. In saving a life, one ascends beyond the seven storeys, bringing us closer to the heavens
3. Da Yu was a legendary monarch of the Xia Dynasty (approx. 2070-1600 BC). China was devastated by massive floods and Da Yu was able to control and direct the flood waters onto the plains
4. Beijing was a manufacturing brand that produced motor vehicles
5. A song written by the poet Ma Zhiyuan (1250-1321) of the Yuan Dynasty. It describes the melancholy of a traveler who longs for his native country

Sixteen

1. Mark 6:31
2. A Chinese encyclopedic dictionary
3. A founding text for the philosophy and religion of Taoism dating back to approximately 600 BC. Its authorship is attributed to Laozi
4. Isaiah 30:15

Seventeen

1. Bing Xin (1900 – 1999) was a Chinese writer of novels, poetry and prose

Eighteen

1. Romans 8:31
2. Li Bai (701-762), Du Fu (712-770), Su Shi (1037-1101) and Xin Qiji (1140-1207) were poets and officials of the imperial court
3. Tao Yuanming (365-427) was also a poet and a civil servant of the imperial court
4. From the poem "Wine" by Tao Yuanming

Nineteen

1. *A Family Guide to Health Care*, edited by Ling Chen, China Textile Publishing House, 1999
2. In Traditional Chinese Medicine, *yuzheng*, or the syndrome of *yu*, means nervous depression

(All the explanatory notes are written by the translator.)

3. *Spiritual Axis* (*Lingshu*): the second part of *Inner Classic of the Yellow Emperor* (*Huangdi neijing*), the earliest book on Chinese medicine, compiled during the Warring States period (475 – 221 BC)
4. "Sickness of the Mind" (*Benshen*): volume II, chapter 8
5. "Verbal Questions" (*Kouwen*): volume V, chapter 28
6. Hua Xiuyun (? – 1753): Chinese physician
7. *Qi*: means energy
8. *Ordering of Patterns and Deciding Treatments* (*Leizheng zhicai*) (1839) was written by the Chinese physician Lin Peiqin (1772 – 1839)
9. *Case Histories That Act as Clinical Compasses* (*Lingzheng zhiyian*) (1746) was written by the Chinese physician Ye Gui (1677 – 1746)
10. The "Carefree Formula" (*Xiaoyaosan*) is a medicinal formula that dates back to 1107. Composition: *danggui* (*Angelica sinensis* (Oliv.) Diels), *chaihu* (*Bupleurum chinense* DC. or *B. scorzonerifilium* Willd.), *baishao* (*Paeonia lactiflora* Pal.), *fuling* (*Poria cocos* (Schw.) Wolf), *baizhu* (*Atractylodes macrocephala* Koidz.), *jiu gancao*: grilled licorice root (*Glycyrrhiza uralensis* Fisch.), *sheng jiang* (*Zingiber officinale* (Willd.) Rosc.), *bohe* (*Mentha haplocalyx* Briq.). Indications: stagnation of the energy of the Liver and Blood, irritability, fluctuating moods, dizziness, irregular menses, nervous depression

Twenty

1. Psalm 27:14

Twenty-one

1. Matthew 5:3-4
2. Cong Fei (1969 – 2006): a Chinese singer and philanthropist who died of stomach cancer
3. *Chongcao*: abbreviation for *dongchong xiacao*. It is a fungus that lives on the caterpillar of certain insects of the Hepialidae family. It is used for its medicinal properties
4. John: 3:19

Twenty-two

1. A therapeutic method in Traditional Chinese Medicine that consists of scratching the skin with a hard metallic object to lower fever and relieve pain

Twenty-four

1. Genesis 50:20

Twenty-five

1. The proverb means "to persevere in a difficult task."
2. Exercises in body posture, movement, breathing and meditation that promotes health and spiritual awareness
3. The magnetic field of someone who practices qigong
4. The character *lan* means "orchid."
5. The character *nan* means "south."
6. *Nangua* means "pumpkin."

Twenty-six

1. Kings 12:24
2. Genesis 50:20
3. Matthew 5:4
4. Psalm 18:1
5. Job 34:29
6. Romans 8:31
7. Philippians 4:6
8. Isaiah 40:29
9. Isaiah 40:31

Twenty-seven

1. Corinthians 12:9
2. Ecclesiastes 1:9

Thirty

1. Psalm 103:3
2. Joshua 1:9
3. *Nanru* peanuts are peanuts cooked in fermented soya and is a specialty of Guangdong province
4. A blind man
5. A blind woman
6. Sweet and savoury cookies made and sold by blind people

Thirty-two

1. Chinese angelica or "female ginseng" (*Angelica sinensis*)
2. Chinese yam (*Dioscorea polystachya*)

Thirty-three

1. Preface to *Life in Shenzhen*, Li Lanni, Shenyang Publishing House, 1996

Thirty-four

1. Erich Fromm, *For the Love of Life*, New York: Free Press, 1986

Thirty-five

1. In the ancient Chinese method of telling time, the night is divided into five sections or *geng*. The time length of a *geng* is two hours. The third *geng* corresponds to the time slot between 1 am and 3 am
2. The fifth *geng* corresponds to the time slot between 5 am and 7 am
3. A saying of Confucius
4. Isaiah 32:15
5. Matthew 12:43-45

Thirty-six

1. Wang Xizhi (303-361): a famous poet and calligrapher. The story goes that a military commander wanted to marry his daughter to Wang Xizhi, so he sent a subordinate to his home. The subordinate was led into the eastern chamber, where he saw Wang Xizhi lying on the bed, eating with his belly exposed

Thirty-seven

1. Gu Hongming, *The Spirit of the Chinese People*, The Peking Daily News, 1915

Thirty-eight

1. Chinese herbal medicine for cardiac problems
2. Psalm 62:5
3. Qiu Jin (1875 – 1907): Chinese revolutionary, feminist and writer
4. *A Doll's House* (1879) by Henrik Ibsen (1828 – 1906)
5. A cultural documentary produced by China Central Television in 2000

Thirty-nine

1. Job 34:29
2. Reform movements launched by Mao Zedong in 1951. The Three-anti Campaign aimed to eliminate corruption, waste and bureaucracy. The Five-anti Campaign aimed to eradicate bribery, tax evasion, theft of state property, cheating on government contracts and stealing state economic information
3. Movement introduced by Mao Zedong in 1963 in an effort to "clean up" on four different fronts: politics, economy, organization and ideology

Forty

1. Philippians 4:6
2. The fox spirit is a mythological creature with magical powers, capable of acquiring human forms. This popular belief is particularly strong and widespread in the north of China

Forty-one

1. Psalm 66:12
2. Huang Xing (1874 – 1916): a revolutionary leader and one of the founders of Guomindang
3. Liu Shaoqi (1898 – 1969): vice president of People's Republic of China (1956 – 1966)
4. Li Lisan (1899 – 1967): and Zhang Guotao (1897 – 1979): two of the founding members of the Chinese Communist Party
5. A resistance movement founded by Sun Yat-Sen in 1905 and later became the Guomindang
6. A military campaign launched by the Guomindang with the purpose of reunifying China
7. Verena Kast, *Vom Sinn der Angst: wie Ängste sich festsetzen und wie sie sich verwandeln lassen*, Herder, 1996
8. The root of *Codonopsis pilosula* (Franch.) Nannf., or "poor man's ginseng"

Forty-two

1. In Traditional Chinese Medicine the Five Organs are the heart, liver, spleen, lungs and kidneys

Forty-three

1. A saying of Confucius
2. Proverbs 9:10
3. Gareth O'Callaghan, *A Day Called Hope: A Personal Journey Beyond Depression*, Hodder Mobius, 2003

Forty-four

1. Mark 5:36
2. *Yueqin* or the moon zither is a traditional Chinese string instrument
3. A song in praise of Mao Zedong that was often sung and played during the Cultural Revolution

Forty-five

1. Meng Jiangnü is the heroine of a folk legend. During the construction of the Great Wall of China, Meng Jiangnü's husband was among the workers put into forced labour. In the depth of winter, she left home to bring him warm clothes. But when she arrived, she found out that her husband had died and was buried under the wall. Her tears and sorrow were so overwhelming that the part of the wall, where his body was buried, collapsed

Forty-eight

1. *Tangshi* fish is a freshwater fish found in the southern regions of China

Forty-nine

1. Matthew 16:23
2. In Traditional Chinese Medicine, some of the symptoms of Stagnation of Energy are distention or soreness. Soft palpable lumps may be present. Psychologically, it gives rise to feeling of being blocked, tense or frustrated
3. In Traditional Chinese Medicine, signs of Stasis of Blood include tumours, lumps and hard immobile masses. Psychologically, it can give rise to feelings of insecurity, suspicion and paranoia

Fifty

1. Sticky rice dumpling. Glutinous rice mixed with various fillings, wrapped in bamboo leaves and then steamed or boiled
2. A goddess in Chinese mythology. She created the first humans on earth and repaired the heavens, which were torn and cracked, with five-coloured stones
3. A legendary archer who shot down nine suns
4. A giant in Chinese mythology who chased after the sun
5. A god of the highest rank in the mythologies of the Chu Dynasty (221 – 207 BC)

6. A mountain goddess
7. Daughter of Emperor Yao, a legendary sovereign

Fifty-one

1. Daniel Schacter, *Searching For Memory: The Brain, the Mind, and the Past*, Basic Books, 1996
2. Wen Tianxiang (1236 – 1283) was a public official of the Song Dynasty. A symbol of patriotism, he refused to yield to the Mongol invaders and was imprisoned and executed

Fifty-two

1. Liu Hulan (1932 – 1947): A symbol of courage and resistance, Liu Hulan was a member of the Communist Party executed by the Guomindang at the age of 14

Fifty-four

1. Luo Wen (1945 – 2002): A Hong Kong singer who died of liver cancer
2. *Dantian*: Literal meaning: cinnabar field. It is an energy centre on the abdomen and an important focal point for meditation and *qigong* exercises

Fifty-five

1. Andrew Solomon, *The Noonday Demon: An Atlas of Depression*, New York: Scribner, 2001

Fifty-six

1. Mount Jihua, located in the Anhui Province, is one of the four sacred mountains of Buddhism in China

Fifty-seven

1. A derogatory term in Cantonese slang for an uncouth and ill-mannered man
2. An expression in Cantonese slang meaning: "Extract as much money as possible from someone"

Fifty-nine

1. Master Wang's medicinal herbal tea. In the southern regions of China, it is taken, during the hot summer months, to dispel heat from the body

Sixty

1. M. Sara Rosenthal, *50 Ways to Fight Depression Without Drugs*, McGraw Professional, 2002
2. *Huanglian* (*Coptis chinensis* Franch.): Chinese medicinal plant used for fever

3. A wall poster written in large characters as a means of protest or to express a political opinion. It was an effective tool used by Mao Zedong during the Cultural Revolution
4. Li Bai (701 – 762)
5. Li Qingzhao (1084 – 1155)
6. "Drunk wine at dusk beside the fence facing east / My sleeves soaked with the delicate fragrance of wine": Extract from the poem "In The Shadows of Drunken Flowers • Fine Mist, Thick Clouds, Days of Eternal Sorrow" by Li Qingzhao

Sixty-one

1. David K. Reynolds, *Constructive Living*, University of Hawaii Press, 1984
2. *The Toilette of Esther* by Théodore Chassériau, 1841
3. Esther 2:15
4. Esther 2:17
5. Esther 4:14
6. Henrietta C. Mears, *What the Bible is All About*, Gospel Light, 1953

Sixty-two

1. *Huoxiang zhenqi* is a mixture of medicinal herbs used for stomach pains and flu-like symptoms
2. Arthur Smith, *Chinese Characteristics*, New York: Revell, 1894
3. Window of the World is a theme park in Shenzhen that has over a hundred reproductions of the most famous tourist attractions in the world

Sixty-three

1. Job 34:29

Sixty-four

1. Psalm 66:12
2. Psalm 46:10
3. Lettie Cowman, *Streams in the Desert: 366 Devotional Readings*. 1925. Revised edition, Zondervan, 1997

Sixty-five

1. A James L. Brooks film with Jack Nicholson, 1997

Sixty-six

1. Susan Sontag, *Illness as Metaphor*, New York: Farrar, Straus & Giroux, 1978

Sixty-seven

1. Isaiah 30:15
2. A red packet is a monetary gift presented in a red envelope. It is given on special occasions such as birthdays, New Year, etc. and, in this case, in appreciation of services rendered

Sixty-nine

1. Elizabeth Swados, *My Depression: A Picture Book*, New York: Hyperion, 2005
2. Susan Sontag, *op. cit*
3. *Idem*
4. *Idem*
5. *Idem*
6. *Idem*

Seventy

1. Cheng Wenchao (2001, July 10). "The Book of Life". *Art and Literature*

Seventy-two

1. In East Asia, the ritual of *zhuazhou* is held on a child's first birthday. Various objects are placed in front of the child and the object he or she chooses will predict the child's profession later in life. For example: picking a calligraphy brush means the child will become an intellectual, writer or painter; money coins, a merchant; a ruler, an engineer
2. A popular saying meaning "be determined to succeed."
3. Ecclesiastes 9:7
4. Ecclesiastes 9:11

Seventy-four

1. A television presenter

Seventy-five

1. Karen Horney, *The Neurotic Personality of Our Time*, New York: W.W. Norton & Co.Inc,, 1937
2. Baruch Spinoza, *A Short Treatise on God, Man and His Well-Being*, (1660), translation by Abraham Wolf, Cambridge University Press, 1905

Seventy-six

1. Karen Horney, *Our Inner Conflicts*, New York: W. W. Norton & Company, Inc., 1945

Seventy-seven

1. An acupuncture point that is located on the top of the head
2. Elizabeth Swados, *My Depression*, translated into Chinese by Wang Anyi, New Star Publishing House, 2007

Seventy-eight

1. It is a unit of length. One *li* is equivalent to 500 metres
2. *Landmine Warfare* (1962) directed by Tang Yingqi

3. Carl Jung, *Memories, Dreams, Reflections*, recorded and edited by Aniela Jaffe, translated from German by Richard and Clara Winston, Vintage Books, Revised Edition, 1989

Seventy-nine

1. Laozi, *Tao Te Ching*, in *Sacred Books of the East*, Vol. 39, translated from Chinese by James Legge, Oxford University Press, 1891

Eighty

1. Psalm 66:12
2. Mother Teresa, *A Gift for God: Mother Teresa of Calcutta*, New York: Harper & Row, 1975

Eighty-one

1. Psalm 118:24
2. From the hymn "Thanks to God for My Redeemer"

Eighty-two

1. Alexandre Dumas, *The Count of Monte Cristo*, London and New York: George Routledge and Sons, 1888. Project Gutenberg eBook

Postscript one

1. Matthew 7:7

ABOUT THE AUTHOR

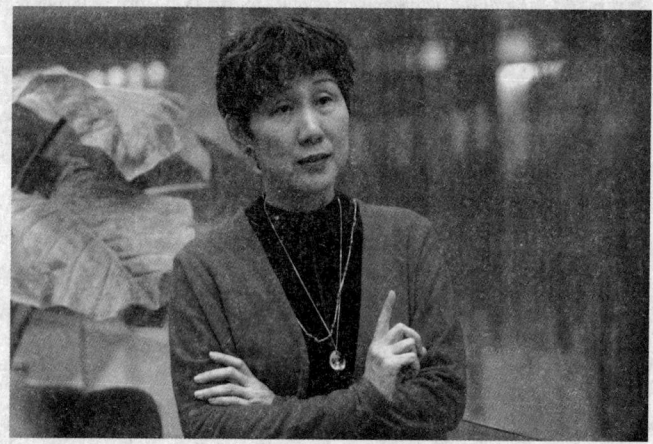

Li Lanni was born in Guangdong province. She grew up on island military outposts and in remote mountainous regions where her parents were stationed in the army. She attended the Lu Xun Literary Institute in Beijing and Nanjing University and worked for several years as a journalist in Shenzhen.

As part of Shenzhen's early migrant population, she witnessed the city's economic development and reforms first-hand. Drawing on her experience with cancer and depression, her work explores mental health issues among the Chinese people of today and the difficulties they face in an increasingly modernised world.

Her writings include novels, essays, film scripts and nonfiction. In 2009, her memoir *A Crowded Silence* was named an outstanding literary work and was selected to be part of the project China Classics International set up by the China News Publication Bureau.